# Theories for Mental Health Nursing

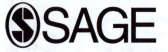

# Theories for Mental Health Nursing

## A Guide for Practice

*edited by*

## Theo Stickley & Nicola Wright

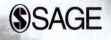

Los Angeles | London | New Delhi
Singapore | Washington DC

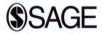

Los Angeles | London | New Delhi
Singapore | Washington DC

SAGE Publications Ltd
1 Oliver's Yard
55 City Road
London EC1Y 1SP

SAGE Publications Inc.
2455 Teller Road
Thousand Oaks, California 91320

SAGE Publications India Pvt Ltd
B 1/I 1 Mohan Cooperative Industrial Area
Mathura Road
New Delhi 110 044

SAGE Publications Asia-Pacific Pte Ltd
3 Church Street
#10-04 Samsung Hub
Singapore 049483

Editor: Alex Clabburn
Assistant editor: Emma Milman
Production editor: Katie Forsythe
Copyeditor: Jane Fricker
Proofreader: Bryan Campbell
Indexer: Silvia Benvenuto
Marketing manager: Tamara Navaratnam
Cover design: Wendy Scott
Typeset by: C&M Digitals (P) Ltd, Chennai, India
Printed and bound by Ashford Colour Press Ltd,
Gosport, Hampshire

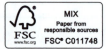
Introduction and editorial arrangement © Theo Stickley and
Nicola Wright 2014
Chapters 1 and 6 © Alastair Morgan
Chapter 2 © Andrew Clifton and David Banks
Chapter 3 © Dawn Freshwater
Chapter 4 © Paul Cassedy
Chapter 5 © Philip Kinsella
Chapter 7 © Fiona McCandless-Sugg
Chapter 8 © Nigel Plant and Aru Narayanasamy
Chapter 9 © Theo Stickley and Helen Spandler
Chapter 10 © Sally Binley and Theo Stickley
Chapter 11 © Tim Sweeney
Chapter 12 © Julie Repper and Rachel Perkins
Chapter 13 © Lorraine Rayner
Chapter 14 © Gary Winship and Sally Hardy
Chapter 15 © Gemma Stacey and Bob Diamond
Chapter 16 © Louise Thomson
Chapter 17 © Margaret McAllister
Chapter 18 © Anne Felton
Chapter 19 © Marie Chellingsworth
Chapter 20 © Patrick Callaghan
Chapter 21 © Ann Childs

First published 2014

**Library of Congress Control Number: 2013932399**

**British Library Cataloguing in Publication data**

A catalogue record for this book is available from
the British Library

ISBN 978-1-4462-5739-5
ISBN 978-1-4462-5740-1 (pbk)

# Contents

# About the Editors and Contributors

**David Banks** Senior Lecturer, Health, Community & Education Studies, Northumbria University.

**Sally Binley** Practitioner Health Lecturer, School of Health Sciences, University of Nottingham.

**Patrick Callaghan** Professor of Mental Health Nursing, School of Health Sciences, University of Nottingham.

**Paul Cassedy** Lecturer in Mental Health, School of Health Sciences, University of Nottingham.

**Marie Chellingsworth** Senior Lecturer, Clinical Education and Research (CEDAR), University of Exeter.

**Ann Childs** Lecturer in Physiotherapy, School of Health Sciences, University of Nottingham.

**Andrew Clifton** Senior Lecturer in Mental Health Nursing, The School of Human and Health Sciences, University of Huddersfield.

**Bob Diamond** Mental Health Adviser, Disability and Dyslexia Support Service, University of Sheffield.

**Anne Felton** Lecturer in Mental Health, School of Health Sciences, University of Nottingham.

**Dawn Freshwater** Professor of Mental Health and Pro-Vice Chancellor, University of Leeds.

**Sally Hardy** Professor of Mental Health and Practice Innovation, School of Health Sciences, City University, London.

**Philip Kinsella** Practitioner Health Lecturer, School of Health Sciences, University of Nottingham.

**Margaret McAllister**   Professor of Nursing, Division of Higher Education, CQ University, Queensland, Australia.

**Fiona McCandless-Sugg**   Lecturer in Mental Health, School of Health Sciences, University of Nottingham.

**Alastair Morgan**   Senior Lecturer in Mental Health, Faculty of Health and Wellbeing, Sheffield Hallam University.

**Aru Narayanasamy**   Associate Professor in Nurse Education, Diversity and Spiritual Health, School of Health Sciences, University of Nottingham.

**Rachel Perkins,** Freelance Consultant and  a member of the supporting recovery through organisational change project. Formerly Director of Quality Assurance and User Experience at South West London and St George's Mental Health NHS Trust.

**Nigel Plant**   Associate Professor of Mental Health, School of Health Sciences, University of Nottingham.

**Lorraine Rayner**   Lecturer in Mental Health, School of Health Sciences, University of Nottingham.

**Julie Repper**   Reader and Associate Professor in Recovery and Social Inclusion, School of Health Sciences, University of Nottingham.

**Helen Spandler**   Reader in Mental Health, School of Social Work, University of Central Lancashire.

**Gemma Stacey**   Lecturer in Mental Health, School of Health Sciences, University of Nottingham.

**Theo Stickley**   Associate Professor of Mental Health, School of Health Sciences, University of Nottingham.

**Tim Sweeney**   Cognitive Behavioural Psychotherapist and MBCT Clinical Lead, Nottingham Psychotherapy Unit, Nottinghamshire Healthcare Trust.

**Louise Thomson**   Senior Research Fellow, School of Sociology and Social Policy, University of Nottingham.

**Gary Winship**   Associate Professor, School of Education, University of Nottingham.

**Nicola Wright**   Lecturer in Mental Health, School of Health Sciences, University of Nottingham.

# Editors' Introduction

## THEO STICKLEY AND NICOLA WRIGHT

This book is written for students of mental health nursing and others who are interested in the topic of mental health. In this sense, it is intended to be an educational book. Each chapter begins with learning outcomes, describes the relevant theory in relation to historical development, offers examples of relevance to practice and ends with a brief summary. We hope students find this book not only helpful to their studies, but also helpful to their practice.

In relation to mental health nursing, theory is pretty useless without practice; mental health nursing (and nursing per se) is necessarily a practical endeavour. Nurses have to attend meetings, write notes, talk to people, give medication, assess risk and monitor physical and mental health and so on. Despite this very practical focus on what mental health nurses do, the thinking behind how these tasks are conducted is influenced by several factors. For example, national policy shapes the services within which nurses work and defines the key areas for development and investment, whereas local policies specific to individual health care organisations describe how medical and nursing records should be kept. However, when developing therapeutic relationships and working face-to-face with service users, the approaches mental health nurses use to guide them are based on a wide range of theories.

In general the term 'theory' uses ideas or concepts to explain individual experience, observations of behaviour and relationships. Traditionally a theory organises concepts so that their relationship to each other is explained and phenomena can be both described and predicted. Theories therefore help nurses to find meaning and to understand experience; to describe knowledge and to raise questions leading to new insights and ways of working. Nursing theories are not new, for example Florence Nightingale used theory to describe what is and what is not nursing. However, the explanations offered by any particular person do not provide the whole truth about a given situation. It is therefore important for mental health nurses to critically assess the usefulness of any given theory against both their own experience and the historical and social context in which they work. This book presents a number of different theories which have been used to underpin and influence mental health nursing practice over the last half a century. Some of the theories presented in this book are quite old, others are quite new. Theories grow and change over time and hopefully you will get this sense from reading every chapter. We have tried to make every chapter relevant to contemporary mental health nursing practice.

The book is not exhaustive; we could have included many more theories than we have and some may argue that we should not have included some of the topics we have chosen for this book. In a way, some of the theories may be regarded as 'competing'. There are those who prefer one kind of theory and approach over and above another because it fits with their beliefs and values. Some people will think one approach is superior to another, and so on. As with so many things in life, we prioritise and warm towards the things that fit with our own view of the world. That is why we begin this book with a chapter on philosophy; because mental health nursing often involves thinking, judging and decision-making about matters that are more related to philosophy than illness. For example, a person believes God is speaking to him and is telling him he is the next Messiah. Any intervention will need to consider the implications of a person diagnosed psychotic and having Christian beliefs. Another person may wish to kill themselves and insists they have a moral right to do this; the nurse needs to consider the ethical implications of this situation and make judgements according to beliefs and values. Another person may question the point of their existence and be enduring a genuine philosophical crisis. So mental health nursing inevitably involves philosophy; a purely medical interpretation of mental illness is woefully lacking.

Mental health nurses also need to understand about psychology, i.e. theories of what it means to function as a person. There are hundreds of psychological theories we could have included in this book. Instead we have chosen some of the major theories to help mental health nurses understand that there are many ways of interpreting human experience and ways to help when things go wrong. Of course, people are not islands and we can only understand and help people in the context of their social lives. Again, there are many social theories we could have included in this book. Understanding of issues such as race, poverty, inequality is vital to mental health nursing practice.

Naturally, it has been a challenge for us as editors to include a balanced view of mental health theories. We have attempted a holistic approach that we could describe as biopsychosocial, but additionally we have included a chapter on mindfulness and issues around the relationship between body and mind.

In the world of health care the word 'evidence' is used a great deal and it might be helpful to make a comment about the relationship between theory and 'evidence'. 'Evidence' often refers to research that underpins practice. For example, if you were unfortunate to be diagnosed with cancer, you would want the very best treatment that was based upon the best research evidence that was available for your illness. The 'best evidence' in the health care world is obtained by conducting rigorous clinical trials with large numbers of people over long periods of time. If we apply this model to mental health nursing however, it falls apart. Very little of what mental health nurses do has been subject to rigorous clinical trials. Does this mean that mental health nursing interventions are therefore worthless? Of course not; it does mean however that the definition of best evidence is inadequate. There is evidence from around the world of high quality and effective mental health nursing. Much of this is learnt from reading journals, books and attending conferences. The best kind of nursing practice is invariably guided by theory and is in turn contributing to theory development.

Our hope is that students reading this book will gain intellectual understanding and will be encouraged and inspired to apply this learning to practice. If they can then share this good practice with others, mental health nursing theory will continue to grow. We make no apology for including in this book theories that some people would describe as ancient and irrelevant to current mental health nursing practice. Apart from anything else, we believe that we can only understand the present in the light of the past; furthermore, in the UK, we have a saying: 'Don't throw the baby out with the bath water'. We think it would be a great foolishness to dismiss the older 'big' theories as irrelevant to contemporary practice because in doing so, we might throw away some of the most precious ideas that have contributed to the development of such an important profession.

# 1

# Philosophy of Mental Health

## ALASTAIR MORGAN

### Learning Objectives

- Understand the importance of philosophical ideas in mental health theory and practice.
- Understand the four main themes of philosophical controversy in mental health care.
- Apply these themes to concrete examples in contemporary mental health practice.

## Introduction

There is a strong case to be made that the discipline of philosophy should be central to all mental health care and practice. What is it about mental health and mental illness that should lead us to philosophical enquiry? Radden (2004) has articulated the centrality of philosophical questions to any interrogation of the concept of mental disorder. She writes that:

> Conceptions of rationality, personhood and autonomy, the preeminent philosophical ideas and ideals grounding modern-day liberal and humanistic societies such as ours also frame our understanding of mental disorder and rationales for its social, clinical and legal treatment. (Radden, 2004: 3)

When we think through questions of what it means to experience mental distress we are immediately confronted with a range of philosophical questions. These can be questions about personal identity, ownership of thoughts and experiences and the nature of the self and its relationship to the world and other people. These can also be questions about how we can classify and label mental health conditions and what our evidence is for labelling them as diseases. How do we understand the biological underpinning of mental illnesses and what is the relationship between the mind and the brain? How are we justified in detaining and treating people with mental illnesses against their will?

Furthermore, the very nature of mental distress and the experiences that accompany it raise questions that are often akin to a process of philosophical questioning. Mental distress can be characterised as a set of experiences that are centrally concerned with meaning and the self in a manner quite different from physical illnesses. Although one might question one's life, identity and relationships when diagnosed with a serious physical illness like cancer, it is not the illness itself that is a repository of such meanings but the impact it has on your life. In contrast, mental illnesses such as depression and psychosis are themselves full of meaning about who one is, how one relates to the world and the significance of one's life and experience. Fulford et al. (2003) argue that the discipline of psychiatry is unique amongst medical specialities in that its central concepts and categories are not only difficult to define but highly contested. A person experiencing psychosis may not label their disorder in medical terms and may actively dispute any medical description of their experience as schizophrenia. Mental distress is thus a field of complex and contested definitions and an experience which itself is a crisis of meaning, identity and relations with the self and the world, hence the centrality of philosophical questions in mental health care and day-to-day practice (Fulford et al., 2003).

## What is philosophy?

The literal meaning of philosophy comes from the Ancient Greek meaning 'love of wisdom'. In the *Theaetetus*, Plato outlines a concept of philosophy as a fundamental questioning of the basis of the world in an attitude of wonder (Plato, 1987). This fundamental questioning leads philosophy to a desire to uncover the foundations of knowledge. This philosophical project is encapsulated in the work of Descartes who wrote in his *Meditations* that his philosophical goal was to uncover the solid and certain foundations for all knowledge (Descartes, [1641] 1984). Interestingly, the method by which Descartes attempted to do this was through a radical scepticism; he doubted everything to try and identify a secure and certain foundation for all knowledge. In this project, Descartes united two key elements of philosophy, a critical and sceptical deconstruction of knowledge, alongside the attempt to provide foundational underpinnings for knowledge.

Later philosophers were critical of this attempt to provide certain foundations for knowledge as the supreme philosophical task. They preferred a more modest description of philosophy as a critical reflection upon the possibilities, justification and limitations of thought. This critical reflection may not produce certainty, only plausible beliefs based upon limited evidence. Hume argues that philosophy cannot provide ultimate foundations for thought and that it can only draw plausible and provisional conclusions based on a critical examination of the evidence of experience (Hume, [1739–40] 2000). This conception of philosophy as critique, as the discipline that outlines the limits and boundaries of rationality became a key task of philosophy in the late eighteenth century and through the nineteenth century.

Philosophy is therefore an abstract enquiry into fundamental questions of existence, knowledge and morality. These areas are often broken down in the following manner as questions of ontology (namely questions about existence – what kinds of things are there in the world), epistemology (questions of knowledge – truth, validity, the limits of reason) and questions of ethics (what is right and what is wrong and how do we characterise a 'good' society). This set of definitions makes philosophy sound very withdrawn from everyday life; however, increasingly philosophers have felt it important to be engaged in applications of knowledge and to try to clarify the concepts underpinning institutions, practices and ways of living.

## Philosophy of mental health

Philosophy is characterised as the threefold investigation into questions of existence, knowledge and ethics. Therefore, philosophy of mental health can be characterised as an enquiry into these questions as they apply to mental health care (Thornton, 2007). In this chapter, I will focus on four main areas of interest for the philosophy of mental health. As Banner and Thornton (2007) argue that any philosophy of mental health needs to be oriented around practice and become a philosophy of mental health care, I will outline a contemporary issue that applies these philosophical questions in practice in each one of these areas.

The four areas for philosophy of mental health are as follows:

- The question of human consciousness, and particularly the relationship between mind and brain. How do we characterise the fundamental nature of human consciousness and what is the relationship between conceptions of the human mind or psyche and its biological underpinning in neurochemical processes in the brain? Can we reduce experiences that are attributed to a person to neurochemical reactions in the brain, or are these fundamentally different levels of explanation?

- The question of mental illness as a disease. Can we classify mental distress as a form of disease or is it better understood as a response to societal and individual pressures rather than a form of illness? Should we classify and label forms of mental distress and can these classifications be validated, or should we dispense with all classification and attempt to understand distress in individual or narrative terms?
- The question of understanding the subjective experience of mental distress. How is it possible to understand and empathise with a mad experience? Should we try to explain it through biological processes or is it possible to empathise and understand the content of madness?
- The ethical issues in psychiatry, particularly the question of coercion and care. The ethical underpinning of mental health practice will be addressed in detail in a later chapter of this book, so here I will just consider briefly a contemporary contested ethical issue in mental health practice.

## Mind and brain

The background to the mind/brain problem in psychiatry is the question of the biomedical model in psychiatry. The biomedical model remains the dominant model in mental health care, but it has been contested right from the origins of psychiatry as an academic and clinical discipline in the mid-nineteenth century (Double, 2003). Fulford et al. (2006) outline the origins of present-day psychiatry in what is often termed its 'first biological phase' from 1850 through to 1910, when the first professor of psychiatry, Wilhelm Griesinger, famously wrote that all mental illness is a disease of the brain (cited in Fulford et al., 2006: 146). The goal of psychiatry was to define an area of illness for mental disorders that could be analogous with that of physical illness. Therefore, the idea was that all mental illness could be shown to have a biological underpinning in terms of a brain disease, and that the underlying basis of mental illness would be either some form of inherited genetic abnormality or a pathological alteration in neurochemistry. Underlying this belief was a larger philosophical claim for biological reductionism. This is the idea that all experiences of the person can be reduced to their determinants in the brain. A strong reductionism will argue that mental illnesses should not be understood as experiences occurring in a person, but only explained as biological abnormalities. The German psychiatrist Kurt Schneider gave a very succinct outline of this form of reductionism when he argued that when we assess a person experiencing psychosis:

> Diagnosis looks for the 'How' (form) not the 'What?' (the theme or content). When I find thought withdrawal then this is important to me as a mode of inner experience and as a diagnostic hint, but it is not of diagnostic significance whether it is the devil, the girlfriend or a political leader who withdraws the thoughts. Wherever one focuses on such contents, diagnostics recedes; one sees then only the biographical aspects or the existence open to interpretation. (cited in Bentall, 2004: 31)

Schneider, here, expresses a central belief of biological psychiatry. Engagement with the content of experiences is of limited importance. These are just surface expressions of an underlying disease process that is ultimately biologically determined and driven.

A variant of reductionism, which could be termed a weak reductionism, will argue that biological vulnerabilities interact with environmental stressors and personal experiences to produce illnesses. The stress vulnerability model in mental health care is a variant of a weak reductionist approach, in that it hypothesises a biological vulnerability that is then only later expressed or developed due to the stresses the person faces (Zubin and Spring, 1977).

The reductionist approach to human consciousness is based on a philosophical argument that all states of human consciousness can be fundamentally explained by their reduction to neurological states. A prominent exponent of such a view is the philosopher Patricia Churchland. She argues that when we want to explore what it means to think, feel and decide then we should not explore the meanings that a person attributes to such activities. Rather we should look at the neural underpinnings of the activities, and it is these neural underpinnings that ultimately explain our behaviour. Churchland (2004) writes that:

> ...what I know depends on the specific configuration of connections among my trillion neurons, on the neurochemical interactions between connected neurons, and on the response portfolio of different neuron types. (Churchland, 2004: 42)

This reductionist argument leads to an emphasis on altering our neurochemical makeup through psychiatric drugs to ameliorate problems in our mental health (Moncrieff, 2008). However, many philosophers are critical of reductionist arguments and want to argue that complex human experience cannot be reduced to brain states and that it does make sense to talk about the mind rather than the brain. The philosopher Alva Noe has written that consciousness can only be understood in terms of an interaction between brains, bodies and environments. The term 'mind' then can be used to refer to what Noe terms a 'living activity' rather than reduced to neural states (Noe, 2009: 7). Neural structures are of course necessary for consciousness to occur, but they are not the whole picture, and consciousness cannot be understood separately from human history, activity and culture, according to this argument. The biomedical model in psychiatry can therefore be seen to reduce minds to brains and to downplay the centrality of experience and society in the construction and causation of mental distress (Double, 2003).

## Mind and brain: contemporary issues in neuroscience

One of the key contemporary interfaces where issues of mind and brain have come to the fore is through the growth of neuroimaging technologies. This is an area which is increasingly being used in mental health research if not in practice. Often subjects of research are asked to perform specific activities whilst having their brains scanned and then the results of such scans are produced and attempts are made to correlate brain activity with specific dysfunctions in people labelled with mental illness. These neuroimaging techniques are termed fMRIs (functional Magnetic Resonance Imaging). The use of the term functional relates to the notion of a research subject performing an activity whilst being scanned. The philosophical basis of much of this research is reductionist; the notion that you can reduce a complex set of behaviours, experiences and meanings to a specific activity that can then be correlated with levels of blood flow in the brain. These technologies that function through the production of images produce a powerful force for reductionist philosophies. As Johnson (2008) writes, these images function through producing a representation of a host of activities as reducible to brain states. These images of 'active brains' are powerful cultural icons of our time. As Fernando Vidal (2009) has pointed out, we are replacing a concept of 'personhood' with a concept of 'brainhood', an identity that ultimately refers all meaning to patterns of activity at a neuronal level. Cohn (2004) has indicated how such neuroimaging remains tied to a notion of reductionism due to its isolation of all activity to a specific, calculable and repeatable set of functions that are then, themselves, only loosely mapped on to the production of chemical activity in the brain. The philosopher and physician Raymond Tallis has termed the dominance of neuroscientific discourse a form of 'neuromania' (Tallis, 2011).

A central irony of this reductionist approach is that it has occurred at the time when biological science is moving away from reductionist models. This is particularly the case in genetics where the idea of defined heritable diseases through specific genetic abnormality is increasingly questioned in what has been termed the 'postgenome era' (McInnis, 2009). Following the complete mapping of the human genome in the early twenty-first century, scientists were shocked to discover that there were far fewer human genes than had previously been hypothesised (McInnis, 2009). This has moved research away from the pursuit of discrete genetic abnormalities that could underlie mental disorders and towards the complex relationship between how genes are expressed and the interrelationship between environment and gene expression. As McInnis (2009) writes, this is a move away from the possibility of reducing complex mental disorders to singular genetic causes.

What this brief survey of current controversies in medical research in neuroscience demonstrates is the continuing relevance and importance of philosophical discussions of consciousness to current understandings and conceptualisations of mental distress. Do we understand mental distress as simply the byproduct of a neurochemical misfiring, or as the complex unfolding of human experience in response to interpersonal and societal stresses? Ultimately, in the absence of clear pathological underpinnings for most mental illnesses, this debate becomes one of philosophical argument and justification.

## Can we classify mental distress as an illness?

A central philosophical question for the practice of mental health care is the ontological status of mental illness itself. When we talk about mental distress are we discussing a disease process that is akin to physical illnesses, or is it better to conceptualise mental distress as a series of responses to life pressures? If we do dispense with a concept of disease then why do we include psychiatry within the medical sciences? If the classification of mental disorders continues to take place in the absence of underlying biological findings then how can we validate diagnoses and guarantee that clinicians are diagnosing correctly, or should we dispense with the whole process of diagnosing mental disorders?

The historical background to this set of questions lies in the absence of biological markers for most mental illnesses. Although biological markers for diseases affecting the older person such as dementia have increasingly been identified, the major classifications for disease within psychiatry have been developed in the absence of identifiable, underlying biological pathology (Read et al., 2004). Therefore, you cannot conduct a simple blood test or brain scan to identify schizophrenia, bipolar disorder, depression or ADHD. Even the fact that there are two classification systems for psychiatric disorders testifies to the contested nature of these illnesses. Not only are there two classification systems, but these classification systems themselves are subject to constant historical revisions, and we are currently in the process of a major revision of diagnostic categories leading to the formulation of the DSM-V which will be published in 2013 (APA, 2000; ICD-10, 2010).

The major categories of mental disorder were constructed discursively through the observation and classification of institutionalised people within asylums. At the end of the nineteenth century the German psychiatrist Emil Kraepelin proposed that we could divide the major mental illnesses into two classifications, and these two distinct classifications developed into the diagnoses of schizophrenia and manic depression (later re-termed bipolar disorder) (Kraepelin, 1919). This classification system still broadly stands over 100 years later, although it is purely based on grouping people into observable signs and symptoms rather than any other biological basis, and this has led many people to question the system.

## What is a disease?

The peculiar case of mental illnesses leads to a philosophical question as to the nature of disease. If we are to claim that mental illnesses are illnesses in the same way as physical illnesses then we need to try and clarify the concept of disease and how it applies to mental distress. One way of defining mental illness is by a so-called 'lesion' model of disease. Disease occurs if we can find some underlying biological abnormality or pathology, some form of damage or lesion to a bodily part, cell or tissue. In the case of mental illness, we would be looking for 'lesions' in the brain (Thornton, 2007). On this model of disease, most mental illnesses would not count as disease as there are no identifiable underlying biological abnormalities that are universally agreed upon as underlying the major classifications of mental illness. This argument led the writer Thomas Szasz to claim that mental illnesses are a 'myth' (Szasz, 1972).

However, other writers have disputed the 'lesion' model of disease. Kendell (1975) argues that there are many diseases that do not fit the simple model of causation by some easily identifiable 'lesion'. We can think of heart disease, diabetes, asthma or high blood pressure as examples. Kendell proposes a concept of 'biological disadvantage' rather than a 'lesion' model as the source for an all inclusive disease concept. Disease must include a deviation from a norm of health that puts the person at a 'biological disadvantage', which Kendell defines in terms of decreased fertility and life expectancy (Kendell, 1975: 311). Although Kendell claims that this concept of disease is value-free it is difficult to agree, in the sense that the definition of what is a biological disadvantage is highly susceptible to evaluations. Even his stress on fertility as a marker of health is itself a value. Why not pick another aspect of human behaviour, such as artistic ability? Kendell argues that his concept of disease can include specific mental illnesses and does escape the critiques of the 'lesion' model, but his own account is prone to problems.

The philosopher John Sadler has criticised notions of disease based on 'dysfunction'. He argues that any notion of 'dysfunction' will be values-based and therefore includes some kind of evaluation of the right way of living. This has implications for defining dysfunction purely in terms of departure from the norm and therefore of not being objective enough to count as a classification of disease (Sadler, 2005).

This general difficulty with defining diseases within psychiatry is even more complex as the very definition of mental disorder itself is highly contested. Pilgrim (2005) identifies an attempt to provide a legal definition of mental disorder by the UK government in the lead up to proposed changes to the Mental Health Act. Pilgrim cites the following definition of mental disorder by the Department of Health:

> Mental disorder means an impairment of or a disturbance in the functioning of the mind or brain resulting from any disability or disorder of the brain, and 'mentally disordered' is to be read accordingly. (cited in Pilgrim, 2005: 435–6)

As Pilgrim (2005) notes, this definition raises a series of irresolvable philosophical problems. He writes that there is a confusion between identifiable neurological disorders and psychiatric problems. There is also a lack of definition of what exactly a dysfunction of 'mind' will be (Pilgrim, 2005: 436).

One proposed solution to these philosophical complexities is to get rid of the whole system of psychiatric classification and diagnosis. Bentall (2006) has proposed a 'complaint-oriented' model of mental illness. Rather than the classification and diagnosis of people according to highly contested diagnostic categories such as schizophrenia, we should simply understand and describe the experiences that people bring when they attend for help such as hallucinations, delusions, mania and disordered communication (Bentall, 2006: 224). Bentall proposes that health care practitioners should help people with their distress but not impose arbitrary medical categories upon their experience. Whilst this appears an attractive proposal and a solution to the problems of defining mental illness, there are two questions for

Bentall's approach. First, it becomes clear that even when attempting to move away from diagnostic categories, Bentall's list of complaints begins to sound stereotypically medical (i.e. he sidesteps the issue of just what is to count as a delusional belief and for whom). Second, is the issue that many people with severe mental distress do not present with complaints in the way that Bentall describes, so how are we to seek out and help these people without a classification system.

## Classifications in practice: should the schizophrenia label be abolished?

This debate about the nature of mental illness and the use of classifications is not only of philosophical interest but it enters into day-to-day practice in mental health care. One example of this is the term 'schizophrenia', which has been used for over a century to define a range of experiences including hallucinations, strange beliefs, poor communication and poor ability to be motivated and make decisions. Boyle (1990) has argued that this grouping of symptoms does not necessarily make a coherent category for a disease or a syndrome. She writes that there is no coherent agreement as to onset of such a putative illness or the course of the illness or a prognosis for its outcome. This becomes particularly problematic in practice as many service users do not want the label schizophrenia and the consequences of such a label are highly stigmatising. Thornicroft et al. (2009) reported a study of people diagnosed with schizophrenia who found difficulty in maintaining jobs, friendship and sexual partnerships due to stigma and discrimination. Such was the stigma facing service users with the schizophrenia label in Japan that there was a campaign which eventually led to the renaming of schizophrenia as 'integration disorder' in 2002 (Sato, 2006).

A key issue in clinical practice was the labelling of all people with psychosis as experiencing schizophrenia, when psychotic experiences can exist across a range of mental health problems and in people who do not have contact with psychiatry (Romme and Escher, 1993). This led to the development of early intervention services working with people with psychosis that explicitly did not diagnose using the classifications of schizophrenia or bipolar disorder but viewed psychotic experience as caused by a range of stressors in the environment that could be worked with psychologically as well as medically (Garety, 2003). Thus, we can see how the debate around disorders and classifications has entered the mainstream of clinical practice and everyday mental health care.

# Understanding madness

If classifying and labelling people with medical diagnoses is an ethically contested and a clinically problematic enterprise, there are also philosophical issues surrounding the possibility of understanding a person who is experiencing strange beliefs or experiences. If somebody is expressing feelings that they have been taken over by an alien force or that parts of their bodies have been taken away, then these statements are very hard to understand. Karl Jaspers (1997) famously argued that schizophrenia could not be understood. His radical claim was that all understanding relates to empathy, and that when confronted with the profound disturbances in schizophrenia, there is a block to empathic understanding. For Jaspers, we cannot empathise with these strange experiences for two reasons. First, they put an immediate block to any project of attempting to understand because we are confronted with statements that we cannot grasp or attach any meaning to, and we are bewildered in the presence of such bizarre statements as someone claiming that their body has been taken over by alien forces. Second, we can't make any sense of such statements in narrative terms, as the feeling that one is occupied by alien forces cannot be linked to previous life events in any clear manner. Jaspers concluded that such experiences are beyond understanding, and therefore we should only try and explain them as symptoms of underlying biological defects that are yet to be discovered. We can never understand schizophrenia, and therefore it can only be explained through biological causes.

This approach became orthodoxy in psychiatry, and to a large extent the lifeworld and beliefs of people with psychotic experiences were ignored, and in clinical training health care practitioners were encouraged not to engage or 'collude' with the strange beliefs of people who were seeking help (Read et al., 2004). However, there is a branch of philosophy termed phenomenology that is explicitly engaged with understanding the meaning of subjective experience. This branch of philosophy was very influential in the development of French and German psychiatry in the twentieth century, and a number of key psychiatrists attempted to understand the experiences and beliefs of 'madness' from the perspective of the person (Blankenburg, 2001; Minkowski, 1958). The psychiatrist Minkowski famously wrote a case study of a patient who he lived with over a short period of time to try to thoroughly understand his experiences which were centred around the belief that the world was coming to an end (Minkowski, 1958).

Phenomenology literally means the 'science of phenomena' and the phenomena being studied here were the thoughts and experiences of people with hallucinations and strange beliefs. Minkowski, for example, focused on alterations in how the person with the catastrophic end of the world belief experienced time and day-to-day existence, and identified concepts of meaning, significance and the particular logical structure of the person's beliefs. Understanding begins here with a patient attentiveness and openness to another person's experience however strange that may be, and this phenomenological tradition in psychiatry was briefly influential in the UK context and was highly important in the early work of the radical psychiatrist R.D. Laing, who tried to understand how people might retreat into psychotic experiences due to overwhelming family and societal pressures (Laing, 1975). However, until the last 15 years, Jaspers' view that psychoses should be explained and treated biologically rather than understood psychologically has held sway. Nevertheless, in the past 15 years, a number of approaches have revived an interest in understanding and working with voices and prioritising the service user perspective on their own experiences.

## Accepting voices: the work of Romme and Escher

A new approach to working with voices was instituted in the early 1990s by the Dutch psychiatrist Marius Romme and his colleague Sandra Escher. There were two strands to this approach. The first was bringing together people who experienced voices in order to share their experiences. Rather than thinking that voice hearing was a meaningless expression of biological disorder this approach quickly demonstrated the therapeutic benefits in terms of peer support from sharing experiences. The second approach was to try and understand the full extent of voice hearing in the so-called 'normal' population; those people who had no contact with psychiatric services (Romme and Escher, 1993). Romme appeared on Dutch television and asked for people to contact him if they hear voices. Many people who heard voices wrote in and many of them had no contact with psychiatry. Romme and Escher (1993) then began to learn about how people lived with their voices and coped with their distressing and positive effects. They described a new way of working with voices which was about accepting the experience of the person as real and then attempting to understand the frame of reference within which people understood that experience (Romme and Escher, 1993).

In many ways, there was a continuity here with earlier phenomenological approaches in psychiatry, in that understanding the person from their own perspective and the significance and meaning they gave to their experience was central, rather than just dismissing this experience as pathological. In 2000, the

British Psychological Society produced a report recommending the use of more psychological approaches working with psychosis, and the latest National Institute for Health and Clinical Excellence (NICE) guidelines on working with schizophrenia recommend a wide-ranging use of psychological therapies (BPS, 2000; NICE, 2010). This demonstrates how a new framework for conceptualising the understanding of unusual experiences can impact upon improved and more person-centred practice.

CASE EXAMPLE

James has been referred to a community mental health team by his GP as his parents have become concerned about him isolating himself from his friends and seeming increasingly preoccupied with martial arts. James is an 18-year-old young man. He has dropped out of Further Education College and lost contact with a number of his friends. When the community mental health nurse visits James he discloses that he started hearing voices six months ago. This happened following a very stressful time in his life when his parents separated and he split up from his long-term girlfriend. He had become very interested in martial arts and the first voice he heard represented to him a 'grand master' who was educating and mentoring him. He found this voice gave him strength and helped him. He then started to hear another voice that was criticising him for his martial arts practice and then started making further derogatory and negative comments about his appearance and how he spoke to people in public. He also began to hear an indeterminate voice that would comment on his activities. Sometimes he didn't mind this, but occasionally this voice joined with the negative voice to make negative comments which James found very distressful.

## Working with James

Of primary importance is trying to understand James's frame of reference for the voices – how does James understand and conceptualise his experience (Romme and Escher, 2000)? James did not accept he had a mental illness and felt the voices represented forces both helpful and harmful to him. He did recognise that at times he became too preoccupied with the voices and might need help in 'tuning out' the voices. It may be helpful at this stage to communicate to James that the startling onset of voices is quite common and is often linked to stressful life events (Romme and Escher, 2000).

The nurse then encouraged James to make a weekly log of his voices (Chadwick et al., 1996). This logged the frequency of the voices, their emotional consequences and how easy James felt he was able to 'tune in' or 'tune out' of the voices.

James reported that the negative voices often occurred when he was in difficult or stressful situations and sometimes became overwhelming so he had to flee from these situations. He was not able to ignore the voices as they were so intrusive. He found that the only way he could get rid of them was by responding to them and speaking directly to them. He was able to 'tune out' the voices that came in a running commentary by distraction techniques such as listening to music or doing some exercise. Occasionally, the 'good' voice would cause him to be too preoccupied with his martial arts activities so the mental health nurse encouraged James to set time aside to 'listen' to the good voice and to undertake his martial arts hobby.

The nurse worked with James's frame of reference and coping strategies, but also assisted James with techniques to manage his anxiety in social situations as this might lessen the onset of his negative voice hearing experiences (Coleman and Smith, 2005).

## Implications for practice

- The nurse did not impose a frame of reference on James's experience but understood and accepted his understanding of his experience. This is central to assisting a person who is hearing voices (Romme and Escher, 2000).
- Helping James to understand he is not alone in hearing voices and the sudden onset of his voices is quite common and often linked to stressful experiences can help to make sense of the experience (Coleman and Smith, 2005). This feeling of shared experience could be helped by encouraging James to attend a group for voice hearers where experiences and coping strategies could be shared.
- It is important to work alongside the person and to understand and utilise their own coping strategies as well as attempting to assess how well these coping strategies work and trying alternative approaches (Romme and Escher, 2000).
- Medication may be used as a tool to help someone alongside other coping strategies but it is not necessarily the first or the only option.

## Mental health and ethics: coercion and care

The final aspect of philosophy of mental health care is the broad aspect of ethics. Ethical conflicts are acute in mental health care as mental health is the one field in which people can be coerced to accept treatment against their will. In all other aspects of health care if an adult refuses consent then they cannot be treated against their will, but in mental health care, subject to particular provisions, forced treatment can and does take place.

# Ethics in practice: Community Treatment Orders

In 2008 in England and Wales amendments to the Mental Health Act 1983 were put in place to provide for a level of mandatory treatment of people with mental health problems in the community. People who had previously been on Section 3 or Section 37 of the Mental Health Act and who had a history of disengaging from mental health services could be compelled to present themselves for assessment in the community. Additional conditions can be applied by a clinician, usually including a requirement that the person remains compliant with medication (DH, 2008). This extension of coercion into the community was a radical change to the Mental Health Act. Previously, individuals could refuse to consent to treatment in the community and could only be coerced into treatment if they met the criteria for an admission to hospital under the Mental Health Act. After these changes, individuals could be recalled to hospital if they refused to comply with the measures under a Community Treatment Order (CTO).

The arguments put forward for Community Treatment Orders were explicitly consequentialist. Proponents of these measures argued that it would enable people to spend more time out of hospital and to be freer to live their lives even though they were living under an 'umbrella' of coercion (Dale, 2010; Molodynski et al., 2010).

Supervised community treatment was introduced in England and Wales against a background of much controversy and a united opposition amongst health care professionals and service users organised through the Mental Health Alliance (Mental Health Alliance, 2005). The background evidence for the effectiveness of CTOs was extensively reviewed by Churchill et al. (2007) and found to be lacking. The restriction of autonomy here is quite extensive and would normally only be considered if someone had committed a crime, and it demonstrates how far consequentialist arguments, backed up by elements of social control, have come in policing the lives of those labelled with mental illness.

The issue of supervised community treatment is just one recent example of how these complex ethical questions are continually and daily negotiated in modern mental health care and practice.

## Summary

This chapter has introduced the reader to the importance of philosophical issues in mental health care. Philosophy has been defined as concerned with issues of existence (ontology), knowledge (epistemology) and what is right and wrong (ethics). Four areas of philosophy and mental health care have been outlined and introduced; mind and brain, classifications and diagnosis, understanding madness and ethical issues in mental health. A contemporary issue within practice and research has been outlined and related to each of these four areas; neuroscience and neuroimaging of the brain, the existence of the schizophrenia label, working with voices and Community Treatment Orders.

# References

APA (American Psychiatric Association) (2000) *Diagnostic and Statistical Manual of Mental Health Disorders* (4th edn, text revision). Washington, DC: American Psychiatric Association.

Banner, N. and Thornton, T. (2007) 'The new philosophy of psychiatry: its recent past, present and future: a review of the Oxford University Press series International Perspectives in Philosophy and Psychiatry', *Philosophy, Ethics and Humanities in Medicine*, 2 (9): 1–3.

Bentall, R. (2004) *Madness Explained: Psychosis. Psychosis and Human Nature*. London: Penguin.

Bentall, R. (2006) 'Madness explained: why we must reject the Kraepelinian paradigm and replace it with a "Complaint-Orientated" approach to understanding mental illness', *Medical Hypotheses*, 66 (2): 220–33.

Blankenburg, W. (2001) 'First steps toward a psychopathology of "common sense"', trans. A. Mishara, *Philosophy, Psychiatry and Psychology*, 8 (4): 303–14.

Boyle, M. (1990) *Schizophrenia: A Scientific Delusion?* London and New York: Routledge.

BPS (British Psychological Society) (2000) *Recent Advances in Understanding Mental Illness and Psychotic Experiences*. Available at: http://dcp.bps.org.uk/dcp/dcp-publications/good-practice-guidelines/recent-advances-in-understanding-mental-illness-and-psychotic-experiences$.cfm (accessed on: 13/1/2013).

Chadwick, P., Birchwood, M. and Trower, P. (1996) *Cognitive Therapy for Delusions, Voices and Paranoia*. Chichester: John Wiley and Sons.

Churchill, R., Owen, G., Singh, S. and Hotopf, M. (2007) *International Experiences of Using Community Treatment Orders*. London: Institute of Psychiatry.

Churchland, P. (2004) 'How do neurons know?', *Daedalus*, Winter: 42–50.

Cohn, S. (2004) 'Increasing resolution, intensifying ambiguity: an ethnographic account of seeing life in brain scans', *Economy and Society*, 33 (1): 52–76.

Coleman, R. and Smith, M. (2005) *Working with Voices II: Victim to Victor*. Lewis, Scotland: P and P Press.

Dale, E. (2010) 'Is supervised community treatment ethically justifiable?', *Journal of Medical Ethics*, 36 (5): 271–4.

Department of Health (2008) *Supervised Community Treatment: A Guide for Practitioners*. London: Department of Health.

Descartes, R. ([1641] 1984) *A Discourse on Method: Meditations and Principles*, trans. J. Veitch. London and Melbourne: Everyman Library.

Double, D. (2003) 'Can a biomedical approach to psychiatric practice be justified?', *Journal of Child and Family Studies*, 12 (4): 379–84.

Fulford, B., Morris, K., Sadler, J. and Stanghellini, G. (eds) (2003) *Nature and Narrative: An Introduction to the New Philosophy of Psychiatry*. Oxford: Oxford University Press.

Fulford, B., Thornton, T. and Graham, G. (2006) *Oxford Textbook of Philosophy and Psychiatry*. Oxford: Oxford University Press.

Garety, P. (2003) 'The future of psychological therapies for psychosis', *World Psychiatry*, 2 (3): 147–52.

Hume, D. ([1739–40] 2000) *A Treatise of Human Nature*. Oxford: Oxford Philosophical Texts.

ICD-10 (2010) *International Classification of Diseases – Reference Manual*. Available at: www.who.int/classifications/icd/ICD10Volume2_en_2010.pdf (accessed on: 17/1/2013).

Jaspers, K. (1997) *General Psychopathology: Volumes 1 and 2*. trans. J. Hoenig and M. Hamilton. Baltimore: Johns Hopkins University Press.

Johnson, D. (2008) 'How do you know unless you look? Brain imaging, bio-power and practical neuroscience', *Journal of Medical Humanities*, 29 (3): 147–61.

Kendell, R. (1975) 'The concept of disease and its implications for psychiatry', *British Journal of Psychiatry*, 127 (4): 305–15.

Kraepelin, E. (1919) *Dementia Praecox and Paraphrenia*, trans. R.M. Barclay. Edinburgh: E. and S. Livingstone.

Laing, R.D. (1975) *The Divided Self*. Harmondsworth: Penguin Books.

McInnis, M. (2009) 'Paradigms lost: rethinking psychiatry in the post-genome era', *Depression and Anxiety*, 26 (4): 303–6.

Mental Health Alliance (2005) *Towards a Better Mental Health Act: The Mental Health Alliance Policy Agenda*. London: Mental Health Alliance.

Minkowski, E. (1958) 'Findings in a case of schizophrenic depression', in R. May, E. Angel and H.F. Ellenberger (eds), *Existence: A New Dimension in Psychiatry and Psychology*. New York: Basic Books.

Molodynski, A., Rugkasa, J. and Burns, T. (2010) 'Coercion and compulsion in community mental health care', *British Medical Bulletin*, 95 (1): 105–19.

Moncrieff, J. (2008) *The Myth of the Chemical Cure: A Critique of Psychiatric Drug Treatment*. Basingstoke: Palgrave Macmillan.

NICE (National Institute for Health and Clinical Excellence) (2010) *Core Interventions in the Treatment and Management of Schizophrenia in Adults in Primary and Secondary Care*. Available at: www.nice.org.uk/CG82 (accessed on: 12/1/2013).

Noe, A. (2009) *Out of our Heads: Why You Are Not Your Brain and Other Lessons from the Biology of Consciousness*. New York: Hill and Wang.

Pilgrim, D. (2005) 'Defining mental disorder: tautology in the service of sanity in British mental health legislation', *Journal of Mental Health*, 14 (5): 435–43.

Plato (1987) *Theaetetus*, trans. R. Waterfield. London: Penguin.

Radden, J. (ed.) (2004) *The Philosophy of Psychiatry: A Companion*. Oxford: Oxford University Press.

Read, J., Mosher, L. and Bentall, R. (eds) (2004) *Models of Madness: Psychological, Social and Biological Approaches to Schizophrenia*. London: Routledge.

Romme, M. and Escher, S. (1993) *Accepting Voices*. London: Mind Publications.

Romme, M. and Escher, S. (2000) *Making Sense of Voices: A Guide to Mental Health Professionals Working with Voice Hearers*. London: Mind Publications.

Sadler, J. (2005) *Values and Psychiatric Diagnosis*. Oxford: Oxford University Press.

Sato, M. (2006) 'Renaming schizophrenia: a Japanese perspective', *World Psychiatry*, 5 (1): 53–5.

Szasz, T. (1972) *The Myth of Mental Illness: Foundations of a Theory of Personal Conduct*. St Albans: Paladin.

Tallis, R. (2011) *Aping Mankind: Neuromania, Darwinitis and the Misrepresentation of Humanity*. Durham: Acumen Press.

Thornicroft, G., Brohan, E., Rose, D., Sartorius, N. and Leese, M. (2009) 'Global pattern of experienced and anticipated discrimination against people with schizophrenia: a cross-sectional survey', *The Lancet*, 373: 408–15.

Thornton, T. (2007) *Essential Philosophy of Psychiatry*. Oxford: Oxford University Press.

Vidal, F. (2009) 'Brainhood, anthropological figure of modernity', *History of the Human Sciences*, 22 (1): 5–36.

Zubin, J. and Spring, B. (1977) 'Vulnerability: a new view on schizophrenia', *Journal of Abnormal Psychology*, 86 (2): 103–26.

# 2

# Social Theories

## ANDREW CLIFTON AND DAVID BANKS

### Learning Objectives

- Understand and critically engage with a range of sociological perspectives.
- Identify the key features of structure and agency.
- Examine the relationship between the structure/agency dualism and mental health nursing.
- Appreciate mental health nursing from a social perspective.
- Consider the extent that mental health nurses enable or constrain the well-being of mental health service users.

## Introduction

Mental health nursing has drawn upon and been shaped by competing social theories. Its history as a cadet profession allied to psychiatry has been heavily influenced by the biomedical model and other psychological theories. Social theories have also provided competing accounts of nursing practice and nurse relationships to service users, other disciplines and health care structures. Rather than focus on a particular social theory we discuss a theoretical perspective of mental health nursing which specifically addresses structure and agency, concepts of power, and equality as expressed through gender, class and race.

This chapter will examine the relationship between the structure/agency dualism and mental health nursing. Throughout the decades mental health nursing has operated within structures sanctioned by the state. Mental health nurses are shaped by these structures and in return they help to reshape them. Fundamental to interpreting and understating the mental health nursing phenomenon is an appreciation of the economic, political, social, legislative and cultural structures and the impact they have on mental health service users. We acknowledge structures can both constrain and enable the well-being of service users. Historically (and arguably even today) service users have not been served well by many of these structures and although individually and collectively mental health nurses have made positive impacts to improve outcomes for service users this is the crux of the structure/agency dualism: the extent that mental health nurses enable or constrain the well-being of mental health service users.

## Historical development

There is no simple, straightforward or indeed universally agreed definition of social theory. Books, chapters and academic papers over the years have written about the elusiveness of a standard definition of the concept (Craib, 1997; Layder, 1994; Scott, 2006; Turner, 2000). To complicate matters further writers often make a distinction between classical social theories (Craib, 1997), contemporary social theories (Turner, 2000) and social theory in the *real* world (Miles, 2001). John Scott (2006) argues the history of social theory can be traced back to the European Enlightenment of the seventeenth and eighteenth centuries when there was a realisation that such a thing as 'society' existed and those 'social' factors such as politics, ethics, psychology and morality and other distinct phenomena could be studied in their own right. Prior to the conceptualisation of society the predominant recognisable features of the day were the economic and military functions of the state and organised religion. Early social theorists began to shed light on and interpret the social domain which was emerging between the private individual and the organised state (Delanty, 2000).

Turner (2000) offers a useful starting point in the search to learn more about the concept: 'Social theory is a diverse and complex collection of perspectives that attempt to understand, to interpret, and to explain social phenomena' (Turner, 2000: xiv). What do we mean by social phenomena? Rather than focusing on individual behaviour, social phenomena are concerned with interpreting and understanding social systems. For example a system could be a small unit, such as a community of young people (in a small rural school), or an organisation like the National Health Service (NHS). Conversely, the system could be something much bigger such as the whole of UK society, if such a thing exists, or even the globalisation concept which encapsulates phenomena and includes several continents, hundreds of countries and *c.* 7 billion people (Coleman, 1990). The social phenomenon we are interested in for the purpose of this chapter is mental health nursing. As you can see from other chapters in this book social theory is just one of many perspectives from which we seek to understand, explain and interpret the phenomenon of mental health nursing and as Turner (2000) points out above, there is no one social theory but rather a complex collection of perspectives which seek to explain any social aspects of our lives.

Therefore this begs the question: Which social theory or perspective can we utilise to explain, interpret and understand mental health nursing as a phenomenon? There are many social theories, some you may have read about including Marxist theory and feminist theory, others such as globalisation theory, rational choice theory, social phenomenology, critical theory or grounded theory or symbolic interactionism you may be less familiar with. Table 2.1 lists and briefly describes a range of such social theories. These theories have been selected to provide an understanding of social theories and to prompt you to seek out other competing but no less valuable theories.

Fundamentally mental health nursing is about people who work and practise as nurses – let's call them agents. These agents tend to provide care, support and facilitate recovery for people with mental health problems. However, they don't work alone, they tend to operate in teams with other clinicians, and these teams are usually part of a service such as a community mental health team which is provided by the NHS. The NHS is a large organisation with *c.* 1.3 million employees and has many policies, procedures and guidelines that drive service delivery. These operational arrangements, or 'structures' as they are often called, can and do impact on the way that individual agents interact with patients and service users. In social theory this is sometimes referred to as the structure/agency dilemma and according to Miles (2001: 10):

> In many ways the structure and agency debate underpins contemporary social theory. It could well be argued that the prime concern of the social theorist is whether the actions of individuals or the broader social structures represent the prime influence in the reproduction of social life.

The structure/agency dilemma boils down to the extent an individual or group (agency) can influence or affect their environment. Structure, according to McAnulla (2002), is the context or the 'material conditions' which define the range of actions available to the agents. Agency implies that individuals behave independently and have the capacity to create, change and influence events depending on the course of action they choose to take (Bilton et al., 1996; Giddens, 1984).

**TABLE 2.1**   Social theories

| | |
|---|---|
| **Functionalist theory** | The functionalist perspective, also called functionalism, is one of the major theoretical perspectives in sociology. It has its origins in the works of Emile Durkheim, who was especially interested in how social order is possible or how society remains relatively stable. |
| **Conflict theory** | Conflict theory emphasises the role of coercion and power in producing social order. This perspective is derived from the works of Karl Marx and Sigmund Freud, the former saw society as fragmented into groups that compete for social and economic resources. Social order is maintained by domination, with power in the hands of those with the greatest political, economic and social resources. |
| **Symbolic interactionism** | The symbolic interaction perspective, also called symbolic interactionism, is a major framework of sociological theory. This perspective relies on the symbolic meaning that people develop and rely upon in the process of social interaction. |
| **Feminist theory** | Feminist theory is one of the major contemporary sociological theories, which analyses the status of women and men in society with the purpose of using that knowledge to better women's lives. Feminist theory is most concerned with giving a voice to women and highlighting the various ways women have contributed to society. |
| **Rational choice theory** | Economics plays a huge role in human behaviour. That is, people are often motivated by money and the possibility of making a profit, calculating the likely costs and benefits of any action before deciding what to do. This way of thinking is called rational choice theory. |
| **Critical theory** | Critical theory is a type of social theory oriented towards critiquing and changing society as a whole, in contrast to traditional theory oriented only to understanding or explaining it. Critical theories aim to dig beneath the surface of social life and uncover the assumptions that keep us from a full and true understanding of how the world works. |
| **Game theory** | Game theory is a theory of social interaction, which attempts to explain the interaction people have with one another. As the name of the theory suggests, game theory sees human interaction as just that: a game. |

*Source*: Crossman (2012).

The capacity to influence an event or intervene in a course of action is indicative of possessing a degree of power (Giddens, 1984). Giddens further stipulates that structures can be both 'constraining' and 'enabling' in the sense that people are not always constrained by structures and individuals do possess the power to alter their own or someone else's course. Miles (2001) points out in relation to the structure/ agency dilemma that there is a danger we perceive 'social structures' as some sort of predetermined framework.

This is of course true, however it cannot be ignored there are times when social structures do constrain our actions. For example in periods of recession and high unemployment it could be argued many people want to work but cannot get a job even though they have tried extremely hard to land one. Some people would say unemployment is an inevitable result of free market capitalism in which businesses around the world compete with each other to provide goods and services and if not efficient enough your company will go bust and your employees will be made redundant. Therefore it could be argued we are locked into a global economic system or 'structure' that is cyclical in nature and results in periods of high unemployment which individual people or 'agents' do not have the power or capacity to counteract.

We acknowledge the structure/agency dilemma is complicated and there is much disagreement and debate around the primacy of this dualism. However, we agree with McAnulla (2002) and Miles (2001) that a central feature of social theory is a consideration of structure and agency, therefore the remainder of this chapter will consider mental health nursing through the theoretical perspective of structure and agency.

## The social theory of mental health nursing

The term mental health nursing is of a fairly recent origin. Historically, people who worked in psychiatric/mental health services have been referred to in various guises, from 'asylum keepers', 'attendants', 'mental nurses', to 'psychiatric nurses'. The term mental health nurse was adopted in the late 1980s in line with a reformed register and the introduction of Project 2000, the preferred UK nursing curriculum of the day (Nolan, 1993). From the asylum keeper of the eighteenth century to the mental health nurse of the twenty-first century the name and role of the nurse has evolved and changed; however, many of the debates emanating in the 1960s from the anti-psychiatry movement around the nature of psychiatry remain relevant today. The following section will discuss these issues with a particular focus on nursing practice and nurse relationships with service users and will address structure and agency, concepts of power, nursing identity and equality as expressed through gender and ethnicity.

When discussing a social theory of mental health nursing it is important to recognise the relationship which exists between the nursing and medical professions. According to Nolan (2000) the history of mental health nursing is inextricably linked with that of psychiatry; mental health nurses have been to a greater or lesser extent subservient to and controlled by psychiatrists, with psychiatry being the hegemonic, or dominant discourse within mental health in western societies (Rogers and Pilgrim, 2011). This discourse is often framed around the 'medical model' or 'illness framework' in which psychiatrists seek to identify an illness (diagnosis), predict its future (prognosis), speculate about causation (aetiology) and prescribe an intervention (treatment) (Rogers and Pilgrim, 2011). In the UK the link between mental health nurses and psychiatrists is well established and as we can see from Table 2.2 there has been a shift away from treating people with mental illness in bespoke institutions to individualised care in the community.

**TABLE 2.2**   State response to mental illness

|  | Period | Nursing role |
|---|---|---|
| Asylums | 1845 Lunacy Act and onwards | *Attendants:* primarily a custodial role by maintaining order and keeping the asylum tidy, attendants were subservient to doctors' so-called knowledge and expertise. |
| Mental hospital/ institution | Mental Treatment Act 1930 | *Mental nurse/psychiatric nurse:* move towards voluntary treatment but the role of nurse was task-orientated and to maintain 'cleanliness and orderliness'. |
| Medicalising mental illness | 1970s onwards | *Mental health nurse:* the shift from institutional care to district general hospitals began in this period and more rigorous forms of mental health nursing training were introduced. |
| Community care | National Health Service and Community Care Act 1990 | *Community mental health nurse:* move towards community care in which mental health nurses offered support and treatment to service users. Individualised care programmes were put in place for service users in the community. |

Mental health practice throughout this period and even today is contentious; according to the medical historian Roy Porter 'the history of madness is the history of power' (Fawcett et al., 2011). The organised state in collusion with the medical profession has created a highly integrated network of doctors, experts, service providers, professional associations and medical journals to disseminate an evidence base for clinical practice (Giddens, 2001). Additionally the state has a long history of introducing legislation to curtail the liberty and freedom of mental health service users culminating in the Mental Health Act 2007, which is already proving to be more punitive and coercive than many policy-makers anticipated in England and Wales (Bates and Stickley, 2012).

Mental health nursing cannot be dissociated from the operationlisation of state power to control and coerce mental health service users. Michel Foucault (1926–84) studied contemporary institutions such as prisons, hospitals and schools to highlight how the state uses these institutions to control and monitor the population (Giddens, 2001) and as we can see from Table 2.2, the ancestors of current day mental health nurses have long featured in the social control of people experiencing mental health problems.

The institutions were created by the state but it was nurses and doctors working in these institutions who shaped the structures in which people were treated. Layder (1994) emphasises that people shape the social institutions that they operate within and are in turn shaped by them. The capacity to shape roles is however a product of power, a property, or in a Foucauldian sense, a relationship that is unevenly distributed. Traditionally nursing has been organised as a hierarchy with nurse managers and nurse educationalists, acting as gatekeepers to the profession, whilst within their respective institutions they act individually and collectively as an officer class, consciously distinguishing themselves from others further down the hierarchical relations of the occupation. As such, they are agents, both shaped and shaping the institutions within which they work and consequently develop their careers. Their formal status specifically allows them to play a more important role in the construction of health care institutions than those within the 'other ranks' of their respective nursing hierarchies.

Hierarchical relations, from age, to educational qualifications and professional accreditation, position individuals in chains of allegiance and dependency. This empowers some to direct others and obliging others to obey. This is predicated on the ability of people being able to collectively identify themselves, as well as others, in terms of both social categorisation and group identification. Both processes exist within a dialectic of collective identification. The categorisation of individuals and populations by government through, for example, psychological assessments and censuses utilises the 'objective' procedures of the social sciences. People are then established as subjects of the state and objects of government through instruments provided by social science disciplines given to proclaiming their own independence, disinterest and scientific objectivity, as exemplified by the emergence of the clinical gaze of modern psychiatry (Foucault, 1973).

> From a Foucauldian perspective power as it operates in the medical encounter is a disciplinary power that provides guidelines about how patients should understand, regulate and experience their bodies. The central strategies of disciplinary power are observation, examination, measurement and comparison of individuals against an established norm, bringing them into a field of visibility. It is exercised not directly through direct coercion or violence (although it must be emphasized these strategies are still used from time to time), but rather through persuading its subjects that certain ways of behaving and thinking are appropriate for them. (Lupton, 1997: 99)

The degree to which mental health nurses coerce service users into behaving and thinking is debatable and for some it might appear inconceivable that nurses have the power to socially control the very people they are supposed to support and facilitate recovery. However, mental health nurses do not work in isolation (Clifton et al., 2012), they are locked into a state-sanctioned legal and organisational structure and to an extent their practice is shaped, formed and dominated by psychiatry.

Despite these structural constraints and alignment with psychiatry the mental health nursing profession has its own identity, particularly the social identity of people working as nurses in the British NHS, which entails for example some engagement with concepts of citizenship and public service. A sense of identity from this perspective emerges from the ways in which people relate to and shape the world around them. So a two-way constructive process emerges between individuals and the work they do. Hence the experience of nursing affects the kind of person a particular nurse is, while the characteristics brought to that work will partially define the nature of that employment. A sociological view of workplace and identity is necessarily concerned with such things as gender, ethnicity, occupational role and status at the institutional level.

Institutionalising identity for Jenkins (1996: 127) occurs through the establishment of patterns of behaviour over a period of time in particular contexts as the 'way things are done'. This echoes Bourdieu's concern with habitus. Collective habit is then a form of institutionalisation, and habit often emerges from individual expression of institutionalised patterns. Such social institutions normalise 'how things are done', or 'the way we do things here' and are an integral part of the way individuals make decisions and direct their attention and behaviour. Still, this is a two-way process. As with identity, institutions are emergent products of what people do as well as being constitutive of what people do. Habitualisation helps the individual accommodate uncertainty through avoiding constant reassessment of interactions, even avoiding the need for predictability in many scenarios when habit creates a substantive and secure social environment that does not even require conscious reflection (Bourdieu, 1977, 1990).

Institutionalisation develops from sharing the above processes to the extent that a common history is acquired, people communicate in the same terms based on a shared sense of that they are performing in the same ways (Jenkins, 1996: 128). Sanctions emerge, but the primary process of social control is established by the very existence of the social institution and the hegemony it imposes – 'the way things are' excludes the possibility of thinking otherwise.

Traditionally the 'way things are' and 'how things are done' have informed nursing practice and underpinned therapeutic nursing relationships with service users. Mental health nursing from this perspective can be viewed as conservative, conformist and maintaining the status quo (Banks et al., 2012) and although recent developments such as the move towards evidence-based practice, recovery focused support and a politicised service user movement (Cowan et al., 2011), the profession remains resistant to change not only in 'how things are done' but also in the nature and makeup of the profession.

The literature shows empirical evidence of occupational segregation by gender by positive correlation of salaries and grade seniority with the proportion of men in the occupation. Women have historically replaced men in feminised occupations (Williams, 1995). Reskin and Roos's (1990) theory of queuing argues that white men are favoured by potential employers, whose capitalist practices are also shaped by patriarchal assumptions. Queuing can be conceived as an imaginary device, a managerial response to a shortage of favoured candidates, white males. This preferred category would usually be selected in preference to other categories of potential worker. They are placed at the front as a discriminatory practice. The presence of women and other minority workers in higher grades of nursing, albeit statistically under-represented, shows this does not operate in all circumstances. Aside from legal requirements to adhere to equality standards, nurse managers are more subtly concerned with 'acceptability' and 'suitability' interacting as selection criteria.

The possibilities for subtle discrimination abound in the determination of criteria for acceptability, or rather, 'who you are'. Managers are likely to wish to select 'one of us', someone who is likely to 'fit in' to the local networks and relationships of the organisation. Given the history of nursing in Britain this seems likely to run the risk of being exercised from radicalised and gendered perspectives. But in both recruitment and promotional practices rationalisation may well operate in either direction, as a mental defence mechanism, in supplying a defence for either rejecting an unsuitable candidate, because they are black and/or a woman, or alternatively opting for them despite their apparently unacceptable status (Silverman and Jones, 1976).

Suitability, as in 'what you are' in the sense of achieved or acquired characteristics, typically competencies, or expressed interests, is more likely to be taken into account when promotion, rather than membership of the organisation, is being applied for. Beishon et al. (1995) found evidence of professional development opportunities being unequally distributed on racial lines. This might take the form of grooming practices, including for example appointment to committees, or funded training that would clearly help develop profiles in terms of suitability, or employability indicators. But access to such opportunities can also depend on access to acceptability criteria.

Organisations are then deeply gendered, jobs are effectively designed for men and women, assumptions about gender and work are embedded within job descriptions, hierarchies and organisational practices. Individual workers also bring in values and expectations that are socially reproduced with regard to gender. This was noted by Williams in relation to way men actively responded to boundary heightening in predominately women's professions. This effectively overturns token theory, which argues all numerical minorities are disadvantaged. The assumed qualities of masculinity override such positioning, as the organisation and men themselves reproduce and accentuate their difference as a resource, one that brings prestige and advantage. Williams argues that minority men in women's work actively redefine their work and recast their participation in this work as consistent with hegemonic masculinity (Williams, 1995: 183). Securing a masculine gender identity propels men up varying career ladders, no matter how feminised the occupation. Managers, including some women, continue to subscribe to masculine values with regard to senior positions. The assumption here of masculinity is a binary position that subjugates the feminine; masculinity emerges from dialectic interplay between the organisational structure and the needs and desires of men. Habitus varies the context of such relations, and Williams highlights the work of Simmel on 'contexts of social interaction' (Williams, 1995: 181), yet the literature points to the consistent ascendancy of men, whatever the context of their employment.

Mental health nurses shape and are shaped by the organisational context in which they work. These structural conditions are determined by political, economic and sociological factors based on past and current policy initiatives implemented by a patriarchal state which has a long history of containing and controlling 'madness'. Theoretically, mental health nurses act as agents of social control. The institutionalisation of a particular identity in mental health nursing has been cultivated by the privileged few social agents. The 'male as norm' syndrome excludes women, people from ethnic backgrounds and those nurses who attempt to challenge the status quo and the 'way things are done'. Psychiatry has provided the 'clinical tools' in which mental health nursing is practised; however, the extent to which mental health nurses, or agents, have the capacity to promote recovery for individual service users remains contested (Clifton et al., 2012).

## Theory applied to practice

Underpinning contemporary mental health nursing practice is the notion of recovery (as opposed to treatment) and although the meaning and operationalisation of the term is disputed the concept has taken centre stage in recent policy developments (Bonney and Stickley, 2008).

> Recovery emphasizes that, while people may not have full control over their symptoms, they can have full control over their lives. Recovery is not about 'getting rid' of problems. It is about seeing beyond a person's mental health problems, recognizing and fostering their abilities, interests and dreams. Mental illness and social attitudes to mental illness often impose limits on people experiencing ill health. Health professionals, friends and families can be overly protective or pessimistic about what someone with a mental health problem will be able to achieve. Recovery is about looking beyond those limits to help people achieve their own goals and aspirations. (Mental Health Foundation, 2012)

Mental health nurses have a role in promoting recovery in conjunction with service users, their friends and families (DH, 2006), however, the extent they can facilitate recovery is very much predicated around the structure/agency dilemma (Clifton et al., 2012). As the Mental Health Foundation point out above, health professionals have been in the past and continue to be overly protective or pessimistic about what mental health service users can achieve.

Arguably part of this negative approach derives from the nature of treatments often prescribed by psychiatrists and administered by mental health nurses, coupled with

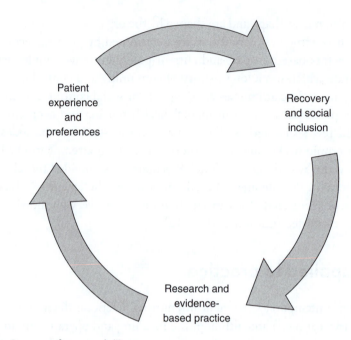

**FIGURE 2.1**    Recovery framework (1)

an unwillingness and failure of the profession to challenge the 'dominant discourse' in mental health (Fawcett et al., 2011). Another feature of contemporary psychiatry is the move towards research and evidence-based practice. Rogers and Pilgrim (2011) argue evidence-based practice is driven by policy-makers to manage the cost of services. Therefore treatment should produce tangible benefits and be cost effective. Figure 2.1 captures the 'new deal' between service users and professionals which is based on different perspectives and research approaches, considers diverse forms of evidence or knowledge and empowers service users to make informed choices about their recovery and/or treatment.

Despite this apparent move towards a more progressive framework for mental health service users, mental health nurses work in a plethora of different services and have competing and often conflicting views on their professional roles:

> Mental health nurses work in multi-disciplinary teams where they experience inequality, lack of integration and an unstable division of labour. They hold differing views about what their work should be; some are concerned with correcting malfunctioning biochemistry, others with reorganizing pathological thinking; some aim to restore the social functioning of their clients and others argue that their work is to help service users achieve purpose and meaning in their lives. (Nolan, 2000: 96)

Additionally mental health nurses have a dominant role in the surveillance of service users. Holmes (2001) characterises this as 'panopticism' (a figure of invisible power), a term used to describe how service users, without their knowledge and consent, are continuously monitored and watched by mental health nurses. In contemporary settings surveillance technologies such as windows, cameras and microphones are utilised to aid and abet the process.

There are wider implications for this therapeutic fragmentation within mental health nursing in relation to structure and agency. Yanos et al. (2007) argue that both structure and agency are important factors which impact on the recovery of people with severe mental illness and optimistically suggest actions such as 'coping', 'goal setting' and 'collective action' by individuals can overcome structures such as poverty, poor housing, inequality and neoliberalism, which is inherently individualistic. In contrast, both Clifton et al. (2012) and Druss et al. (2010) highlight the lack of power and resources some service users have in overcoming these structures.

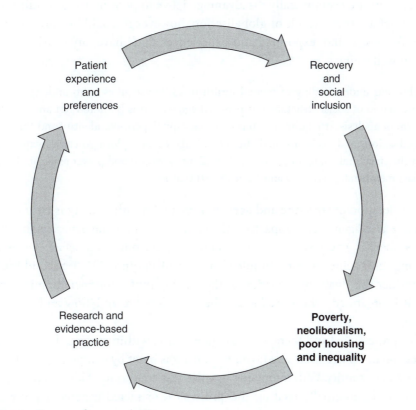

**FIGURE 2.2** Recovery framework (2)

If we revisit our recovery framework (Figure 2.2) and include some of the structural constraints (poverty, neoliberalism, poor housing and inequality) which service users/ mental health nurses need to overcome to achieve recovery, it sheds a different light on the process.

Overcoming these structural constraints requires power, which more often than not mental health nurses (and service users) do not possess. The power to decrease inequalities, confront and tackle poverty and provide appropriate housing is often held in the hands of the state. Furthermore it is posited many of these social and economic structures are the cause of mental ill health in the first place. 'Basically the poorer a person is the more likely they are to have a mental health problem' (Rogers and Pilgrim, 2011: 51). We can therefore appreciate the structure/agency dilemma. That is not to suggest mental health nurses cannot and do not co-produce or enable recovery. Many mental health nurses in co-production with service users have in the past and continue to produce positive outcomes for service users. It would be patronising and wrong to suggest all mental health service users are economically disadvantaged, live in poor housing conditions and cannot get a job as a result of globalisation, however it would be naïve to think a person's background, exposures and experiences don't have any bearing on their mental well-being.

> Thus our understanding of mental health in society requires us to understand the interaction of social structure and personal agency – it is both/and not an either/or form of analysis. It requires notions of social capital, personal identity and the situated actions and decisions made by individuals, when exploring health inequalities in the structural context of a material gradient of wealth and power associated with class membership. (Rogers and Pilgrim, 2011: 50)

A consideration of structure and agency in mental health nursing is twofold. First, structure and agency can impact on the chances of someone experiencing mental illness: there is a very strong correlation of people from lower social classes experiencing schizophrenia, for example (Rogers and Pilgrim, 2011). Second, we have to consider this dualism in relation to the nursing profession including its identity, how it is organised, who it excludes, what its values are and 'how and why things are done'.

This professional and therapeutic fragmentation within nursing does neither the profession or service users any favours. Nursing is beset by competing ideologies of professional identity. Within nursing practice this confusion of ideas is traditionally fended off by internally reciting the 'principles', or sacred canons of professional identity (Strauss, 1966). Reflection becomes a useful tool here in curriculum defence of these canons of identity/knowledge. The confessional act is a central construct operating on the premise that knowledge is revealed as parables – powerful and enlightening. These parables appeal to local knowledge and relationships, drawing in effect on anecdotes to illustrate desired and undesirable practice. This appeal to local knowledge and relationships serves another function in reducing anxiety concerning uncertainty in practice, or performance, and enabling practitioners to reject or downplay other sources of knowledge. Established practitioners can claim role competence through approbation of their local peers.

Unsurprisingly, such localism depends on knowing 'who's who' and being known within this network of work, a habitus which is unexpressed, or rather not formalised. Despite current attempts to persuade or impose the development of evidence-based practice (DH, 1997, 1998, 2000) a cosmopolitan ideal, local nursing hierarchies sustain and reinforce authority resting on established local orders. This poses problems for outsiders seeking to negotiate their way into the habitus established there. So mentor roles and clinical supervision in nursing are often hierarchically imposed; negotiation may often be impractical if a nurse wished to reject a supervisory relationship with a senior team colleague.

In this section I have not utilised a specific social theory to illuminate mental health nursing practice; rather I have considered a sociological perspective underscored by structure and agency. This structure/agency dualism can both enable and constrain mental health nursing practice. Mental health nursing has a historical legacy of being constrained by psychiatry and the 'medical model' of illness although recovery principles aligned to evidence-based practice have gained much currency in some contemporary settings. Covert and open surveillance remains a significant feature of practice and mental health nurses remain divided in the emphasis they place on biological, psychological or sociological interventions; the Mental Health Act 2007 is a powerful reminder of state-sanctioned control measures. Many mental health nurses have degrees and advanced clinical practice skills, others are initiating and undertaking research to improve outcomes for service users. There are now nurse consultants and many nurses are trained to be nurse independent prescribers. Nursing has become a graduate profession and in higher education institutions mental health nurses hold senior academic positions such as lecturers, readers and professorships.

Despite these professional advancements mental health nursing remains embedded in structures sanctioned by the state which are designed to retain power over the powerless. We have to question the extent to which mental health nurses (agents) can facilitate recovery given their alignment to psychiatry and the economic and political constraints of the state. Historically the profession has been exclusionary, with women and people from different ethnic backgrounds finding it difficult to progress in a white male dominated profession. Challenging the status quo was/ is frowned upon and the dominant discourse in practice has been driven by local networks of knowing 'who's who' and fitting into established 'norms'.

CASE EXAMPLE

Stephen is a 36-year-old man who lives alone in a rented room, is unemployed, has lost contact with his immediate family and has several friends but they tend to meet regularly in the pub. Although he likes to meet them there he finds it increasingly expensive and seems to be spending more and more time on his own.

Ten years ago he was given a diagnosis of paranoid schizophrenia and was prescribed antipsychotic medication which he has taken on and off over the years. He is in touch with a community mental health nurse who he meets with regularly in his home. His consultant psychiatrist is keen to increase Stephen's medication.

He would like to find a job, but feels he lacks energy and volition due to the medication. The last time he had an interview he thought his prospective employers realised he had a mental health problem and therefore made it difficult for him during the interview. He wasn't employed in this instance.

Stephen has firm beliefs about what his recovery should entail but often thinks they are completely different from his mental health nurse and other professionals from mainstream health and social care services.

As a community mental health nurse part of the job is to work with Stephen to engender a notion of recovery which he is comfortable with and has control over. From a structure and agency perspective consider some of the issues we have discussed in the chapter, including:

- The nature of state power and social control in how mental illness is managed.
- What economic and social structures might impede the ability of Stephen to find a job?
- How could the state or the community mental health nurse facilitate Stephen's recovery?
- As an individual agent what is the role of the community mental health nurse in advising Stephen on increasing his medication – to discuss, coerce, offer advice or leave it up to him?
- Does the nature and culture of the mental health nursing profession have any impact on Stephen's recovery?

## Summary

Mental health nursing has had a chequered history. Allied to psychiatry the profession was/is embedded in state-sanctioned structures which have disempowered many service users down the years. A particular professional identity emerged which was conformist and failed to challenge the status quo, with the profession favouring white males to the detriment of significant 'others'. From a sociological perspective these factors need to be considered through the lens of the structure/agency dualism. Many of these structures were created by governments of the day often responding negatively to political and social discourses around the treatment of 'madness'. Many service users are now empowered and have been given a voice. In an age of evidence-based practice they can often express their therapeutic choices and preferences to enable their own recovery. The profession has responded by creating a more representative and diverse workforce who have advanced skills and higher educational qualifications. Many are at the forefront of generating research and promoting evidence-based interventions which are non-biomedical. Nonetheless, the structure and agency dilemma remains. Structures are both enabling and constraining. I finish by asking the question posed at the beginning of this chapter and from a social perspective, is fundamental to the type of profession mental health nursing will become in the twenty-first century: To what extent do mental health nurses enable or constrain the well-being of mental health service users?

# References

Banks, D., Clifton, A.V., Purdy, M.J. and Crawshaw, P. (2012) 'Mental health nursing and the problematic of supervision as a confessional act', *Journal of Psychiatric and Mental Health Nursing*. doi: 10.1111/j.1365-2850.2012.01959.x.

Bates, L. and Stickley, T. (2012) 'Confronting Goffman: how can mental health nurses effectively challenge stigma? A critical review of the literature', *Journal of Psychiatric and Mental Health Nursing*. doi: 10.1111/j.1365-2850.2012.01957.x.

Beishon, S., Virdee, S. and Hagell, A. (1995) *Nursing in a Multi-ethnic NHS*. London: Policy Studies Institute.

Bilton, T., Bonnett, K., Jones, P., Skinner, D., Stanworth, M. and Webster, A. (1996) *Introductory Sociology* (3rd edn). London: Macmillan.

Bonney, S. and Stickley, T. (2008) 'Recovery and mental health: a review of the British literature', *Journal of Psychiatric and Mental Health Nursing*, 15 (2): 140–53.

Bourdieu, P. (1977) *Outline of a Theory of Practice*. Cambridge: Cambridge University Press.

Bourdieu, P. (1990) *In Other Words: Essays Toward a Reflexive Sociology*. Stanford, CA: Stanford University Press.

Clifton, A., Repper, J., Banks, D. and Remnant, J. (2012) 'Co-producing social inclusion: the structure/agency conundrum', *Journal of Psychiatric and Mental Health Nursing*. doi: 10.1111/j.1365-2850.2012.01953.x.

Coleman, J.S. (1990) *Foundations of Social Theory*. Cambridge, MA: Harvard University Press.

Cowan, S., Banks, D., Crawshaw, P. and Clifton, A. (2011) 'Mental health service user involvement in policy development: social inclusion or disempowerment?', *Mental Health Review Journal*, 16 (4): 177–84.

Craib, I. (1997) *Classical Social Theory*. Oxford: Oxford University Press.

Crossman, A. (2012) *Sociological Theories: A List of Sociological Theories and Frameworks*. Available at: http://sociology.about.com/od/Sociology101/tp/Major-Sociological-Frameworks.01.htm (accessed on: 20/8/2012).

Delanty, G. (2000) 'The foundations of social theory: origins and trajectories', in *The Blackwell Companion to Social Theory* (2nd edn). *Blackwell Companions to Sociology*. Malden, MA and Oxford: Wiley-Blackwell.

Department of Health (1997) *The New NHS: Modern and Dependable*. London: HMSO.

Department of Health (1998) *Quality in the New NHS*. London: HMSO.

Department of Health (2000) *The National Plan*. London: HMSO.

Department of Health (2006) *From Values to Action: The Chief Nursing Officer's Review of Mental Health Nursing*. London: HMSO.

Druss, B.G., Von Esenwein, S.A., Compton, M.T. et al. (2010) 'A randomized trial of medical care management for community mental health settings: the primary care access, referral and evaluation (PCARE) study', *American Journal of Psychiatry*, 167 (2): 151–9.

Fawcett, B., Weber, Z. and Wilson, S. (2011) *International Perspectives on Mental Health: Critical Issues Across the Lifespan*. Basingstoke: Palgrave/Macmillan.

Foucault, M. (1973) *The Birth of the Clinic: An Archaeology of Medical Perception*. London: Routledge.

Giddens, A. (1984) *The Constitution of Society: Outline of the Theory of Structuration*. Berkeley: University of California Press.

Giddens, A. (2001) *Sociology* (4th edn). Cambridge: Polity Press.

Holmes, D. (2001) 'From iron gaze to nursing care: mental health nursing in the era of panopticism', *Journal of Psychiatric and Mental Health Nursing*, 8 (1): 7–15.

Jenkins, R. (1996) *Social Identity*. London: Routledge.

Layder, D. (1994) *Understanding Social Theory.* London: Sage.

Lupton, D. (1997) 'Foucault and the medicalisation critique', in A. Petersen and R. Bunton (eds), *Foucault, Health and Medicine.* London: Routledge.

McAnulla, S.D. (2002) 'Structure and agency', in D. Marsh and G. Stoker (eds), *Theory and Methods in Political Science.* Basingstoke: Palgrave Macmillan.

Mental Health Foundation (2012) *What is Recovery?* Available at: www.mentalhealth. org.uk/ (accessed on 20/8/2012).

Miles, S. (2001) *Social Theory in the Real World.* London: Sage.

Nolan, P. (1993) *A History of Mental Health Nursing.* London: Chapman and Hall.

Nolan, P. (2000) 'History of mental health nursing and psychiatry', in R. Newell and K Gournay (eds), *Effectiveness in Mental Health Nursing.* London: Harcourt Brace.

Reskin, B. and Roos, P. (1990) *Job Queues, Gender Queue.* Philadelphia: Temple University Press.

Rogers, A. and Pilgrim, D. (2011) *A Sociology of Mental Health and Illness* (4th edn). Maidenhead: Open University Press.

Scott, J. (2006) *Social Theory: Central Issues in Sociology.* London: Sage.

Silverman, D. and Jones, J. (1997) *Organizational Work: The Language of Grading, the Grading of Language.* London: Collier Macmillan.

Strauss, A. (1966) 'The structure and ideology of American nursing: an interpretation', in F. Davis (ed.), *The Nursing Profession: Five Sociological Essays.* London: Wiley and Sons.

Turner, B.S. (ed.) (2000) *The Blackwell Companion to Social Theory* (2nd edn). Oxford: Blackwell.

Williams, C. (1995) *Still a Man's World: Men Who Do Women's Work.* London: University of California Press.

Yanos, P.T., Knight, E.L. and Roe, D. (2007) 'Recognizing a role for structure and agency: integrating sociological perspectives into the study of recovery from severe mental illness', in J. McLeod, B. Pescosolido and W. Avison (eds), *Mental Health, Social Mirror.* New York: Springer.

# 3

# Psychodynamic Theories

## DAWN FRESHWATER

---

### Learning Objectives

- Understand the fundamental principles of psychodynamic theories and how these inform our understanding of human relations.
- Identify ways in which psychodynamic practices can be used to develop a therapeutic relationship to develop insight and facilitate change.
- Explain the relevance of psychodynamic theories to mental health nursing practice.

---

## Introduction

In this chapter I will examine psychodynamic theories (originally referred to as psychoanalytical theories) and the way in which they can help to guide and understand the development of a facilitating relationship in mental health nursing. Many psychological theories have generic components which can be taught and practised without emphasis on a particular theoretical model. They can also be applied and adapted to suit a diversity of health care contexts and settings. However, psychodynamic theories and the associated therapies, aside from the generic and transferable principles of the theory itself, have a specific relational perspective that demand a deeper knowledge and experientially based understanding than many other psychological theories. This is an important context for this chapter, given the requirement for insight and reflective practice by practitioners of psychodynamic therapies, in which the intention is not only to develop intentionality and to make the unconscious conscious, but also for individuals, therapist and patient alike, to be better able to articulate their espoused theories and how they enact them in daily life.

# Historical development of psychodynamic theories

## Sigmund Freud and the topographical model of the psyche

Psychodynamic approaches were pioneered by Sigmund Freud, whose method of psychoanalysis is seen as the starting point for all future work developed in the field of psychotherapy. Freud's theories and concepts have been modified and adapted over the years by a large number of theorists including Carl Jung, Melanie Klein, John Bowlby and Donald Winnicott. McLeod (1993), over two decades ago, identified three distinctive features of the psychodynamic approach. These are that the client's difficulties have their ultimate origins in childhood experiences; that the client may not have a conscious awareness of their true motives or impulses behind their behaviour; and that the use of dream analysis, interpretation and transference in counselling may help the client to become more conscious.

## Freud's pioneering work

Sigmund Freud was born in 1856 in Moravia and lived in Vienna until he was 82, when he was forced to seek asylum in London, and where he died the following year, 1939. He began his career as a neurologist; then, in his thirties, he studied under Charcot and became interested in psychology. During 10 years of clinical work with Breuer, he used hypnotic treatment for hysterics and published *Studies on Hysteria*. Moving from hypnosis to free association, Freud gradually developed his ideas on psychoanalysis, based on his own and his patients' analyses. He arrived at the fundamental discovery of the unconscious forces as influencing our everyday thoughts and actions, and finally developed his theory on personality and psycho-sexual development. What began simply as a method of treating neurotic patents by encouraging them to talk about their dreams ('the royal road to the unconscious') and fantasies, and to free associate, grew into an accumulation of theory about workings of the mind in general, whether sick or healthy.

Freudian views of the human personality propose that it consists of three systems, the id, ego and super-ego. People, according to Freud, operate on three levels of consciousness, the unconscious (repressed), preconscious (unknown) and conscious. Much of our behaviour Freud saw as a result of unconscious motives and drives and it was the aim of the psychoanalysis to gain access to these through free association, working through resistances, the interpretation of dreams, transference and counter-transference.

The notion of conscious and unconscious processes were born out of Freud's (1915) early topographical model in an attempt to understand the mind. He later developed this model to include a structural model (Freud, 1923). The main tenets of these models can be seen in Tables 3.1 and 3.2.

The human psyche is seen as an energy system, the energy, libido, being instinctual and sexual in the sense that it drives us to reproduce as a species. It works psychodynamically between the ego, id and super-ego. Cathexes are charges of instinctual energy seeking discharge and anti-cathexes are energy which blocks that discharge. The id has cathexes only with the ego and super-ego have both. Freud also argued that humans have two main drives, these being eros (life/pleasure drive) and thanatos (death/aggression drive).

It is worth exploring the structure of the psyche in more detail to facilitate a better understanding of the application of theory to mental health nursing practice. The id can be defined as a cauldron of seething emotions without a clear sense of good and evil, and with no conscience or morality and which is motivated by gratifying instinctual needs, operating primarily from the pleasure principle. Freud

**TABLE 3.1**   Freud's (1915) topographical model of the psyche

| | |
|---|---|
| **The conscious** | Contains ideas and feelings in awareness at any particular time. |
| **The preconscious** | Contains acceptable ideas, feelings and experiences which can become conscious through the process of reflection. |
| **The unconscious** | Contains unacceptable ideas and feelings, experiences and repressed needs which may be recalled under certain therapeutic conditions. |

**TABLE 3.2**   Freud's (1923) structural model of the psyche

| | |
|---|---|
| **The id** | Contains inherited drives and is governed by the pleasure principle. |
| **The ego** | Maintains the psychic balance between the demands of the id, the superego and external reality. Governed by the reality principle. |
| **The super-ego** | Attempts to inhibit the id and influence the ego by setting moralistic values internalised from parental, cultural and social influences. |

believed that this was all a baby is born with, the modus operandi being from the id until such time as the ego is developed. The ego is a portion of the id, which is, through developmental processes, modified by the real world. In this sense the ego acts as the intermediary, using reason and common sense, between the id and the real world. This reality principle of the ego struggles and gets into tension with the pleasure principle of the id. Ego processes are secondary and include perception, problem-solving and importantly, repression. The ego also includes preconscious and unconscious material. The super-ego is part of the ego formed by parental and other significant influences including culture, society and, critically, family, friends and teachers, as well as other close significant others. In the early phases of development the super-ego develops in the child as an internalised form of authority, with moral commands such as 'ought', 'should', 'must', by identifications and repressions as the human struggles but also strives towards the higher side of human life, termed ego ideal and conscience. Growing awareness of the struggles and tensions of the id, ego and super-ego leads to movement of energy, thoughts and feelings across the unconscious, preconscious.

Anxiety is a reaction to dangers, some of which are external and realistic, experienced by the ego. However, Freud argued that anxiety is also a reaction to danger experienced through internal struggles and reactions to moralistic situations (experienced by the super-ego) and neurotic reactions to unconscious impulses (experienced by the id). Freud believed that the unconscious impulses and wishes of individuals can be defended against, and that defences help us to cope with anxiety.

In other words, defence mechanisms develop as part of the socialisation necessary in human societies to inhibit and cope with the often conflicting demands of the id and super-ego.

Anxiety is of course something that many of us experience and is one of the main reasons for individuals presenting themselves at their general practitioners (the other is depression). It is often when defences cease to function effectively that a person seeks help, for example presenting in general practice; this is sometimes because anxiety and other feelings are expressed through physical symptoms. In mental health practice, defence mechanisms are part and parcel of everyday encounters and are what many mental health nurses and therapists are working with as the mainstay of their therapeutic practice. Practitioners naturally employ and survive using their own defence mechanisms, which they become more aware of through reflection and supervision, which is also addressed in this book.

Denial is an example of a defence mechanism frequently employed in order to avoid facing distressing situations, causing thoughts, feelings and perceptions to be distorted. Examples of this include people who are dealing with their anxiety by obliterating it with intoxicants such as alcohol or drugs and who eventually suffer physical deterioration as a result. Other examples include people who deny that they have any mental health concerns, and those who believe that they can manage and cope with more than they can, i.e. mental health professionals! Isabel Menzies-Lyth (1988) for example, in her seminal research, discovered that health professionals use defence mechanisms, such as denial, as a way of managing the anxiety that they encounter on a daily basis through relating to the patient, their families and their obvious distress. The following example illustrates how denial may lead someone to a visit to their general practitioner with physical symptoms.

**CASE EXAMPLE**

Kate, a 29-year-old mother, recently lost her second child during the final stages of labour. Desperate to get back to normal and to continue with the routine of taking care of Daniel, her two-year-old son, Kate determined to 'get on with it' after the burial of her daughter. Despite repeated attempts by the health visitor and midwife to offer support to Kate and her husband, Kate insisted that she was coping well. Over time Kate's husband, Dave, became increasingly concerned about Kate's mood and her difficulty in sleeping at night. He was particularly concerned about the amount of alcohol she was consuming to 'help her get to sleep', but was unable to persuade her to seek help. Unable to face food in the morning on waking, Kate soon got into the habit of not eating for long periods of time, finding that when she did eat she experienced some abdominal discomfort and acid regurgitation. Kate eventually presented to her doctor with what she thought was a stomach ulcer, which she said was waking her up in the night.

Other defence mechanisms include:

| | |
|---|---|
| Repression: | Involuntary exclusion of a painful or a conflicting thought, impulse or memory from awareness, ego censorship, this is the most common defence. |
| Sublimation: | Instinctual sexual activity is repressed and re-emerges as socially acceptable activities such as sport or art, the most satisfactory way to deal with id impulses and essential to civilised culture. |
| Reaction formation: | The ego acknowledges impulses contrary to the one by which it feels threatened. |
| Fixation: | The libido is stuck at an earlier stage of development. |
| Projection: | An instinctual impulse is externalised. |

The defence mechanism of rationalisation is also commonly employed and is an example of how individuals can find reasons to justify their behaviour, even unhealthy and self-destructive or behaviours harmful to others, as illustrated in the following example.

Stan, a 49-year-old man with circulatory deficits brought about by smoking had recently undergone a below knee amputation of his right leg following severe necrotic changes in his feet. Despite being advised to stop smoking, Stan continued to believe that his circulatory problem was caused by an accident he had when he was younger. He told himself that he needed to smoke because he had asthma; and when he had tried to give up in the past, he had found that this had exacerbated his asthma as he developed a cough. He was provided with evidence that a cough is a symptom that the lungs are repairing the damage done to them following years of smoking, but he chose to deny the evidence, stating that smoking helped him to breathe more easily.

CASE EXAMPLE

Defence mechanisms are also played out through the unconscious mechanisms known as transference and counter-transference. Transference occurs in a relationship when one individual responds to another individual as if they were a significant person from the other's past. These feelings are likely to be present in any situation but are often evoked or exaggerated in cases where the individual is vulnerable, for example in the experience of physical illness, mental distress or hospitalisation (Rolfe et al., 2001). Counter-transference refers to feelings, behaviours and attitudes of the individual, for example, the mental health nurse, to the transference of a client or colleague. These responses may result from unresolved conflicts in the nurse's own life. Originally viewed as an impediment to the therapeutic relationship, counter-transference is now seen as a valuable indicator of what is happening between the client and therapist.

As Freud's work continued, he came to believe, as a result of his growing experiences of working with patients, that the secret cause of neurosis lay in sexual factors. In 1896, he stunned a scholarly audience and shocked Viennese society by declaring that infantile sexuality was normal and he further asserted that the origin of hysterical disorders was in the incestuous seduction of young children. For reasons about which there is still speculation, Freud later revised his initial theory to arrive at the Oedipus complex, where the fantasy of seduction came to play as important a role in development as his earlier notion where seduction was a reality.

Freud's theories and propositions have been criticised on many levels and at various junctures, as theories of psychological development progress and change. Criticisms include arguments that Freudian theories are not testable and therefore unscientific, relying too heavily on clinical data from a small, select sample (mainly Viennese 'neurotic' females). This challenge is one that would not hold so much credibility in the current research climate, in which clinical data, case studies and small sample narrative research continue to grow in stature and credence. Claims have also been made that the theories are sexist; it is easy to see why such challenges have been made! Nevertheless, Freud's contribution is important, as is evident from its popularity. Neo-Freudians such as Erikson, Horney and Fromm have modified and extended his work considerably, and his contemporaries such as Jung, Reich and Adler went on to develop their own theories. We will briefly examine the main theorists whose work was derived from Freud's original thesis; however before moving on to think about the contribution that Adler and Jung made to psychodynamic theories, let us look at the therapeutic style associated specifically with Sigmund Freud.

## Traditional therapeutic style of Freud

As has already been mentioned the aim of Freudian therapy is to enable people to function better by making the 'unconscious conscious' through creating a safe and neutral environment for the patient. To do this the therapist must adopt a formal approach, subordinating his/her own personality. In brief the key elements of this approach can be summarised as creating a stable environment, using anonymity, being passive and neutral and allowing attention to be free-floating. A stable environment is created by providing structured therapy sessions, which, ideally, must be of a set duration and frequency. Arriving late for or missing a session is considered relevant to the treatment. In order to preserve anonymity, Freud posited that the therapist should not exist as a person, but as a 'mirror' for the patient. No personal information, therefore, is brought to the session by the therapist. A Freudian therapist will, generally, only speak when interpreting and there are long periods of listening without interpretation. There is no attempt to create a social environment within the analytical space – the therapist does not reassure, persuade or reproach the patient, rather they remain passive. To encourage free-floating attention, the therapist attempts to let him/herself go whilst listening to the patient. The therapist actively avoids analysing the content of the patient's disclosure with the aim of hearing the overall tone.

## Alfred Adler and the theory of man as a social being

Alfred Adler was born in Vienna in 1870 and died in Scotland in 1937 while on a lecture tour. Having obtained his medical degree in Vienna and after a period of general practice, Adler became a psychiatrist. He joined the Vienna Psychoanalytic Circle, founded by Freud, in 1902 but by 1911 he had begun to establish his own theories and founded the Society of Individual Psychology in 1913. After the war he became interested in child guidance and inspired the establishment of an experimental school in Vienna which applied his theories of education, developing a strong and abiding interest in socialism and sexual equality.

Adler's basic concepts include theories that individual personalities are a unique configuration of motives, traits, interests and values. Social interest is inborn, although the specific types of relationships with people and social institutions which develop are determined by the nature of the society into which a person is born. The person's creative self searches for experiences which will aid in fulfilling the unique style of life and if these experiences are not found in the world, 'the self' tries to create them. According to Adler the human being is aware of inferiorities and conscious of the goals for which she/he is striving and is capable of planning and guiding actions with full awareness of their meaning for his/her own self-realisation.

Other more well-known Adlerian assumptions include the notion that individuals are motivated primarily by social urges and they are inherently social beings; in other words, Adler believed that many of people's problems were social in origin and, as such, are basically rooted in interactions with others. Adler differed from Freud in that he believed that humans are indivisible, which is in direct contrast to Freud's theory that divides the personality into segments.

Adler focused on life as a movement, and one that is directed towards striving from a felt minus to a perceived plus; hence people are self-determining and creative in the way in which they move through life. An Adlerian view of our behaviour is that behaviour is goal-directed and purposive; that as individuals we are not pushed by causes, but rather pulled by goals and our own dynamic strivings. This then sets the basic premise for the therapeutic style of the Adlerian therapist; causes of pain and difficulties cannot usually be changed but goals, once they are recognised, offer the individual a choice to change or not. Individuals, Adler suggested, look for a pattern, but not in the same way as Freud spoke about pattern recognition or pattern repetition, but a pattern into which details of our experiences will fit; this pattern is called Life Style.

Adler identified several key life tasks that would facilitate the individual's experience of wholeness: these included finding a suitable occupation and being able to adjust to all forms of obligation and responsibility; contributing to society and friendship, where one tries to find a position amongst others and being able to cooperate with them. Living as a sexual and loving being we accommodate ourselves to the fact that we live as two sexes and that the continuance of humanity depends on our love life, including struggles with intimacy, sexual identification, role values, performance and adequacy.

Adler did not, however, completely deny the influence of childhood and childhood experiences on the emerging person. His research and interests were primarily concerned with the impact of the order of birth on personality, early memories and childhood experiences. Specifically, he is most remembered for his work on inferiority and superiority and spoilt and neglected children. These conditions, namely organic infirmity, pampering and rejection, according to Adler, are erroneous conceptions of the world, resulting in a pathological style of life.

## Therapeutic style of Alfred Adler

The aim of Adlerian therapy is to enable individuals to modify self-defeating behaviours, to facilitate the making of effective decisions and in doing so help people to solve problems efficiently. As already discussed, Adlerian therapists subscribe to a theory of people as social, creative, active, decision-making beings moving towards unique goals and influenced by unique beliefs and perceptions. An individual seeking Adlerian therapists will find themselves in an empathic relationship and one that prizes a collaborative relationship between equals, in which therapist and client are active partners working towards mutually agreed goals. The primary function of an Adlerian therapist is to help the client recognise mistaken ideas and to understand their genesis, i.e. to develop insight. While the therapist is empathic and accepting, confrontation may also be necessary. Adlerian therapists believe that insight may occur through confrontation and encouragement as well as interpretation and other techniques. Insight must be put into action and active techniques may be used to promote movement. Attention is directed towards seeing alternatives and making new choices. Encouragement is seen as a prime factor for stimulating change in the client, generating the self-confidence and self-esteem that enable a person to act upon his/her concerns. Clearly stated specific goals and purposes foster the client's involvement and commitment to change.

## Carl Jung and man's growth towards individuation

Carl Gustav Jung (1875–1961) earned his medical degree from the University of Basel, reading extensively in the fields of philosophy, language and theology. After working in Burgholzhi mental hospital and lecturing in Zurich, Jung devoted his time to his writing and private practice and joined the Vienna Psychoanalytic Circle in 1907. He eventually broke with Freud seven years later, as had Adler, to pursue his own approach to psychoanalysis. Jung continued to practise and write until he died, travelling extensively, particularly in Africa, with the aim of studying different cultures.

For Jung, mental health was characterised by unity and wholeness and the development of personality is aimed at integration. Jung applied the ideas of psychotherapy to the insane and introduced concepts such as complex, collective unconsciousness, extrovert, introvert, archetype and individuation. Jung considered that people's most urgent task is to deflect their gaze from the conquest of the external world towards the study of their own nature. Jung described his way of working as analytical psychology (also known as depth psychology).

Jung then, held a differing view of the ego, conscious, unconscious and psyche to that of Freud, hence the eventual split. Jung used the term psyche to define the whole psychological state of the person. Jung's theories of the mind placed the ego at the centre of the conscious mind, with the primary function and goal of making and preserving consciousness and of creating a sense of personal identity and continuity. Consciousness is described as a state of being awake, aware and importantly, self-aware. Jung then separates out the personal unconscious from the collective unconscious. The personal unconscious being the part of the psyche that contains repressed material, impulses, fears, wishes and memories. The collective unconscious being defined as the communal heritage of humankind, containing the all important archetypes. Archetypes and symbols formed a critical part of Jung's thesis. Symbols act like a bridge, linking conscious to unconscious, past to present and future, and the fragment to the whole. This view contrasts with Freud, who saw symbols as more of a sign for something else. Archetypes are universal symbols; inherited patterns of the psyche, derived from instincts. The archetypal themes can appear in myths, folklore, art, and are personified in images such as the wise old man, the clown, the divine child and the shadow. This last mentioned archetypal image is perhaps one of the most well-known aspects of Jung's theory, representing as it does, the unknown side of the self, the dark and seemingly negative, often denied or repressed, aspects of the self and a community or culture.

No discussion of Jung's theories would be complete without reference to his theory of psychological types and the importance of dreams. The psychological types include the dominance of either an introvert or an extrovert way of relating to the world; and ways of perceiving the world through four predominant areas: thinking, feeling, intuition and sensory. Dreams were of course significant to Freud's understanding of the psyche, and both Freud and Jung viewed dreams as a normal psychic phenomenon that transmit unconscious reactions or spontaneous impulses to consciousness. Dreams can be interpreted with the help of the dreamer, who provides both the associations to and the context of the dream image. Both Jung and Freud would take this view. However, Jungian therapists in their work with individuals take the stance that the dreams are replete with archetypal images and symbols and as such are representative of both the personal and the collective unconscious.

## Therapeutic style

The aim of the Jungian approach is to enable people to function better by helping them to attain a balance between their internal and external worlds. Both therapist and patient are seen as being in the therapeutic relationship together, both having something to learn. Self-awareness is a fundamental necessity for a Jungian therapist, who must be aware of his/her own responses and be able to adapt them to the demands and needs of the patient. Jungian therapists avoid prescribing a rigid format to the session, actively encouraging an endurance and acceptance of the unknown in both patient and therapist. The aim of this is to demonstrate to the patient that uncertainty can be contained and tolerated in the search for integration and individuation. Individuation was regarded by Jung as unique to a person's psychic development; he believed that we have an innate tendency towards personal growth and towards becoming aware of all aspects of our personality; towards wholeness and the bringing together of opposites. For Jung then, the relationship between patient and analyst/therapist is all important, but is not only limited to the transference/counter-transference, as both patient and therapist participate in the process and change towards individuation. As part of the therapeutic encounter, the patient is likely to be persuaded to examine and reflect on the split of emotions (known as complexes) and meaningful coincidences linking events in time (synchronicity). In summary, the role of the Jungian analyst is to draw together material presented by the patient, to offer translations and interventions using their knowledge of archetypal structures, symbolism and current themes in the patient's life.

Whilst I have attempted to provide a broad overview of the main psychodynamic theorists, it should also be acknowledged that Freud's original work has been substantially developed and progressed since his early thesis. Neo-Freudians have proposed and evidenced theories of object relations (see for example Melanie Klein), attachment and loss (John Bowlby), theories of personality development (Erik Erikson) and theories of dependence and independence (Donald Winnicott), to name a few. It is not possible to extend or deepen the analysis or understanding of the psychodynamic field within this chapter, however, I would recommend further reading for those interested, and have included some suggestions in the references section at the end of this chapter.

## Relationship of psychodynamic theories to mental health nursing

Hildegard Peplau was an outstanding leader and pioneer in psychiatric nursing, whose career spanned many decades and whose model of therapeutic practice was developed with a group of women experiencing depression. Peplau majored in psychodynamic theories, viewing anxiety as a crucial influence in health and illness: positive anxiety she linked to healthy mental energy and productivity, and negative anxiety she associated with symptoms such as headaches, depression and insomnia. Kirby (1999) suggested that Peplau's model presents the nursing response to this dynamic tension as one which 'involves the nurse–patient relationship as a vehicle for assisting the client toward resolution of this dilemma. That is, toward the unbounding of anxiety and the achievement of personal growth' (1999: 413). Nurses, then, are well placed to act as a mediator between the person who was and the person who is in the process of becoming someone different. Whilst ill health (physical or mental) is often an unwelcome experience, for many individuals it can also provide the opportunity, if facilitated appropriately, for growth and integration.

It is fair to assume that for many individuals the experience of ill health, physical, mental or both, brings about a regression; that is to say that the person goes back to an earlier state of emotional development. Not least this is because the individual is suddenly forced into a position of dependency and reliance upon others. It is not surprising then that many clinical situations evoke transference and counter-transference responses in the patient together with the opportunity for the carer to assist the patient in managing themselves and their relationships differently. This potential was the subject of a research study conducted 20 years ago, Palmer et al. (1992) argued that workers in mental health settings were in a unique position to help women who were sexually abused as children to regain their confidence and self-esteem. Citing a study that identified that one in two women who sought help from the mental health services remembered being sexually abused in childhood, Palmer et al. argued that nurses should have access to opportunities for training and supervision to explore professional and personal responses to sexual abuse (Palmer et al., 1992; Sayce, 1993).

## Practical and relational aspects

A central tenet of the psychodynamic approach to working with people is that the therapeutic relationship be characterised by the anonymity and the objectivity of the counsellor/therapist, so that the client can project feelings and experiences on to them. The focus is on working through defences and the interpretation of transference and counter-transference as a means of understanding the client and enabling the client to expand their view of themselves. In this way the client is moved towards developing insight into their motives and patterns, and into reasons behind symptoms, emotions and impulses. Links are established between the past and the present and between the external and internal world of the patient.

In practical terms an understanding of the parallel processes between client–counsellor, client and significant others (past and present) can be obtained by analysing the interaction between transferential and counter-transferential responses. Peplau saw this as being as relevant to therapeutic relationships in mental health nursing as in therapist–client relationships. She viewed the therapeutic situation as a highly structured one and coined the term 'professional closeness' to describe a professional working relationship which is also based on intimacy and closeness. This may be one reason why practitioners often find the psychodynamic way of working uncomfortable, as the focus is on self-awareness and the therapeutic use of self. This can be quite demanding in that the practitioner needs to know and understand themselves in relation to others, including their counter-transferential responses and their own uncaring aspects (Rolfe et al., 2010).

## Summary

Nurses, doctors, psychiatrists, mental health nurses and other health professionals are engaged in a great deal of counselling, in its broadest sense. The use of basic counselling skills, in conjunction with a sound theoretical understanding of the dynamics of the psyche as explained here, can assist the mental health nurse in gaining an awareness of the person as well as the problem; in promoting the ability to communicate and empathise with people from a variety of diverse backgrounds; in recognising patients' anxieties including the anxiety they are almost bound to have regarding their health status. Frameworks for guiding the practitioner in the use of their skills can provide a set of pathways for the nurse–patient interaction, as well as a means of assessing the effectiveness of the therapeutic relationship. Psychodynamic theories provide a structured and meaningful way of understanding the workings of the psyche and importantly, a structure, that when held lightly by the mental health practitioner can inform and support the development of a deep and supportive therapeutic alliance.

# References

Freud, S. (1915) *The Unconscious.* Standard Edition, Vol. 12. Harmondsworth: Penguin, pp. 159–204.

Freud, S. (1923) *The Ego and the Id.* Penguin Freud Library, Vol. 11. Harmondsworth: Penguin.

Kirby, C. (1999) 'The therapeutic relationship', in L. Basford and O. Slevin (eds), *Theory and Practice of Nursing: An Integrated Approach to Nursing Care.* Cheltenham: Stanley Thornes.

McLeod, J. (1993) *An Introduction to Counselling.* Milton Keynes: Open University Press.

Menzies-Lyth, I.A.P. (1988) *Containing Anxiety in Institutions.* London: Free Association Books.

Palmer, R.L., Chaloner, D.A. and Oppenheimer, R. (1992) 'Childhood sexual experiences with adults reported by female psychiatric patients', *British Journal of Psychiatry*, 160 (2): 261–5.

Rolfe, G., Freshwater, D. and Jasper, M. (2001) *Critical Reflection for Nursing and the Helping Professions* (2nd edn). Basingstoke: Palgrave.

Rolfe, G., Jasper, M. and Freshwater, D. (2010) *Critical Reflection for Nurses and the Caring Professions.* Basingstoke: Palgrave.

Sayce, E. (1993) 'Given a voice', *Nursing Times*, 89 (36): 48–50.

# 4

# Humanistic Theories

## PAUL CASSEDY

### Learning Objectives

- Understand the historical development of person-centred theory and its key principles.
- Understand Carl Rogers' (1951) development of self-concept and self-actualisation.
- Differentiate between positive regard, unconditional positive regard and conditions of worth.
- Acknowledge the core conditions, congruence, empathy and unconditional positive regard as necessary for therapeutic relationships.
- Understand Abraham Maslow's (1970) theory of motivation and the hierarchy of needs and as it applies to nursing practice.
- Acknowledge the key principles of the person-centred approach as applied to mental health nursing.

## Introduction

Person-centred theory, which developed from the humanistic movement in the twentieth century, has become one of the most popular theories of counselling and therapy. The underpinning principles and philosophy of this approach are also transferable to many, if not all, aspects of mental health nursing. The theory places great emphasis on viewing people as essentially trustworthy, social and creative and are motivated towards reaching personal potential. However, and for whatever reason, there are times in our lives that this natural healthy state of being becomes thwarted and help is needed. This can be a challenge for mental health nurses and calls for us to vacate the role of being the expert and begin to recognise the person's innate ability and inner resources to move in positive directions.

The approach focuses on holistic care that addresses and treats the human person, rather than their illness, condition or a collection of ailments. We need to recognise and tolerate individual differences and the unique potential in each person. In doing so the mental health nurse needs to be able to perceive the world from another's perspective.

The emphasis of a humanistic approach is to work in the here-and-now, to listen attentively and enter into an equal relationship. Rather like becoming a companion on the individual's journey, facilitating further understanding on their road to controlling their own lives with a positive outcome.

This chapter will consider the historical development of person-centred theory. The key theory, concepts and principles are described. The chapter will focus on the qualities of the helping relationship and providing the right conditions for positive growth and development. Implications for nursing are outlined, while also considering some of the limitations – when using a person-centred approach may not be the most immediate or appropriate course of action.

## Historical development

Although Abraham Maslow is often considered to be the founder of the humanistic movement, Carl Rogers is very much the influential figurehead. His journey through life influenced the scope and direction, and became antecedents, to this theory of human development and subsequently to person-centred therapy. Rogers was born in the USA in 1902. His family were prosperous and strict Protestants, working tirelessly to keep society from corrupting their children. They uprooted from suburban life to a farm and held many farming values, such as pioneering attitudes towards independence and self-sufficiency (Rogers, 1990). He developed a keen observation of the natural world around him and a scientific interest in the cultivation of the farmland. At university he studied agriculture and became fascinated in the growth and development of plant life, which would later influence his theories on the nature of human growth. Pursuing his own personal development, his journey led him into religious work and studies. However, conflict and doubt arose when he was required to believe in certain doctrines that conflicted with his own beliefs that people were equal irrespective of what faith they followed. He decided against the life of a preacher: 'I wanted to find a field in which I could be sure my freedom of thought would not be limited' (Rogers, 1990: 10). He went on to study clinical psychology and subsequently psychotherapy, counselling and education.

Developing the learning and insights from his career path, it was in the 1940s that he began to form his own distinctive ideas and philosophies and joined the humanistic movement of the 1950s (Rogers, 1942). Psychoanalysis and behaviourism were the two major forms of psychological treatment and diagnosis at the time and humanistic psychology began to emerge as a reaction to these and is often referred to as the third force in psychology.

The psychoanalytical/psychodynamic and behavioural approaches are essentially deterministic; this means that all behaviour has a definite cause; people are driven by forces beyond their control. These approaches emphasised that the clinician was the expert, rather than the client; the clinician directed treatment programmes and would hypothesise and interpret what was best for the client. The focus of the therapy would be on the origins of childhood development and problems (psychodynamic) or establishing new patterns of behaviour for the future (behavioural). Rogers began to question these theories. Humanists believed that the client was the expert on themselves and ultimately had control over their own destiny; people were unique, essential good and could be trusted. If a safe psychological environment existed, then all people would naturally move towards mental health, have greater awareness and be more able to develop their full potential. He first used the term *client-centred* to describe this approach to therapy but would later change the term to *person-centred* as he saw it applicable to all persons and as a way of being human. In essence, person-centred theory and therapy are frameworks for mental health rather than mental illness.

Abraham Maslow (1908–70) was born in New York. He described his childhood as unhappy and lonely, and spent much of his time in libraries immersed in books. He studied law and psychology and like Rogers, became dissatisfied with the established schools of thought. Maslow (1962) argued that Freud had supplied the 'sick half' of psychology and now was the time to fill it with the 'healthy half'. He felt at the time that all psychology portrayed humans pessimistically because it centred on their animalistic and negative aspects. His desire was to formulate a theory that took away from focusing on the unconscious forces from within (psychodynamic) and the stimulus and reinforcement forces from without (behaviourism) that control the person's actions. Rather than focusing on the negative aspects of childhood and all that could go wrong, he sought to strongly emphasise the more positive qualities that were evident, especially in those children who were respected and loved by their parents (Hough, 1998). Maslow's research was unique for the time, as most psychology focused on why people became mentally ill. His interest and studies were how psychologically healthy people motivated themselves and what gave them meaning, purpose and success in life. Success is defined in this context as becoming a fully functioning human being and to reach self-actualisation. His ideas were similar to those of Rogers and the concept of self-actualisation was common to both of them.

Rogers never sought wide fame or publicity. By and large his name is not publicly well known, which fits in entirely with his philosophy that the client is the expert, not the therapist. Yet he is ranked very high indeed as one of the most influential psychotherapists in the world.

Carl Rogers' ideas have influenced and continue to influence millions of individuals in professional and non-professional settings. The concepts and methods he proposed and developed are used in an eclectic fashion by many different counsellors, therapists, helpers, educationalists, teachers and coaches who work in a humanistic way. His democratic and libertarian ideas have been adopted by those who have a concern and passion for human relationships in general and for a humanitarian society as an ideal. Therefore a person-centred approach can be applied to all aspects of life and living.

It was in the 1970s and early 1980s that this person-centred approach began to have an impact on mental health services in the UK. As the large psychiatric institutions were being phased out and services gravitated towards community and day care, nurses had the need and opportunity to develop new skills. The skills of promoting more independent living were used in helping the patient develop his/her own inner resources, and to develop and maintain a state of psychological well-being, and were well suited to person-centred theory. As nurses began to adopt a more non-directional approach, the utilisation of counselling skills and the overall philosophy of the person-centred approach became more widespread. A fundamental requirement for this philosophy of promoting self-growth and ultimately the self-actualisation of individuals is for the helper to provide the right conditions. These core conditions will be focused on later in this chapter.

# Rogers' person-centred theory

## The actualising tendency

Through his research, Rogers found that an actualising tendency was evident in all organic and human life; he postulated that it was the only motivating force that drives the human organism. As all plant life has an innate tendency to grow from seed to flourish and bloom to its full potential, the same is true of human beings. The concept of the actualising tendency is essential in mental health nursing as it underpins the idea that individuals have the necessary resources for growth and development. So the person-centred helper begins from the premise that each individual has an inherent and natural tendency for growth and development. Rogers viewed this tendency as a trustworthy and motivational force. The only way it can be destroyed is if the organism itself is destroyed. McMillan (2010: 2) states: 'It is not something that requires anything doing to it in order for it to work – it just is.' This strong life force continues throughout life, so therefore we are always in a state of being and becoming (Rogers, 1961). As we have this gift of the actualising tendency, we are programmed to survive. We have the necessary resources for dealing effectively with our own problems and to do as well as we possibly can, if external forces allow us to do so. If as nurses we believe this philosophy, we are more likely to respect and value those we help, with the belief that ultimately the person can bring about change themselves. It is therefore primary to any consideration of how change occurs. If you think of the many problems human beings encounter in their lives, we overcome most on our own, we use our inner resources or create supportive measures when we need help. If at any time and for any reason the self-actualising tendency becomes dormant, for example due to mental illness, Rogers' view is that it can be reactivated. This can be achieved in nursing when the conditions of congruence, unconditional regard and empathy are present (more about these later).

You may view this actualising tendency as a pathway of maturity that leads and motivates us to reach our full potential physically, emotionally and spiritually. The person-centred philosophy places a high value on the uniqueness of each individual and hence fully acknowledges that we develop in different ways according to influences from our environment, culture and the construct of our personalities.

So the underpinning assumption is that the person is the catalyst for his/her own healing. We are able to discover our own capabilities, have the power to heal ourselves and find solutions to our own problems. The potential is there, however there are many of life's obstacles, hindrances and roadblocks in the way.

From birth we are unable to escape everyday life experiences and interactions with others, so this natural tendency is subject to the many influences of life on life's terms. Our growth and development for well-being can be distorted or overcome by our subjective reality and the demands of society, so our actualising tendency may become distorted. Central to understanding some of the distortions that take place we need to consider Rogers' viewpoint on personality development, the meaning of self and self-concept.

## The self-concept

Self-concept is the perception we have about our self and can also be described as an awareness of being (Rogers, 1980). The self-concept develops through interactions with others. Two primary sources that influence our self-concept are childhood experiences and evaluation by others. It is therefore formed from all the acquired learning and messages we receive from significant others and the outside world. To have a positive self-concept we need positive regard, which refers to the acceptance, approval and love by our significant others. Thorne (2011: 149) notes that 'the need for positive regard or approval is overwhelming and is present from early infancy'. Dryden and Mytton (1999) add that as the child grows it becomes aware of the evaluations of others, which will be at times positive and other times, negative. We attach values to these childhood messages and interactions with others and often that will be whether we feel good or bad as a result of the experiences (Frankland and Sanders, 1995). For our own safety and security we need messages of what is right or wrong, safe or dangerous. So the development of the self-concept is heavily dependent on the values and attitudes of parents, parental figures and significant others in our lives. Some messages, however, can be distorted and cause conflict and anxiety with the core self and actualising tendency. The young boy who falls over and cries is maybe told to stop crying like a baby, when what he needed was a big hug; a young girl is maybe told off for being covered in paint, when she wanted praise for being creative. The child's experiences, and evaluations, as he or she interacts with significant others will at times be positive – 'well done' – or negative – 'stop doing that'. So during the child's interactions with the environment and significant others he or she will start to build a picture of themselves. If these experiences are often negative the development and growth of the self-concept in adulthood can also be negative (Hough, 2002). Fortunately rejection and disapproval can be fleeting and we get over it. However difficulties can arise when it is more continuous and there is a conflict with what we truly believe about ourselves, and the conditions others place upon us of what we should and should not do. Patients in our care will often have a poor self-concept and hence poor self-esteem; they may have been judged frequently in their past, and their actualising tendency has been distorted as their own choices and decisions have been taken away from them. The positive or conditional regard we receive from others is significant in the development of the self-concept.

## The need for positive regard

Rogers believed that as human beings we need love and acceptance, which he maintained was essential for the healthy growth of the individual. He believed in unconditional positive regard, implying valuing the person, regardless of the behaviour. While it should be possible to value the person without implying you accept all their actions, distinctions can be difficult for both the giver and the receiver. When you are criticised it is hard not to take it personally; when you are doing the criticising how often do you accuse the person, rather than his/her actions?

We all have a desire to seek positive regard from others. Integrated within this desire is a need for positive self-regard, which is the love and acceptance of our own self and is important for our self-concept. We are more likely to feel good about ourselves if others feel good about us. A child's behaviour is shaped by the need for approval and will do things to please parental figures even to the extent of ignoring his/her own inner feelings of the core self (Dryden and Mytton, 1999). We perhaps received messages of not to get angry, when we felt like shouting, and that we should keep calm and quiet. So we begin to please others and recognise which behaviours will receive positive regard and which ones will not. Regard that is only given for certain standards of behaviour Rogers referred to as conditional positive regard; the problem here is that it often leaves people feeling it is their self, not their behaviour that is unacceptable.

When we feel we are only worthy of affection on our desirable behaviour or receive messages such as 'I will only love you if …', this conditional positive regard is known as conditions of worth.

## Conditions of worth

Conditions of worth is a phrase used to describe a major way the child's self-concept is shaped by parental influences (McLeod, 2003). It is the belief that we will only feel valued by others if we behave in ways which fulfil their expectations of us. So we only have acceptance of self when it meets the expectations of others. For a child at a certain level conditions of worth are not a bad thing, we seek to satisfy, want to be loved and please others and gain positive regard. However, as we grow rules may change, the conditions of worth become more complex and demanding or do not match our own values and beliefs. Our developing self-concept can become confused and distorted when the conditions of worth are overused or place huge demands on us.

Over time, conditions of worth become more ingrained in how we see our-selves in the world; we adopt them as our own and they block our own true values and beliefs of who we really are. Rogers' view was that conditions of worth or conditional positive regard are detrimental to health and development. Anxi-ety and depression can result as we feel lost and confused about who we really are and are leading a life that does not satisfy our real needs and wants. When positive regard is conditional only on pleasing others and this is invariably still not good enough, feelings of disapproval, worthlessness and rejection arise. The self-concept will however strive to preserve itself and we may take on measures to protect ourselves from distress. For example, selectively taking in conditions of worth experiences into our consciousness, distorts them in some way or denies them completely. Therefore a fine balancing act is needed for a healthy indi-vidual, trusting our own values and choices of right and wrong and what is good and bad for our own development, alongside the values and approval imposed upon us by others. The task of the mental health nurse is to remove any condi-tions of worth from the relationship with the patient, so the patient can be free to consider his/her own lives and decisions. By offering unconditional positive regard the patient's own true values can emerge and he or she can consider once again who they want to be.

## The core conditions

From the conditions that Carl Rogers proposed as being necessary and sufficient for therapeutic change to take place, promoting self-growth and ultimately self-actualisation, three have become known as the core conditions. These conditions, often referred to as qualities, are known as congruence, unconditional positive regard and empathy. They are the main ingredients for the therapeutic relationship and the main techniques of person-centred therapy.

We will consider the following conditions in more depth here while noting that the words in parentheses are often used interchangeably with those terms. It is also important to note that although they can be described separately they are inter-linked; to have one quality without the other is not possible.

- Congruence (genuineness)
- Unconditional positive regard (acceptance, respect, warmth)
- Empathy.

## Congruence (genuineness)

The condition of congruence has in more recent times been termed as genuineness. This quality and attitude is a willingness of the nurse to be authentic in the relationship with the patient, with a reference to expressing one's own thoughts and feelings; the nurse is being real and being his/herself in the helping relationship. This means not being false or putting on a facade – for example, not feeling and thinking one thing while saying something different. It does not mean putting aside our role as the nurse, but being ourselves within that role. There needs to be harmony in our thinking and feeling while expressing our views and behaviour in relation to the therapeutic relationship and helping goals. By being open and honest we are conveying that we and our patients are on the same journey. Therefore a degree of trust can be gained. By communicating our genuineness, interest, acceptance and curiosity in the patient, this can help in exploring difficult and painful issues. Being congruent does not mean we have to express all our thoughts and feelings, but make sure the ones we do express are authentic and in the best interest of the patient.

Freshwater (2003: 22) posits that 'congruence is not always easy to achieve in everyday nursing practice', pointing out that nurses are often in a position of authority and will often have access to knowledge and information that is not available to the patient for whatever reason. Mental health nurses may also need to communicate with caution at times, having also to consider the needs of the family, other professionals and ethical codes of practice (Ruddick, 2010). This makes it difficult at times to respond to patients' requests and questions from a position of equality and total honesty. This requires a great deal of self-awareness for the nurse in knowing ourselves and our limits.

To hear patients' statements, such as the following, indicates congruence and genuineness:

'I felt the nurse was always honest with me.'

'I never felt that the nurse gave the wrong impression to me.'

'When it really mattered, the nurse would show her feelings.'

Frankland and Sanders (1995) use the term 'harmony' as an interpretation of congruence in a helping relationship. Some examples of how a harmonious attitude may be displayed are as follows:

- When saying 'how are you today, good to see you' is this reflected in your body language, tone of voice and how you really feel?
- Make sure your gestures and expressions are congruent with what you are saying.

- While saying you are interested in what the patient wants to talk about your words should be consistent with your feelings.
- Be spontaneous, but not impulsive.
- Avoid being defensive.
- Your own values and beliefs towards helping the patient are evident in the relationship.
- Congruence, along with acceptance and empathy, will help develop a trusting relationship in which the patient feels safe enough to share difficult feelings.

## Unconditional positive regard (acceptance, respect, warmth)

The condition of expressing unconditional positive regard is also known as conveying acceptance, respect and warmth. It is a quality that mental health nurses must endeavour to hold, to some degree, to be effective and therapeutic in their work (Dexter and Wash, 1997). Having and holding unconditional positive regard is being able to respond to the patient so that they feel valued and accepted, in whatever they are thinking and feeling. The advantage to the relationship is that the patient will feel the nurse does not judge, hold any ridicule or rejection. This will help create an atmosphere of safety and for the patient to be more open and honest in the relationship. The theory is interwoven with Maslow's hierarchy of needs (discussed later); the need to feel accepted, respected and loved and thus motivating us to reach our own acceptance of self and self-actualisation. In a nursing context we need to demonstrate this attitude by putting aside our own values, beliefs and any prejudices regarding the patients' behaviour, accept patients for whom they are, and to try and understand their values and beliefs. There will be occasions when we need to distinguish between the patient's behaviour and the person. We may not agree or like what they are doing, be opposed to their values and beliefs, but we still need to care for them and value them as a person. We need to demonstrate the difference between not liking the person and not liking the behaviour. As nurses we work with patients from a diverse range of social backgrounds and cultural differences. Add, also, differences in beliefs and value systems towards health and towards other human beings, it is a big ask to dispense with our judgements, preconceived ideas and criticisms.

To hear patients' statements such as the following indicates acceptance:

'Whenever I have felt really low it does not seem to affect the way the nurse feels towards me.'

'No matter how I feel I always have a sense that the nurse respects me.'

'Whatever I have said, not said or done the nurse's attitude towards me is friendly and caring.'

'I never felt put down or was made to feel bad about myself.'

'Through all my struggles, the nurse made me feel I was worth it.'

## Empathy

Empathy is perhaps the most important quality the helper must own for a helping relationship to be therapeutic. A simple definition is the ability to understand the patient's circumstances, experiences, thoughts, feelings and their inner world. However, perhaps not so simple is to communicate this to the patient in an accurate and meaningful way and not for it to be superficial. Rogers (1961) adds importantly that empathy is the ability to sense the other person's world as if it were one's own, without losing the 'as if' quality. The 'as if' quality means not getting lost in the state of the other's world, otherwise when a patient is in distress we may be pulled in and would be of little help to anyone. Empathy is different from sympathy, which is feeling for the other person. This can affect us emotionally and can lead to overidentification and feeling sad or sorry for the patient unless we are able to contain our own feelings. Although sympathy is an expression of caring feelings such as sorrow or dismay it can encompass pity and judgement and can place the nurse in an 'us and them position'. When the nurse communicates sympathy the patient perceives their feelings as justified, but does not necessarily build a therapeutic relationship with the nurse for the purpose of change. Empathy is saying 'I'm here with you; we'll deal with this together.' It helps to create equality in the relationship. Empathy is a willingness to listen and to put aside the label or diagnosis and find the human being in there. By communicating your empathic understanding you can help the patient move beyond feelings of despair and negativity. They will begin to understand their feelings, feel less alone, feel motivated and focus on moving through the situation. Nurses spend a significant amount of time interacting with patients, and although many relationships may be transient and brief, you should adopt a manner that would befit your own children or parents. This can make the patient feel wanted and heard. McCabe and Timmins (2006: 72) cite several research findings on the importance of empathy in nursing and rightly state that 'if nurses fail to empathise with their patients, then they cannot help them to understand or cope effectively as individuals with their illness'.

To hear patients' statements such as the following indicates empathy:

'There were certain moments when the nurse was able to put my thoughts into words.'

'At times the nurse was able to read my mind.'

'After talking to the nurse I felt warmed by her quiet attention to my words, for once I really felt I was listened to, and I really felt she understood how I felt.'

## Implications for nursing

Although Rogers was referring to counsellors offering therapy to clients for therapeutic change, these necessary conditions are very much transferable to all nurse–patient relationships, in particular when the emphasis of the relationship is to be of a therapeutic and restorative nature. Many relationships in nursing will be transient; for example in an acute hospital setting; yet there is still ad hoc opportunity for the nurse to enter into the spirit of the encounter and engagement with these conditions in mind. Rogers argued that it is the qualities exhibited by the counsellor and experienced by the client in the therapeutic relationship which will form the building blocks of that relationship (Green, 2010). As nurses we can take that sentiment from Rogers and exhibit it in our nursing care. I agree with Watkins (2001), who adds that these sentiments are not something that can be turned on and off if they are to be genuine. We can also consider them to be a way of being in the world and a way of being, both in our personal and professional lives. Mearns and Cooper (2009) poignantly and accessibly point out that an effective way of being with someone experiencing mental ill health is to work at relational depth, meaning engaging fully in a congruent, accepting and empathic way.

In true person-centred theory there would be no restrictions on who can benefit. However we need to distinguish here between person-centred therapy and a person-centred approach. While therapy may not be the first choice of treatments for those experiencing more severe and enduring mental ill health, the sentiments of the nurse should always have elements of the person-centred approach. To help patients feel safe and secure and free from the threat of judgement can enable them to make their own choices and decisions about their life.

## Person-centred theory: Maslow's hierarchy of needs

Abraham Maslow's most well-known contribution to humanistic psychology is the hierarchy of needs (Maslow, 1970), which is a theory of understanding human motivation and personality. The basic premise behind this hierarchy is that we are born with certain needs. Without meeting these initial needs, we will not be able to continue our lives moving upward in the hierarchy. The hierarchy can provide a set of theoretical guidelines for understanding the concerns of people suffering from physical illness, mental illness, disabilities and other life problems. A need can be defined here as something that is essential to the emotional and psychological health and survival of human beings. We all strive to meet basic needs at any given time and these needs may be met, unmet or partially met.

This hierarchy is most often displayed as a pyramid (Figure 4.1). The lowest levels of the pyramid are made up of the most basic needs, while the more complex needs are located at the top of the pyramid. The concept is widely acknowledged and used today in many settings such as psychology, education, management, nursing and allied health professions.

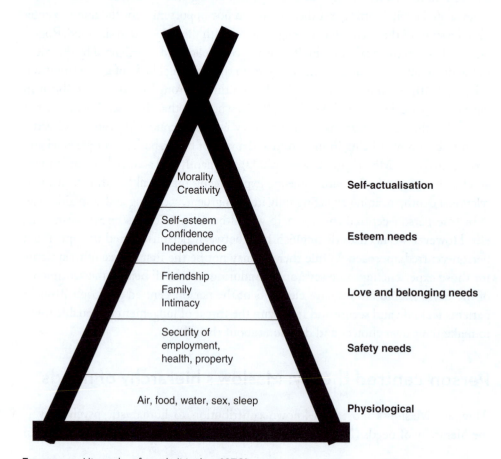

**FIGURE 4.1**  Hierarchy of needs (Maslow, 1970)

The first four levels, physiological, safety, belonging and esteem needs, Maslow calls D or deficiency (deficit) needs; these needs arise due to deprivation. If we don't have enough of something, we feel a deficit and therefore feel a need (Brammer and MacDonald, 1999). Satisfying these lower level needs is important for survival and to avoid unpleasant feelings. The highest and last level of the pyramid, self-actualisation, is somewhat different. Maslow (1970) termed this 'growth motivation', in contrast to 'deficit motivation'. These growth needs are also known as being-needs or B-needs. They do not stem from a lack of something, rather from a desire to grow and achieve as a person.

One must meet, at least at a minimum level, the lower level basic needs before progressing on to meet higher level growth needs. Once these needs have been reasonably satisfied, one may be able to focus attention on the pinnacle need of self-actualisation.

## Physiological needs

Physical needs are inherent in all human beings and are the basic needs and requirements for human physical survival. They are the first and foremost needs and are vital for survival. They include essentials such as oxygen, food, water, shelter, sleep and procreation to assure the continuation of human existence. When these needs are unmet, human beings will focus on satisfying them and will ignore higher needs. Physiological needs must be met at least minimally for life to continue.

## Safety needs

Once the individual's basic physiological needs are met, the need for safety emerges. This need is also important for survival but not as demanding as the physiological needs. Safety is both physiological and psychological. We need not only a safe physical environment, with a sense of security and protection, such as a safe home in a safe neighbourhood, but also the feeling of psychological safety that can offer stability and predictability in the world, such as permanent work with some financial security.

Children and adults alike feel a sense of security and hence safety in having a routine and an element of sameness in their lives. A child may feel insecure and anxious if there is a lack of consistency, injustice, unfairness or negative messages coming from parental figures. Physical, sexual, verbal abuse, divorce or a death within the family unit can cause more serious threats to security. Maslow thought that inadequate fulfilment of safety needs might explain, in some people, neurotic behaviour and other emotional problems, such as anxiety, fear and stress. To help us feel safe we need regular contact with people we trust, can identify with and have empathic understanding for us. The nurse needs to create both the environment and a relationship so the patient feels safe and avoids danger.

## Love and belonging needs

When our physiological and safety needs are met, needs for love and belongingness emerge. The security we gain from love and belonging enhances the feeling of safety. Making friends and finding a partner for a loving and affectionate relationship and starting a family will enable this need for belongingness. There may also be a hunger or need to belong to a group, a church, a club or gang, to feel accepted and be part of a community.

We want to feel part of something enduring, to feel accepted, respected, wanted and most of all loved. Hence we seek mutually meaningful relationships with other people. Maslow emphasised that these needs involve both giving and receiving love. When these needs are not fulfilled key implications can be loneliness and social anxieties leading to sadness and depression. A caring and compassionate nurse can offer the fulfilment of these needs within the therapeutic relationship. Patients need to feel accepted and respected. By being compassionate and communicating warmth, empathy and genuineness we can help the patient to feel wanted and valued. Love and belonging and the following esteem needs are required for the maintenance of good health.

## Self-esteem needs

This need is for the achievement of self-esteem, derived largely from the feeling that we are valued and respected by those around us. Esteem needs include both self-esteem and the esteem of others. We feel good about ourselves when the people who are important to us express acceptance and approval. We feel worthwhile, competent and independent when others respect and appreciate us. Self-esteem also comes from within; it is related to the assessments of our own adequacy and performance. As our awareness of our own self-worth grows, we become more self-assured and competent regarding our deeper thoughts, feelings and values and are less reliant upon others' judgements of our worth. There are major implications here for the nurse. Developing and maintaining the therapeutic relationship can encourage, motivate and facilitate patients to think, plan and problem-solve for themselves.

## Self-actualising needs

This last level differs as it does not arise from deficiencies (as the previous needs do) but from a higher motivating growth-force which Maslow called self-actualisation. This term refers to the innate tendency of all human beings to move forward, grow and reach their fullest potential. Brammer and MacDonald (1999) propose that these fifth level needs are the most difficult to define and describe, as this level functions best when the other four lower level needs are in the process of being satisfied.

The concept of self-actualisation focuses on our strengths rather than our deficiencies. The process of self-actualisation continues throughout life as we become more aware of what we are capable of being, to be all that we can be and our interests are focused on fulfilling that potential (Maslow, 1962).

## Implications for nursing

The theory provides a useful framework for understanding people with whom we work and emphasises the nurse's role in helping them to meet their physiological and psychosocial needs. It is valuable in the organisation of care by focusing on initial priorities and further assessment of needs. You will find descriptions of Maslow's needs hierarchy in many textbooks of nursing, as it is applied to various nursing models and interventions. In the context of mental health nursing we need to be aware that some patients, due to their illness or condition, may be a danger, or are struggling to remain conscious of their basic needs. In such situations the nurse needs to prioritise meeting the physiological and safety needs first.

Joe is a 58-year-old man who has been referred to a psychiatric day unit; this follows his discharge from hospital following an attempted suicide. He lives alone in the same house he grew up in with his parents. He worked in his father's furniture store and inherited a large sum of money following the death of both his parents over the past five years. He has now retired and has no financial worries. His parents were hardworking and strict with Joe. Love and affection were not overtly displayed in the family and Joe, an only child, was often criticised for being overweight, being lazy and not being a high achiever. He grew up with a sense of worthlessness. He has few friends and describes himself as a loner. He was being treated for depression by his GP. The family house still holds many of his parents' belongings, clothes and memorabilia. He has been unable to move on in his life since his mother died two years ago and feels life is not worth living.

CASE EXAMPLE

A person-centred approach to Joe's care by the nursing team would involve the following:

- A team approach with a shared philosophy that is practised by the team and carries the spirit and culture of person-centred care.
- Getting to know Joe as a person and not a diagnosis or label.
- An assessment of Joe's physical condition.
- A risk assessment.
- Getting to know Joe's values, beliefs and aspirations, health and social care needs and preferences.
- Care planning with Joe, enabling him to make decisions based on informed choices about ways to move forward with his life, therefore promoting independence and autonomy.
- Shared decision-making with Joe regarding follow-up services, rather than control being exerted over him; enabling choice of specific care and services to meet his health and social care needs and preferences.
- Ongoing evaluation.

Emma was assigned as Joe's key nurse. She spent time getting to know Joe and developed a therapeutic relationship built on trust and honesty. Emma used active listening and responding to convey her genuineness, unconditional regard and empathic understanding. While at first Joe would look to Emma for direction, the emphasis was on Joe to make his decisions and choices. This was difficult for him at first as Joe had absorbed, over time, messages called conditions of worth, believing that he was only worthwhile if he did what he was told and pleased his parents. He found it difficult to identify his own opinions and choices, a reason why his parents' belongings still dominated the house where he lived. Over time Emma helped and encouraged Joe to focus on his feelings. He expressed that no one in his past had really listened to him; he had always felt that his needs and wants would only be rejected. This had made him feel helpless, unable to make decisions and take direction with his own life. Working with Emma, Joe began to feel accepted and valued in his own right. For Joe to become more fully functioning as a person, he needed to get in touch with his self-actualising tendency. This was gradually acquired as Joe began to believe he was a person of worth. As his image of himself became more positive, so did his self-concept. As Joe became more motivated his needs of feeling that he really belonged in the world and his self-esteem needs were able to develop. He was then able to choose the best course of action for himself and set goals. He began to dispose of many of his parents' belongings, and he planned to use the space to build a studio and study room. He had always been a keen birdwatcher, liking to sketch and then paint his sightings. With a new sense of belief in himself, Joe felt he could pursue this interest.

## Summary

This chapter has focused on person-centred theory. The history and background of the two main psychologists, Carl Rogers and Abraham Maslow, are important as this paved the way for their contributions to the humanistic movement in the 1950s. This became known as the third force in psychology and unlike earlier approaches, the emphasis is on personal responsibility and choices. They believe this is because we are born with a motivational force, known as the actualising tendency; this force moves us towards constructive growth. Mental ill health can occur when the actualising tendency has become thwarted. It is important to understand the development of self and the effect of conditions of worth placed on the individual, as a damaged self-concept greatly hinders progress towards self-actualisation. Rogers placed great significance on the existence of the therapeutic relationship in order for any change to occur. The core conditions are known as congruence, unconditional positive regard and empathy. These qualities, along with a facilitative environment, can enable the nurse to help nurture the patients' well-being and movement towards their own personal growth and development. While Rogers argued for the importance of the core conditions in meeting self-actualisation needs, Maslow's viewpoint was that self-actualisation is achievable when lower needs are satisfied and self-esteem is positive, even when faced with rejection from others. The hierarchy of needs is important as it presents a framework for mental health nurses to understand how patients' motivations and behaviour can change during crises, and therefore prioritise the nature and order of help.

## Acknowledgement and gratitude

In loving memory of my mother, Joan Cassedy, who passed away as this chapter was finally being completed.

## References

Brammer, L.M. and MacDonald, G. (1999) *The Helping Relationship: Process and Skills*. Boston: Allyn and Bacon.

Dexter, G. and Wash, M. (1997) *Psychiatric Nursing Skills: A Patient-centred Approach* (2nd edn). Cheltenham: Stanley Thornes.

Dryden, W. and Mytton, J. (1999) *Four Approaches to Counselling and Psychotherapy.* London: Routledge.

Frankland, A. and Sanders, P. (1995) *Next Steps in Counselling.* Ross on Wye: PCCS Books.

Freshwater, D. (2003) *Counselling Skills for Nurses, Midwives and Health Visitors.* Maidenhead: Open University Press.

Green, J. (2010) *Creating the Therapeutic Relationship in Counselling and Psychotherapy.* Exeter: Learning Matters.

Hough, M. (1998) *Counselling Skills and Theory.* London: Hodder & Stoughton.

Hough, M. (2002) *A Practical Approach to Counselling* (2nd edn). Harlow: Prentice Hall.

McCabe, C. and Timmins, F. (2006) *Communication Skills for Nursing Practice.* Basingstoke: Palgrave Macmillan.

McLeod, J. (2003) *An Introduction to Counselling* (3rd edn). Buckingham: Open University Press.

McMillan, M. (2010) *The Person-centred Approach to Therapeutic Change.* London: Sage.

Maslow, A.H. (1962) *Toward a Psychology of Being.* New York: D. Van Nostrand Company.

Maslow, A.H. (1970) *Motivation and Personality* (2nd edn). New York: Harper and Row.

Mearns, D. and Cooper, M. (2009) *Working at Relational Depth in Counselling and Psychotherapy.* London: Sage.

Thorne, B. (2011) 'Person-centred theory', in W. Dryden (ed.), *Handbook of Individual Therapy.* London: Sage.

Rogers, C.R. (1942) *Counselling and Psychotherapy.* Boston: Houghton Mifflin.

Rogers, C.R. (1951) *Client Centred Therapy.* London: Constable.

Rogers, C.R. (1961) *On Becoming a Person.* Boston: Houghton Mifflin.

Rogers, C.R. (1980) *A Way of Being.* Boston: Houghton Mifflin.

Rogers, C.R. (1990) 'This is me', in H. Kirschenbaum and V.L. Henderson (eds), *The Carl Rogers Reader.* London: Constable.

Ruddick, F. (2010) 'Person-centred mental health care:myth or reality', *Mental Health Practice,* 13 (9): 24–28

Watkins, P. (2001) *Mental Health Nursing: The Art of Compassionate Care.* Boston: Butterworth-Heinemann.

# 5

# Cognitive Behavioural Theories

## PHILIP KINSELLA

### Learning Objectives

- Understand how cognitive behavioural therapy (CBT) arises from psychological research, originally on classical and operant learning, and more recently on cognitive processes.
- Consider the importance of the interaction between thoughts, feelings, physiological states and behaviours for the theory and practice of CBT.
- Understand CBT procedure: for example that it is focused on the here-and-now, is structured and it teaches patients to be their own therapist particularly in applying new ways of thinking and acting.

## Introduction

James is an 18-year-old man, and although he is rather shy, he has a number of good friends. He was out in a bar one night with a close friend and some other people he did not know. He did his best to join in the conversation, and even tried to tell a joke at one point, that fell rather flat. Since that night six months ago, his friends have been ringing him up and asking him to go out for a drink, but he's been refusing, avoiding all social contacts, and more recently not answering the phone. Why is this? Can the theory of cognitive behavioural therapy help explain it?

Cognitive behavioural therapy (CBT) is a way of understanding psychological experiences in a scientific way. At a basic level it tries to explain the link between cognition, emotion, physiological states and behaviour. So, for example, it was subsequently discovered that James has developed social phobia. His anxiety in the pub became so extreme that he left the pub early, and then became very avoidant of social situations. At a cognitive level he was thinking 'my friends don't want to see me … I'm boring'; this threatening thought would then influence his emotional state, leading to anxiety, and he would experience the physiological state associated with anxiety particularly dry mouth and shaky hands. Not only would this emotional state intensify his negative thinking, but it and the negative thinking would encourage him to avoid social situations, thus depriving him of any opportunity to learn that his thoughts are exaggerated (or that he could cope with some people not liking him).

The cognitive behavioural therapist that he later saw applied his knowledge of the cognitive and behavioural mechanisms that maintain mental disorders to the patient's actual presentation of social phobia, thus helping both of them understand how the social anxiety problem was being maintained by avoidance strategies. From this understanding the therapist then discussed various strategies to overcome the problem, mostly based on facing fears, to learn a more helpful and realistic perspective on his anxieties.

## Historical development

Cognitive behavioural therapy has developed from research in psychology, and the most influential initial research was on behavioural processes. Pavlov (1927) described experiments that are now called classical conditioning experiments, most famously demonstrating that two stimuli can become closely associated: for example an animal that would naturally salivate in response to food could be made to salivate in response to a bell that has been rung when the food was presented, the food and the bell becoming associated. This became relevant to CBT later on when an attempt was made to understand how phobias developed. It was argued that a strong emotion of anxiety could not only be produced by certain objects or creatures, for example snakes and spiders (this would be quite common in the population), but this fear would also be triggered by objects the creature is associated with, such as long grass in the case of the snake, and dusty garages with the spiders.

An important development in the 1930s and 1940s was the work of Skinner (1938) and others on operant conditioning. Skinner demonstrated that reinforcements (rewards) would increase a behaviour, punishments would reduce it, and the reduction of rewards would reduce a target behaviour. This may seem fairly obvious, but Skinner was one of the first people who were able to demonstrate this scientifically, and to work out the optimum schedules of rewards and punishments that most powerfully influenced these animal and human behaviours.

This work became influential in helping to understand psychological problems, particularly phobias, through the work of Mowrer (1939). He built on the idea from Pavlov that people could develop anxious reactions to stimuli such as snakes and spiders and that this could generalise. He then argued that people were more likely to develop phobias when they escaped from or avoided the phobic stimuli, as it did not then allow for the process of habituation. Habituation means that repeated exposure to the stimuli reduces the anxious response. This avoidance of and escape from the situation lead to a huge reduction of anxiety which is powerfully rewarding, thus increasing the avoidance behaviour, and stopping the natural habituation. This major development in the theoretical understanding of anxiety led to the treatment of exposure for phobias and this was applied to other anxiety problems. This advance has been one of the most important in mental health, in that it has led to the successful treatment of anxiety disorders for many people (Marks, 1987).

Because the avoidance was stopping the natural process of habituation it was argued that patients, in clinical practice, need to be exposed to their feared stimuli (e.g. the garage and the spiders). Treatments were developed along these lines and proved to be remarkably successful (Marks, 1987). It took various experiments (clinical trials) to discover the optimal way to do this. It was found that the best way to do exposure is to do it gradually (to face a stimulus at the lower end of the hierarchy); prolonged (so that the fear that initially rises in response to the stimulus has a chance to go down, as it naturally does with time passing); regularly (so that each time the person does the exposure he or she feels less anxious); and focused (that the person does not distract him/herself from the benefits of the exposure).

So a behavioural approach, as described above, would consider the following explanation for James's problems: the environmental situation of the pub led to James feeling anxious, the situation would be seen as an unconditioned stimulus, and his anxious response would be an unconditioned response. The theory would suggest that he was predisposed to have these responses because of his temperament, and also because of earlier conditioned responses, like becoming upset in similar social situations. His escape from the situation would be a powerful negative reinforcer of further escape and avoidance behaviour. A behavioural approach to his problems would be to encourage exposure to all avoided stimuli, in his case this would be avoided social situations.

Around the same time that these behavioural treatments were being developed in the 1960s, there was some feeling that cognitive processes were being neglected. Aaron Beck (1967) and Albert Ellis (1962) separately developed cognitive therapies that tried to take these more into consideration. The cognitive processes considered were primarily the content of thinking, 'I'm useless . . . I'm a failure . . . I can't cope', but also thinking processes like worry, rumination, memory, imagery and logic. Beck developed a theoretical model of depression which has been influential, and he and other clinicians have developed models of other disorders such as obsessive compulsive disorder (OCD), social phobia, health anxiety, generalised anxiety disorder, bulimia nervosa and psychosis. Ellis's approach with his strong emphasis on irrational thinking has a less strong evidence base and support.

There has been a considerable amount of research since then looking at the validity of cognitive processes in terms of how they link to dysfunctional emotional states and unhelpful behaviours.

Historically CBT has valued a scientific approach to resolving theoretical and outcome issues, such as whether to see the stressful situation or the response to the stressful situation as most important, and one hopes that this continues to be the case.

## Theory of cognitive behavioural therapy

CBT theory has become quite influential in terms of mental health practice. For example in the UK there has been a development called Improving Access to Psychological Therapies (IAPT), in which investment has been made in helping people get evidence-based therapies, which are predominantly CBT. The CBT approach is also taught in medical and nursing courses at undergraduate level. Therefore, many mental health professionals are aware of, or have an allegiance to this approach.

It should be said, however, that there is not a specific CBT theory to describe, but various schools of CBT theories and practices, for example behaviour therapy, Beck's cognitive therapy, Ellis's rational emotive behavioural therapy, acceptance and commitment therapy and various others. Clinicians have allegiances to different brands of CBT, often depending on where they were trained, and who their supervisors and mentors are.

What do these brands of CBT have in common? Fundamentally, a position that the interaction between the environment, cognition, emotions, physiological states and behaviour is important in understanding mental ill health, and that it is important to understand this interaction from a scientific perspective, and to understand how this perspective leads to treatments that can be objectively evaluated.

Rather than trying to describe the theory behind every brand of CBT, I will focus on describing Beckian cognitive therapy, because I personally find it most persuasive, it is commonly used and there is a lot of evidence to support its theory and application. It may even be able to integrate aspects of behaviour theory and practice into its approach.

The best description of Beck's cognitive therapy is in Alford and Beck (1997):

1  The central pathway to psychological functioning and dysfunction is the meaning-making function, called the schema. These schemas can be understood best as strongly held beliefs. James's key schemas are 'I'm boring . . . other people don't like to be with me . . . the world in general is critical'. These schemas are latent, in that they are not active in the person's awareness until a pertinent activating event occurs. With James it was an incident in a pub when he tried to tell a joke and it fell very flat. His thinking process went from 'that joke was a disaster' to 'they think I'm boring' to 'I am boring'.

2  The purpose of this meaning-making function is to control the various psychological systems (behavioural, emotional, attentional and memory). This control occurs both deliberately and automatically. For example, if a person had a schema that 'my work is more important than my friends', then this would influence their behaviour (choosing working over spending time with friends), emotions (being more anxious about not completing a piece of work than not being able to meet a friend for a coffee), attentional (paying more attention to work than friends) and finally memory (having a stronger memory of work-related problems than friend-related problems).

3  These systems are interactive: being anxious about a work-related issue leads to more attentional focus on the threat of the work issue, more behavioural effort in trying to complete it. The behavioural effort may have a positive or negative effect on the anxiety about work.

4  The meaning is correct or incorrect in terms of a specific context or goal. James's belief that he is not liked is incorrect, because the evidence (from the phone calls for example is that his friends do like him). It is also unhelpful in that it discourages him from socialising, which is one of his goals.

5  Many mental health problems such as anxiety, depression and eating disorders arise from maladaptive meanings regarding the self, one's experiences and the future. All three components are interpreted negatively in depression. In anxiety the self is seen as inadequate, the experience threatening and the future uncertain. With anger and paranoia, the self is seen as mistreated and the experience as unfair.

6  The schemas are activated by situations that are congruent with the schema. So with James his schema is activated (brought more strongly into awareness) by triggering events that are congruent with the schema: for example, interpersonal rejection, critical comments, someone viewing him as boring and so on.

There are a number of assumptions that underlie the theory of Beckian cognitive therapy. One is the objectivist position that there is a real external world that can be referred to. Thus, if a person with social phobia believes he has no friends then it is possible to interrogate the environment to see whether this is actually the case.

Another assumption is that psychological disorders do actually exist, social phobia, depression, OCD, etc., which are driven by the processes outlined above. It is generally accepted in CBT theory that it is useful to categorise mental disorders and use diagnostic categories, because these disorders do exist, and are sufficiently different from one another to make the categorisation worthwhile. For example, bulimia nervosa is sufficiently different from schizophrenia that it would be unhelpful to just lump these together as 'mental health problems'. The other advantage of categorisation is that it does allow for careful research into the psychopathology of the condition. However, it is accepted that labelling/categorisation can be a problem because of potential discrimination against the person concerned, but it is thought that the advantages of diagnosis outweigh the disadvantages. In the spirit of CBT the truth of this statement is open to empirical investigation.

A further assumption is that mental processes can occur out of awareness (this could be called the unconscious), but that normally through the use of questioning these processes can be made more explicit. If James is carefully asked what's on his mind, he should be able to identify that he is worried that people don't like him and that he is boring.

It may be possible to integrate a behavioural learning theory perspective with a Beckian cognitive therapy perspective (Alford and Beck, 1997). A Beckian perspective on James's problems is as follows: temperamentally he is rather shy: this is not a problem, as this is a normal personality variable, and patients only come to clinical attention when their problems impact on their lives. Unfortunately, he had a number of experiences as a young person that made him more vulnerable to social phobia. His father died when he was eight, and he lost this guide and role model. His father's death led to him being moved around schools which stopped him having a very settled set of friends. These experiences reinforced his schema 'I'm boring . . . other people don't want to be with me'. These uncomfortable thoughts led him to be anxious at times. Everyone has a number of *rules for living* which are beliefs usually framed as statements like 'if . . . then . . .' or 'I must . . .'. James's *rules for living* were: 'if I avoid social situations I'll be safe', and 'don't speak out if you can avoid it'. James has evolved these rules as ways of coping with the world, especially to help him avoid the activation of his underlying schemas of being boring, and of people not liking him. One can see that if he generally follows a rule to avoid social situations, or does not say much in them, he is unlikely to be exposed to a sense of himself as boring; so this is how he tends to behave in a general sense. The disadvantage of this is that he lives a rather limited existence, has fewer friends than he would like and also has less opportunity to practise normal social skills, leaving him somewhat deficient in this area. In terms of cognitive therapy theory, the early experiences and the *schemas* and *rules for living* would be viewed as *predisposing factors* for the development of social phobia.

There were a number of *precipitating factors* that led to James having the disorder: starting his first job in which he had to interact more with the public, and also attempts he was making to be more sociable by going out with a wider range of people. These *precipitating events* brought his schemas more to the forefront of his awareness, and led to what is termed *the maintenance cycle* (Figure 5.1). This term is used to explain that although many shy people may have the *predisposing and precipitating factors*, they may never experience social phobia, which is characterised by significant anxiety in social situations and avoidance to a degree that is impacting on the person's life. In James's case when he was in the pub he started thinking 'this joke's boring . . . they don't like me . . . I'm being boring'. These *negative thoughts* in situations represent specific manifestations of his underlying schema. People don't just think in words but also in images, which often are more emotionally laden. James's images are of people laughing at him, and he can see this powerfully in his mind's eye. This image is related to a terrible experience he had at school when he unfortunately wet himself and a couple of people noticed and did laugh at him. Cognitive theory would suggest therefore that it is not just the triggering event that causes the unhealthy anxious emotion that is felt, but the way someone interprets and perceives it through these cognitive processes. The theory would suggest that James's reaction to social situations is excessively anxious in proportion to the actual threat. When the anxiety escalates there is a switching in attention in that there is focus on the threat, and on one's own experience of anxiety, and this attentional shift can get in the way of normally engaging in the social situation. The theory is that when we are anxious we engage in *avoidance* and also *safety seeking behaviours*. It is not hard to see why James would want to avoid social situations, and the negative impact that would have. Safety seeking behaviours are behaviours that persons actively engage in during the social interaction, and believe will help them avoid their worst scenarios, but have various negative effects that powerfully maintain the problem. In James's case he tends to sit at the back of the group, avoid eye contact, not say much, rehearse excessively in his mind what he is going to say. These behaviours are counterproductive in that they get in the way of normal engagement

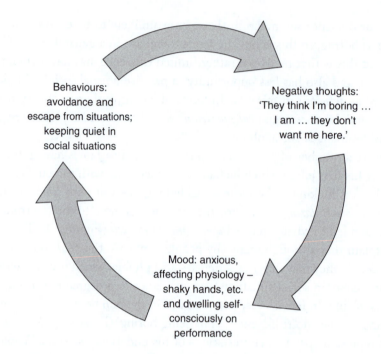

Behaviours: avoidance and escape from situations; keeping quiet in social situations

Negative thoughts: 'They think I'm boring … I am … they don't want me here.'

Mood: anxious, affecting physiology – shaky hands, etc. and dwelling self-consciously on performance

**FIGURE 5.1**  Diagram of James's maintenance cycle using the Beckian CBT model (triggering event: experience in pub)

in the social situation and may indeed lead others to think that the person is quiet, even boring, and they stop the person learning that the worst fears of people laughing and calling him boring are very unlikely to occur. The theory would suggest therefore that these behavioural processes are extremely important in keeping the maintenance cycle of disorder, in this case social phobia, in place.

In summary, individuals because of their temperament and early experiences develop schemas, and these may make them vulnerable to disorder. When these schemas are activated in stressful circumstances they lead to a vicious circle of cognitive processes which lead to an unhealthy emotional state such as anxiety, depression, anger, jealousy and so on, that would be called a disorder. The mechanism for this in social phobia has been described. In other anxiety disorders the mechanism is similar. For example in health anxiety there are schemas around vulnerability to ill health, in OCD around responsibility (Hawton et al., 1989), and in generalised anxiety disorder more general schemas around vulnerability to harm and need for control (Dugas and Robichaud, 2006). With depression the schemas are often very self-critical, for example 'I'm useless ... I'm a failure', which are activated in the face of experiences of loss or failure (Beck, 1967). The vicious circle is typically the activation of these beliefs and the activation of a process of rumination on them, leading to a depressed mood and the various physical manifestations of poor sleep and appetite, and a pattern of significant avoidance that maintains the depression.

CBT does face criticisms, and the most common ones are that: it pays little heed to impoverished environments; it inadequately considers the therapeutic relationship; it is too rationalistic and objectivist in a world that is fluid and constructed; the strong evidence base for its effectiveness can be challenged. These interesting debates can be followed up in other publications (House and Loewenthal, 2008).

## Theory applied to practice

As a theory of mental health applied to nursing, CBT has become increasing influential. In the 1960s, token economy rewards, using behavioural principles, were often administered by mental health nurses (Hall et al., 1976). More recently nurses in their education have been exposed to CBT or behavioural principles, and may have used them in their practice. A number of nurses in the UK, including myself, were trained to an advanced level in behavioural theory and technique (Newell and Gournay, 1994). Very recently many nurses have trained in CBT in specialist courses and in particular through the IAPT initiative (Clark, 2012). It is likely that CBT will be increasingly influential in the mental health nursing field.

So how is the theory applied in practice? Most commonly now it will be through individual practitioners, often CBT trained nurses, treating patients in outpatient and inpatient settings, who have both common mental disorders such as anxiety and depression, and more complex disorders such as somatisation and schizophrenia. (It is also applied in practice through the supervision and training that CBT trained mental health nurses give to other nurses, and which then influences those nurses in their general work.)

Initially, when using CBT, nurses will conduct a detailed structured assessment of a patient to try and understand the *precipitating, predisposing and maintenance factors*, share this understanding with the patient, and determine whether the person is willing to engage in a CBT treatment programme.

The therapy is focused on current problems, but it does not ignore past difficult experiences, and in some instances as with post-traumatic stress disorder, the understanding and addressing of a past trauma is viewed as being essential in dealing with current difficulties.

The application of the theory is strongly scientific (this is apparent in the programme of scientific research that has been conducted into the postulated mechanisms that maintain the disorders, and the best ways to conduct treatments). The scientific approach is also applied to individual patients in that a hypothesis is developed about what maintains the specific problem for the patient, and individual patient data are collected to support or refute that view. Often questionnaires and measures are used to aid this, and also to objectively measure patient response. These data can also be used in research.

There is a strong emphasis on homework, and patients learning to become their own therapist. The argument here is that progress is made through learning techniques in session and applying those to situations outside: these techniques would involve learning to face fears and tackle avoidance, adopting a more rational and constructive attitude to negative thoughts, shifting attention off threats and on to day-to-day functioning, doing behavioural experiments, changing images, reducing rumination, reducing and stopping safety seeking and reassurance seeking behaviours. Homework is agreed in the session collaboratively, and should follow from the logic of the session, it should be clear why the patient has been encouraged to do it, and any difficulties in doing it should be addressed. The homework and the learning that arises from it is always reviewed in the next session, and taken forward to the next level (Hawton et al., 1989).

There are a number of things that are commonly done to aid memorising and engaging with the CBT approach: these would include taping the session; therapist and patient summarising the key learning points; using written records of homework, formulation and 'problems and goals'; encouraging the patient to use self-help books and materials.

Structure is important in CBT's application. It is likely that an agreement would be made with the patient as to how many sessions would be needed (perhaps 8–12 sessions with a straightforward problem). A clearly defined set of 'problems and goals' would be agreed at the beginning of therapy, and significant progress should be made towards these by the end. The sessions would be highly structured in that an agenda for the session is agreed at the beginning, how the person has been is evaluated, homework is reviewed, other issues are addressed, homework is set. Towards the end of the therapy relapse prevention is done by helping the person consider what has been helpful, what could cause a setback in the future and what needs to be done to address setbacks and generally maintain progress.

Although there is a high degree of structure there is also a high level of collaboration. The person is seen as an expert in his/her own life and personal resources are built on, the formulation and problem and targets statements are done collaboratively, the person helps to set the agenda for the session. The therapist brings his/her theoretical understanding of why the problem is occurring (Hawton et al., 1989).

Most of the time this works well but it does require each person to play a role in the process and this may not always happen. For example the patient may not agree with the view of the therapist as to why the problem is occurring, or may struggle to agree on problems and targets. Although this can occur, the most common problem is that the patient finds it difficult to do the homework tasks that are agreed. The person is often being asked to face situations that he or she is terrified of in anxiety disorders, and to activate him/herself when depressed despite feeling worthless and lacking in energy. A key skill of the therapist is to help the person engage with the tasks. Therapists can help the person see that the task is valuable, they can break the task down into smaller components to make it easier to do, they can help individuals engage with their motivation to overcome the problem, they can engage relatives to help, and so on.

James's mental health nurse, who was trained in CBT, conducted a very detailed assessment of the *predisposing, precipitating and maintenance factors*, trying to evaluate whether her initial sense that James had social phobia was correct, but also considered other diagnoses. After the assessment she collaboratively drew out a formulation diagram identifying the negative thinking, self-focused attention and unhelpful avoidant and safety behaviours that were maintaining the problem and James felt this was credible. It was agreed to follow a protocol to treat the disorder: this is a type of CBT that has been found to be helpful for a specific disorder (Clark and Wells, 1995). The structure of the protocol is used to guide therapy, but is applied flexibly and sensitively to the individual. In early sessions James was further encouraged to see that his self-focused attention and safety seeking behaviours were counterproductive. This was done by getting him to interact in a (staged) social situation first using poor eye contact and over-rehearsing what he was going to say, whilst focusing on his own feelings of anxiety. In the second condition he stopped doing this. The therapist measured three things after each condition: his level of anxiety, his performance in the situation and his self-consciousness. Broadly, as is expected from CBT theory, his scores were better not using the safety mechanisms, and placing his attention on naturally engaging with the conversation. Another experiment was to videotape him in a social interaction, making predictions beforehand as to how he would come over. He was surprised to find that his predictions that he would stutter, shake and 'look boring' were exaggerated, although it was agreed that he did not always look completely confident.

The next challenge in therapy was to agree behavioural experiments of going into social situations of increasing difficulty, and reducing the safety seeking behaviours and self-directed attention. He bravely tested out worries that people would laugh at

CASE EXAMPLE

*(Continued)*

*(Continued)*

him; he would shake and stutter; people would find him boring; he could only relax if he had an alcoholic drink. He did various things to evaluate this: talking more and evaluating people's reactions; not drinking alcohol; maintaining eye contact with others; speaking more spontaneously and not rehearsing his comments so much; speaking to people he didn't know. He learned that people were pleased to see him again, he could interact with others and engage their attention, and although he was not the life and soul of the party, he could live with that. He worked on two more things: one is a technique called 'Assertive defence of the self' (Padesky, 1997) in which he, in the session, role played the possibility of someone calling him boring or laughing at him, and he developed an assertive response, 'Please don't say that to me . . . If you're not interested in what I've got to say you don't have to listen.' He also deliberately and bravely exaggerated things he was worried about like shaking, to see if anyone noticed or he could cope with the reaction if they did.

The therapy had its challenges, and he could easily retreat back into avoidance if he felt someone was hostile or critical. Towards the end he worked a relapse prevention strategy mainly based on continuing to face social situations without the use of safety seeking behaviours.

---

# Summary

Cognitive behavioural therapy (CBT) is a way of understanding psychological phenomena in a scientific way, particularly the link between thinking, emotion, physiological states and behaviours. It is based on leaning theory, which has explained how phobias develop and are maintained, and cognitive theory, which has increased understanding of the role of thinking processes in mental disorders.

In practice the style is collaborative, structured, with a focus on here-and-now problems. Patients learn ways to alter unhelpful thinking and behaviours which they apply between sessions.

CBT theory has become quite influential in terms of mental health practice, this is due to a strong evidence base for its effectiveness, and its impact on mental health nurses' training and practice, particularly through IAPT.

# References

Alford, B.A. and Beck, A.T. (1997) *The Integrative Power of Cognitive Therapy.* New York: Guilford Press.

Beck, A.T. (1967) *Depression: Clinical, Experimental, and Theoretical Aspects.* Philadelphia: University of Pennsylvania Press.

Clark, D.M. (2012) 'The English Improving Access to Psychological Therapies Programme (IAPT)', in K.R. McHugh and D.H. Barlow (eds), *History and Progress in Dissemination and Implementation of Evidence-based Psychological Therapies.* Oxford: Oxford University Press.

Clark, D.M. and Wells, A. (1995) 'A cognitive model of social phobia', in R.G. Heimberg, M.R. Liebowitz, D.A. Hope and F.R. Schneier (eds), *Social Phobia: Diagnosis, Assessment and Treatment.* New York: Guilford Press.

Dugas, M. and Robichaud, M. (2006) *Cognitive-behavioral Treatment for Generalized Anxiety Disorder: From Science to Practice (Practical Clinical Guidebook).* New York: Routledge.

Ellis, A. (1962) *Reason and Emotion in Psychotherapy.* New York: Birch Lane Press.

Hall, J.N., Baker, R.D. and Hutchinson, K. (1976) 'A controlled evaluation of taken economy procedures with chronic schizophrenic patient', *Behaviour, Research and Therapy,* 15 (3): 261–83.

Hawton, K., Salkovskis, P.M., Kirk, J. and Clark, D.M. (1989) *Cognitive Behavioural Therapy for Psychiatric Patients: A Practical Guide.* Oxford: Oxford University Press.

Hayes, S.C., Strosahl, K.D. and Wilson, K.G. (2004) *Acceptance and Commitment Therapy: An Experiential Approach to Behavior Change.* New York: Guilford Press.

House, R. and Loewenthal, D. (2008) *Against and for CBT: Towards a Constructive Dialogue.* Ross on Wye: PCCS Books.

Loewenthal, D. and House, R. (2010) *Critically Engaging CBT.* Maidenhead: Open University Press.

Marks, I.M. (1987) *Fears, Phobias and Rituals.* Oxford: Oxford University Press.

Mowrer, O.H. (1939) 'A stimulus-response analysis of anxiety and its role as a rein- forcing agent', *Psychological Review,* 46 (6): 553–65.

Newell, R. and Gournay, K. (1994) 'British nurses in behavioural psychotherapy: a 20-year follow-up', *Journal of Advanced Nursing,* 20 (1): 53–60.

Padesky, C.A. (1997) 'A more effective treatment of social phobia', *International Cognitive Therapy Newsletter,* 11 (1): 1–3.

Pavlov, I.P. (1927) *Conditioned Reflexes,* trans. G.V. Anrep. New York: Liveright.

Simos, G. (2002) *Cognitive Behaviour Therapy: A Guide for the Practicing Clinician.* Hove: Brunner Routledge.

Skinner, B.F. (1938) *The Behaviour of Organisms: An Experimental Analysis.* Oxford: Appleton.

Wolitzky-Taylor, K.B., Horowitz, J.D., Powers, M.B. and Telch, M.J. (2008) 'Psychological approaches in the treatment of specific phobia: a meta-analysis', *Clinical Psychology Review,* 28 (6): 1021–37.

# 6

# Critical Theories in Mental Health Care

## ALASTAIR MORGAN

### Learning Objectives

- Understand the ideas and purpose of critical theory.
- Identify the history of critical ideas and movements in mental health practice.
- Understand the relevance of critical theory to dilemmas occurring in mental health practice.

## Introduction

What exactly is it that makes a theory critical? What does the addition of the word critical or critique add to the concept of a theory? There are two key aspects to critical theories. First, a critical theory examines and explores the central claims of a practice or set of ideas and institutions to try to identify whether those central claims are internally coherent. For example, as we will see, psychiatry claims to be treating something called mental illness. However, we might ask what the concept of illness means and whether when we examine mental health problems they meet the criteria of illnesses. Critical theorists term this procedure an immanent critique (Sabia, 2010). We take the claims of a practice at face value and then critically explore whether the practice upholds its central claims. One of the key voices in critical psychiatry, Thomas Szasz, argues that mental illness does not meet the criteria for an illness at all and therefore the basis for the critique of psychiatry is that it fails to uphold its own central claims as a medical practice (Szasz, 1972). This is a good example of an immanent critique.

However, immanent critique is only the first step in the process of a critical theory, as this critique has the purpose of a larger goal which we could broadly term emancipation. Many theorists will have different perspectives on what constitutes emancipation, but all critical theorists aim to critique existing institutions as they think that these institutions are in some way oppressive, exploitative or demeaning for individuals. The purpose of an immanent critique is to protest against injustice and to open the space for a better world. As Karl Marx, the great nineteenth-century critic of capitalism and the originator of critical theory, famously wrote:

> The philosophers have only interpreted the world, in various ways, the point is to change it. (Marx, 1988: 158)

The focus of Marx's original critique was the manner in which capitalism failed to uphold its own values of free exchange and was instead a system that operated through the exploitation of the working class. In the early to mid-twentieth century a number of thinkers in Germany developed Marx's ideas to critique a range of institutions including culture and the arts, psychoanalysis and psychiatry, journalism and education (Jay, 1996). This group of theorists are known collectively as the Frankfurt School and their approach to developing a broad critique of institutions, practices and the consciousness of individuals in society became highly influential and spawned a number of further developments in critical theory (Held, 1989). Some key movements here were critiques of gender relations and the oppression of women and the fight against racism within society. Whereas Marx had linked all exploitation to that based on class, these theorists argued that there were multiple sites of oppression and that oppression could be 'personal' as well as political (Younge, 2011). These movements based around personal liberation have often been termed forms of 'identity politics', and the claim to liberation was based around an assertion of a previously oppressed or excluded identity. There were liberation struggles for women, minority ethnic groups, colonised people, gay, lesbian and transgender people and importantly, disability rights movements.

## Critical theories in mental health care: historical development and relevance

What is the relevance of critical theory for the history of mental health care? If we take the initial route of an immanent critique, then psychiatry has always had an unstable basis because of its central claim to be a medical discipline based on the identification and treatment of illness.

In 1845, the first Professor of Psychiatry, Wilhelm Griesinger, boldly claimed that all mental illnesses would be identified ultimately as brain illnesses (Kendell, 2001). Griesinger's hope was that psychiatry would be able to disentangle itself from a history of associating madness with spiritual or demonic possession and to establish a scientific grounding for psychiatry on the basis of the classification of mental illnesses or diseases. Initially, this modern endeavour 'struck gold'. In the late nineteenth and early twentieth century researchers identified the physical causation for two mental illnesses. An illness termed general paralysis of the insane, which was previously thought to be a psychiatric disorder, was linked to syphilis infection (Fulford et al., 2006). Second, in the early twentieth century, using techniques of brain dissection, Alois Alzheimer identified the neurological deficits associated with the disease that was to later take his name – Alzheimer's disease (Andreasen, 2001). These two successes encouraged a model for all mental illnesses, that eventually scientific exploration would uncover the physiological abnormalities underlying the disorders.

However, this did not happen, and the classifications of all major mental illnesses occurred in the absence of any identification of underlying pathology. Depression, bipolar disorder, schizophrenia were all classified as illnesses at the beginning of the twentieth century, but the classification occurred through a process of observation and description of behaviours as abnormal rather than a scientific identification of physical alterations in the brain (Porter, 2002).

This produced two main problems for psychiatry. It claimed to be a medical discipline, but unlike other medical specialities it had no physical basis for its identification of disorder. Furthermore, the treatments available and used were often crude, harsh and punitive and without any understanding of how they might cure the supposed illnesses (Moncrieff, 2008). The second issue is that the process of the classification of diseases occurred through the observation of 'abnormal' behaviours. The definition of abnormality here was laden with the values and beliefs of the observers. This meant that abnormality often equated to behaviours that were not culturally acceptable, such as supposed sexual promiscuity in women or homosexuality in men. Homosexuality was classified as a mental illness by the American Psychiatric Association until the early 1970s, and it only removed the classification due to demonstrations by gay and lesbian activists (Kutchins and Kirk, 1997). The value-laden nature of diagnosis meant that the definition of abnormality could easily lead to oppression and long-term incarceration in a period where the labelling of someone with a mental illness often meant long stays in institutional asylums. The most terrible incidence of this association of values, oppression and diagnosis occurred in Nazi Germany where those people diagnosed with mental health prob- lems were first sterilised and then put to death, due to the Nazi belief that they were 'polluting' the racial heritage of the German nation (Torrey and Yolken, 2010).

This very brief history indicates why psychiatry has been particularly susceptible to a critique. If we follow an immanent critique initially, we can see that the claims of psychiatry to be a medical discipline like any other do not stand up, due to the absence of identifiable biological markers for a range of mental health problems. Second, we can see that this claim to be a medical discipline often means that psychiatry has functioned as an agent of social control, by policing the parameters of what counts as normal behaviour, sometimes with terrible and devastating consequences for indi- viduals who become labelled as 'mentally ill'.

## Critical mental health care: the 1960s and critical psychiatry

The critique of the presuppositions and practices of psychiatry reached a boiling point in the 1960s, with a group of thinkers from diverse perspectives and back- grounds who have often been termed the 'anti-psychiatry' movement. In many ways this is a poor description, and one that many of the participants refused to accept (Szasz, 2010). Indeed, many of the protagonists in this critique of psychiatry were themselves psychiatrists. It would be more accurate to term this group as critical psychiatrists. What they shared was a critique of psychiatry as a medical disci- pline – they all believed that mental health problems could not be defined in a straightforward manner as physical illnesses that could easily be treated medically, but rather they should be considered as expressions of mental distress due to a range of social and environmental factors. This led some to argue that the whole concept of mental illness is a 'myth' (Szasz, 1972), whilst others argued for a redefinition of our understanding of mental distress towards a more social understanding of the determinants of mental ill health (Basaglia,2004; Laing, 1990).

Alongside this shared critique of a reductive view of mental distress, all of these thinkers shared a critique of the manner in which people become labelled and insti- tutionalised as mentally unwell. A significant focus of their critique was on the damage done to people through the overuse of medication, the institutionalisation of people and the removal of their rights (Goffman, 1973; Scheff, 1975). This led some to argue for the dismantling of institutions and others to try and set up alter- native or more humane institutions.

Despite these shared positions, many of the thinkers and activists in the 1960s and into the 1970s often had quite divergent perspectives. They all shared a core immanent critique of psychiatry, but their perspectives on emancipation and what emancipation might mean differed significantly. It is worthwhile to look briefly at some of the main protagonists of this first wave of critical psychiatry.

## Thomas Szasz and the myth of mental illness

Thomas Szasz is an American psychiatrist and academic who has argued in numerous publications that mental illness is a myth (Szasz, 1972, 1976). He argues that diseases can only be defined as such if there is an identifiable pathology or lesion underlying the disease, and if this is not the case, as in most mental illnesses, then we cannot use the term disease. When we observe patterns of behaviour and term these mental illnesses we are constructing myths that are more analogous to witchcraft than to scientific understanding. What is worse for Szasz is that this labelling of mental illness leads to the withdrawal of people's rights in an illegitimate manner. As we label someone mentally ill, then we can put them in hospital against their will and treat them against their will. Szasz is a libertarian – he believes that as long as your actions do not interfere with another person's rights then you should be free to do as you please. Controversially, he has argued that all mental health counselling and support should take place through private contractual agreements rather than state or national health services, as these tend to take away a person's rights. He has been criticised for this view, and for being a right-wing libertarian, as some have argued that this position takes away the necessary support and treatment of vulnerable people (see Parker et al., 1995; Sedgwick, 1982). However Buchanan-Barker and Barker (2009) have argued that Szasz's emphasis on contracts is not an emphasis on private contracts, but rather refers to a free and autonomous exchange between individuals. Szasz has consistently argued against any involuntary hospitalisation and treatment of those who are deemed to be mentally ill, and has argued against the use of psychiatry in the criminal justice system. He does recognise that there are significant health problems that occur due to attempts to deal with issues in our lives, but believes that these should not be described in a medical manner.

Szasz has been criticised for his too clear and simple distinction between physical and mental illness. In an early critique, Sedgwick (1982) argued that many physical illnesses such as asthma are diseases that are identified on a continuum of normality and abnormality and that we cannot easily distinguish between a physical illness and mental illness. Bracken and Thomas (2010) criticise Szasz for these too easy distinctions, and also criticise his adherence to a capitalist free market approach to health care. Szasz's critique of mental illnesses as myths is very straightforward and consistent, but there is a worry that it neglects the social pressures on those deemed to be mentally unwell and the costs of abandoning them to a lack of treatment and care.

## R.D. Laing and critical psychiatry

R.D. Laing (1927–89) was a Scottish psychiatrist who developed a series of influential critiques of formal psychiatric practice throughout the 1960s and 1970s whilst still working within psychiatry and accepting mental distress as an experience that needed care and support. Laing was deeply influenced by a tradition of existential psychiatry that attempted to understand the meaning and context within which mental distress developed. It was not enough to simply label mental disorder, but it was more important to understand the context and life situation in which mental distress occurred (see May et al., 1958). Laing's first book was a study of the life-world of people who were diagnosed with schizophrenia, entitled *The Divided Self*, and published in 1960. Laing did not here dispute that mental distress occurred or that people experiencing mental distress needed care and support, but his goal was to try to understand as much as possible the strange utterances of those subject to psychosis. In a series of penetrating and brilliant analyses, he renders seemingly odd and bizarre behaviours and speech understandable in terms of the life situations of individuals, and their responses to existential crises (Laing, 1990).

Whilst this early work concentrated on individuals, Laing moved on in the mid-1960s to explore the importance of family dynamics in the production of psychosis. Working alongside Aaron Esterson, Laing studied the dynamics of communication within families that produced a situation in which there was no way out for the individual who flees into psychotic experience as a form of escape (Laing and Esterson, 1964). Laing and Esterson were deeply influenced by the work of Bateson and his colleagues in developing a theory of what they termed 'double bind' communication systems. These 'double bind' communication systems occur when contradictory emotional messages are given simultaneously, whilst at the same time no questioning of these contradictory messages is allowed. For example, a parent might verbally express love and support whilst acting in a cold and withdrawn manner (Bateson, 1972). Laing and Esterson (1964) studied families to try and uncover these patterns of communication that resulted in forms of psychosis as ways of escaping these systems of family dynamics. Although very influential at the time, this work was highly criticised later for blaming families and particularly mothers for producing mental illness (Harrington, 2012). Although it is debatable whether this is an accurate critique of Laing's work, or more of a mixing up of Laing's approach with a history of psychoanalytic approaches to family work in schizophrenia, it is true that there is a tendency that can stem from this work that could blame families rather than support them. However, it is equally implausible to suggest that family dynamics do not play any role in people developing psychotic experiences. Recent guidelines on working with schizophrenia explore the importance of psychological approaches and family interventions in working with psychosis and stress the range of social factors that can contribute to the development of psychotic experiences (National Collaborating Centre for Mental Health, 2010). A more pertinent critique of Laing's work on the family was the manner in which it did not look at other social contributory factors to psychosis, which have become clearer as time has moved on, such as the stresses of migration, racism, poverty and unemployment.

Laing's clinical practice developed in the 1960s alongside his theoretical critique of psychiatry, and led to the famous development of alternative institutions for caring for people experiencing mental distress. There is a key difference with Szasz's work here, as Szasz wanted nothing to do with any institutional approach to psychiatry and has explicitly criticised Laing's attempt to set up alternative institutions of care as remaining coercive (Szasz, 2008). Laing and colleagues set up an alternative institution in East London in the 1960s called Kingsley Hall, where people could come and experience their madness with minimal medications and with alternative approaches to therapy. Laing also set up the Philadelphia Association, which continues to offer courses and alternative crisis accommodation to people with mental distress (see www.philadelphia-association.co.uk/index.htm). As Parker et al. (1995) point out this process was a reinvigoration of a tradition of trying to provide genuine caring and supportive asylums for people that goes back to the foundation of the York Retreat by the Quaker family the Tukes. Critical analysis of the work at Kingsley Hall may well show contradictions and problems in its practice (Crossley, 1998), but the attempt at a more equal and less coercive form of care inspired a number of imitations. The key point of such alternative institutions was to allow a space for people to express their mental distress, with minimal medical interventions and to flatten the hierarchy and differentials between staff and service users. In the US, the psychiatrist Loren Mosher developed a form of alternative care in a programme that he termed Soteria (the Ancient Greek for salvation) that worked with lay people as staff and minimal medication approaches, to enable supportive and understanding therapeutic communities, and demonstrated some efficacy in outcomes with this approach (Calton et al., 2008).

Laing's work developed in the late 1960s into a more concerted attack on how those with mental illness were labelled and controlled by society. Famously, he questioned the sanity of many of the goals of society and claimed that by comparison with a militaristic and money-driven society, many people with mental illness could be deemed 'sane' (Laing, 1967). In 1967, Laing spoke at a famous conference at the Roundhouse in London, called the Dialectics of Liberation, in which critics of the capitalist system protested against all forms of violence including that perpetrated by the psychiatric system (Cooper, 1968). By the end of the 1960s the struggle against psychiatry had fundamentally linked itself to a series of struggles against capitalism and imperialism worldwide, and Laing's work had moved from his initial concern with the existential situation of the individual to a more thorough and wide-ranging critique of society at large. Nowhere was this radical critique against psychiatry carried through as completely as in Italy, and it is to the work of Franco Basaglia and his movement of democratic psychiatry that we now turn.

## The fight against the institutions

A key critique of psychiatry in the 1960s was that the asylums which were set up to supposedly care for people were actually places in which people were neglected, humiliated and forgotten. In his highly influential study of the processes of institutionalisation amongst inmates (and this *is* an appropriate word here) of asylums, Erving Goffman had already detailed the damage done to people by the institution of the asylum (Goffman, 1973). Goffman showed the way in which people were stripped of their identities, rights and their humanity by the institution and through a series of rituals were transformed into a new and lesser way of life. In many ways, Goffman argued it was the institution of the asylum that created mental illness, rather than the asylums being a place in which illnesses were treated. This critique of institutions was supplemented by a critique of the process of the labelling of people with mental illness. The sociologist Thomas Scheff argued that the labels applied to people with mental illness were ways of controlling so-called 'deviant behaviour' and that once these labels were applied to people then they learnt to behave in accordance with the labels that had been ascribed to them (Scheff, 2009).

The critique of the arbitrary nature of labelling and the manner in which institutions stripped people of their rights and social roles was supported by a famous study conducted by the sociologist David Rosenhan in the early 1970s (Rosenhan, 1973). Rosenhan and a number of research students presented themselves at psychiatric hospitals up and down the US and all repeated the same word to assessing psychiatrists, namely the word 'thud'. Apart from that they all acted sanely; they were all admitted, given diagnoses of schizophrenia or manic depression, and stayed in hospital for months. Rosenhan's study was widely criticised and many psychiatrists claimed that they would have been able to identify the 'fake patients' (Rosenhan, 1973). Rosenhan thus publicly declared that he would repeat his experiment, and psychiatrists claimed to have identified several 'fakes'. Rosenhan then admitted that he had not sent out any new researchers. This study showed the arbitrary nature of diagnostic categories and how easy it was for people to be admitted and treated as ill in psychiatric hospitals.

The result of these critiques was that to really challenge the way that society deemed people to be mentally ill meant a challenge to the institutions that controlled, labelled and incarcerated those with mental illness. The most systematic attempt at challenging these institutions was carried out in the Italian city of Trieste, where the psychiatric institutions were under the directorship of the radical psychiatrist Franco Basaglia. Like Laing, Basaglia was steeped in the work of existential psychotherapy and psychiatry and was also convinced that the asylums needed to be dismantled for a move to a more human and community form of psychiatry (Ramon and Giannicheda, 1989). The radical approach that Basaglia took was to dismantle the asylum from within. As Basaglia argued, the first therapeutic step was a dismantling of the hierarchies and regimes within the asylum (Basaglia, 2004). First, all physical coercion within the hospital was discontinued, including physical restraints and the use of ECT. Following this, Basaglia encouraged the dismantling of the asylum itself and opened it up to the community, alongside the building of new community support facilities. The role of the mental health worker was no longer as a custodian or simple carer, but someone who intervened politically within the family, the welfare system and society to improve the lot of those who were deemed to be mentally ill. Basaglia's approach was supposed to challenge the realm of control over the person with mental illness, not only within the asylum but beyond it, and it resulted in a law passed in Italy in 1978 that produced the first mass move towards de-institutionalisation, although the results of this move were widely felt to have negative elements in terms of the abandonment of the mentally ill alongside the positive elements of the move into community care (Burti, 2001).

## The second wave of critical psychiatry and the psychiatric backlash

The first wave of critical psychiatry in the 1960s was conducted in the context of a system of formal state health care and established institutional care, namely the extensive network of asylums that were first built in the nineteenth century. Many of the demands of the first wave of those critical of psychiatry were structured around the freedom of the individual to live their life free of institutional diagnosis and care. Bracken and Thomas (2007) have noted the limitations of this critique in its emphasis on individualism and its limited concept of power as purely that of a domination of individual capacities for freedom. These limitations were further exposed when there was a move towards the closing down of institutions within mental health care that did not necessarily lead to a more inclusive and less coercive system. Indeed, many observers argued that the move to 'community care', which was occurring at the same time as cutbacks to the welfare state, in many countries led to an abandonment of those with mental illness and a lack of care in the community (Goodwin, 1997). It is false to argue that the complex notion of community care across various jurisdictions led to one outcome, rather than acknowledging the many benefits to the move to community care (Killaspy, 2006). However, this change in the provision of care led to a move to change the nature of critique.

Highly influential here was the work of the French theorist Michel Foucault (1926–84). Foucault argued for a complex notion of power, stating that power is not only about repression but also productive of new identities and new forms of knowledge. In his book *Madness and Civilization*, he writes an alternative history of the treatment of mental illness. The standard history views the move from the demonisation of the mentally ill in the Middle Ages, through to asylum care in the nineteenth century and on to therapeutic approaches in the twentieth century as one of increasing enlightened care. Foucault (1993) argues that all of these are just stages in representing and dealing with what gets termed as mental illness. These are different forms of power that produce different constructions of what mental illness and reason are, due to the frameworks of knowledge and understanding in each moment of history, and not necessarily a progressive and increasingly enlightened approach to care.

This critique led theorists to argue for different approaches to mental illness. Rose (1986: 83) argues for a critical psychiatry that focuses on what he terms a 'proliferation' of sites for psychiatric knowledge. The discipline of psychiatry penetrates a diverse range of institutions and disciplines and can no longer be exclusively dealt with in terms of the encounter with madness in the asylum. Indeed, Rose argues that one of the distinctive features of modern psychiatry is the way in which more and more behaviours become pathologised and treated across a wide number of sites. Increasingly, it is not a matter of defining abnormality, but rather a matter of producing and policing what counts as normality. Miller and Rose (1986) argue for a focus that moves away from an obsession with madness itself, towards a focus on the practice and discipline of psychiatry and how this practice produces forms of power and individual responses to these forms of power.

This critical move was also a response to a psychiatric backlash against the ferment of the 1960s and 1970s. This backlash was most clearly represented in a manifesto written by Gerald Klerman, who argued for clear boundaries between illness and health and that mental illnesses could be treated like physical illnesses (Klerman, 1978). This backlash also contributed to the new diagnostic system of classification of mental illnesses drawn up under the leadership of Robert Spitzer and published in 1980 (Bentall, 2009). This new system of classification produced a checklist of symptoms that was supposed to codify and clearly validate diagnosis. The idea was that psychiatrists who used the checklist would always agree on their diagnoses, and in this way, the *Diagnostic and Statistical Manual of Mental Disorders-III* (DSM-III) was a direct response to the critics of psychiatric labelling. Psychiatry aimed to reassert its ability to assess and treat mental illness medically, but this was still in the absence of identifiable biological markers for most mental illnesses.

A significant critical response to this psychiatric backlash that grew out of radical work in the 1960s and 1970s was the service user/survivor movement. The survivor movement viewed themselves as survivors of the damage done by psychiatry and radically challenged the status of psychiatry (Chamberlin, 1978). However, this movement coexisted with other service user groups which had a more consumer focus and often contradicted the survivor perspective by demanding access to treatment and medication (Speed, 2006). There was a multiplicity of voices that challenged the system, but often from very divergent perspectives. The radical critique of psychiatry survived in a service user movement that criticised coercion and overuse of medication and labels, whilst at the same time a consumer-driven movement led by self-described patients and carers argued for access to services and medication. This split was encapsulated in the different non-statutory charities and lobby groups in the UK, with Mind representing the more radical position and groups like SANE arguing for a more medical approach.

## Postmodernism and psychiatry

In the last 10 years or so a highly influential form of critique of psychiatry has been an approach that argues for what is termed a 'postmodern' critique of psychiatry. Lewis (2000) has characterised the move from a critique based on the principles of modernity to a critique based on postmodern ideas in the following manner. Rather than searching for one objective truth that will underpin our criticism, we should open ourselves to multiple and different narratives. These narratives might represent a variety of different methods or ways of seeing the world, each of which have equal validity. Finally, we should not see ourselves as moving towards an ultimate goal of emancipation, but instead accept that there are many different truths for different people. Muir Gray (1999) argues that a postmodern medicine will be equally concerned with values as well as disease, and will welcome working with service users who are well informed. Bracken and Thomas (2007) have argued for a form of postpsychiatry, that is concerned not with diagnosis and treatment, but with understanding, peer support and care.

This move to a pluralistic approach is most clearly represented in the current context of mental health care by the principles of recovery (Repper and Perkins, 2003). The principles of recovery focus on the person defining their own needs and forms of support, and being enabled to choose their pathway to managing their mental health. It is an emphasis not on cure, but on self-management and true recovery, which often means coping with persistent life problems with support either medical or not.

Whilst the radical critique survives in some adherents to a recovery approach, the difficulty with this move to postmodern ideas and pluralism is that it often downplays the continuing exercise of power by psychiatric authorities and does not take any position on the central questions that were disputed by the first wave of critical psychiatrists. For example, adherents of a recovery approach are explicit that it is not important to develop a theory about the origins of mental illness (Repper, 2012). In many ways, this is a strength in that it allows people to make their own choices, but it does not always recognise the levels of coercion and dominance that exist within a medical conceptualisation of mental illness.

## Critical theories and mental health nursing practice

What is the relevance of these disputes in psychiatry to everyday nursing practice? Are these just abstract issues that we can read about and have no impact on our working practice? There are a number of concrete ways in which the issues we have discussed in this chapter impact on our practice.

- An awareness of coercion in psychiatry and how nurses work within a coercive system. It is vital to reflect on our beliefs and feelings around formal coercion in the mental health system as many of us will work in settings where coercion takes place. This is even more significant given the extension of coercion with the creation of enforced community treatment in the revision of the Mental Health Act of 2007.

- An awareness of alternatives to formal psychiatry and to a medical approach. As nurses we can build links and alliances with service user groups and use a range of skills to provide social and non-medical care to people with mental health issues.
- An understanding of the history and abuses of psychiatry and a commitment to work in a way that involves people and supports their fundamental rights.
- An acknowledgement that working in mental health is as much about values as it is about scientific understanding or evidence, and that we need to respect values and understand our own values and how they impact on practice (Fulford and Woodbridge, 2004).
- An understanding of the impact of psychiatric labels on people's lives.
- An awareness of the importance of peer support in mental health and our role as nurses to facilitate and encourage self-management and peer support where possible.
- An understanding of the political determinants of mental ill health and how we can intervene politically to demand improvements in people's lives.

**CASE EXAMPLE**

When you spend time on a placement or working on an acute ward, try to think of the role the institution plays in shaping the responses and needs of the service users and staff. Ask yourself the following questions:

- What are the rituals for entry into this environment for both service users and staff?
- What happens to the person admitted to the psychiatric ward – do they retain their roles and identity and are their rights respected?
- What kind of treatment approaches are offered – are there a range of options available for people, both medical and non-medical?
- How do the staff attempt to understand the experience of the service user? What opportunities for discussion and debate are there about the meaning of mental distress? Are alternative viewpoints encouraged and respected?
- How is the institution structured on a day-to-day basis – how involved are the service users in their own care?

These questions and the answers you develop will enable you to reflect on how life in an institutional setting has changed for the current user of mental health services, and how much of the radical critique of psychiatry remains relevant.

## Summary

This chapter has introduced the reader to the recent history of critical theories in mental health care. The reader has been introduced to the concept of critical theory and its relevance and appropriateness for mental health care. Three historical approaches to criticising psychiatry have been outlined. It has been acknowledged that these are broad outlines, and that there are often multiple viewpoints within these approaches. First, the first wave of critical psychiatry from the 1960s and 1970s was outlined through the critique of labelling, the concept of illness and institutional care. Second, the importance of a more fluid concept of power was outlined and how this applies to a changing context for psychiatric care in the move from the asylums to the community. Third, the idea of postmodernism and multiple perspectives was briefly introduced and its relevance for the concept of recovery was outlined. Finally, the reader has been encouraged to think through the practice implications of these critical theories. What does it mean to work effectively and critically as a mental health nurse in a culture often marked by coercion and the withdrawal of human rights? The reader has been encouraged to reflect on their own practice experience and to think through ways in which practice can be both supportive and critical.

# References

Andreasen, N. (2001) *Brave New Brain: Conquering Mental Illness in the Era of the Genome*. Oxford: Oxford University Press.

Basaglia, F. (2004) 'Breaking the circuit of control', in D. Ingleby (ed.), *Critical Psychiatry: The Politics of Mental Health*. New York: Free Association Books.

Bateson, G. (1972) *Steps to an Ecology of Mind: Collected Essays in Anthropology, Psychiatry, Evolution and Epistemology*. Chicago: Chicago University Press.

Bentall R. (2009) *Doctoring the Mind: Why Psychiatric Treatments Fail*. London: Penguin.

Bracken, P. and Thomas, P. (2007) *Postpsychiatry: Mental Health in a Postmodern World*. Oxford: Oxford University Press.

Bracken, P. and Thomas, P. (2010) 'From Szasz to Foucault: on the role of critical psychiatry', *Philosophy, Psychiatry and Psychology*, 17 (3): 219–28.

Buchanan-Barker, P. and Barker, P. (2009) 'The convenient myth of Thomas Szasz', *Journal of Psychiatric and Mental Health Nursing*, 16 (1): 87–95.

Burti, L. (2001) 'Italian psychiatric reform 20 plus years after', *Acta Psychiatrica Scandinavica*, 104 (s410): 41–6.

Calton, T., Ferriter, M., Huband, N. and Spandler, H. (2008) 'A systematic review of the Soteria paradigm for the treatment of people diagnosed with schizophrenia', *Schizophrenia Bulletin*, 34 (1): 181–92.

Chamberlin, J. (1978) *On Our Own: Patient Controlled Alternatives to the Mental Health System*. New York: Hawthorne.

Cooper, D. (ed.) (1968) *The Dialectics of Liberation*. Harmondsworth/Baltimore: Penguin.

Crossley, N. (1998) 'R.D. Laing and the British anti-psychiatry movement: a socio-historical analysis', *Social Science and Medicine*, 47 (7): 877–89.

Foucault, M. (1993) *Madness and Civilization: A History of Insanity in the Age of Reason*, trans. R. Howard. London: Routledge.

Fulford, K.W.M. and Woodbridge, K. (2004) *Whose Values? A Workbook for Values-based Practice in Mental Health Care*. London: Sainsbury Centre for Mental Health.

Fulford, K.W.M., Thornton, T. and Graham, G. (2006) *Oxford Textbook of Psychiatry*. Oxford: Oxford University Press.

Goffman, E. (1973) *Asylums: Essays on the Social Situation of Mental Patients and Other Inmates*. London: Penguin.

Goodwin, S. (1997) *Mental Health Policy: From Institutional to Community Care*. Thousand Oaks, CA: Sage.

Harrington, A. (2012) 'The fall of the schizophrenogenic mother', *The Lancet*, 379 (9823): 1292–3.

Held, D. (1989) *Introduction to Critical Theory: Horkheimer to Habermas*. Cambridge: Blackwell.

Jay, M. (1996) *The Dialectical Imagination: A History of the Frankfurt School and the Institute of Social Research: 1923–1950*. Berkeley: University of California Press.

Kendell, R.E. (2001) 'The distinction between mental and physical illness', *British Journal of Psychiatry*, 178 (6): 490–3.

Killaspy, H. (2006) 'From the asylum to community care: learning from experience', *British Medical Bulletin*, 79/80 (1): 245–58.

Klerman, G.L. (1978) 'The evolution of a scientific nosology', in J.C. Shersow (ed.), *Schizophrenia, Science and Practice*. Cambridge, MA: Harvard University Press.

Kutchins, H. and Kirk, S. (1997) *Making us Crazy: DSM: The Psychiatric Bible and the Creation of Mental Disorders*. New York: Free Press.

Laing, R.D. (1967) *The Politics of Experience and the Bird of Paradise*. London: Penguin.

Laing, R.D. (1990) *The Divided Self*. London: Penguin.

Laing, R.D. and Esterson, A. (1964) *Sanity, Madness and the Family: Volume 1, Families of Schizophrenics*. London: Tavistock.

Lewis, B. (2000) 'Psychiatry and postmodern theory', *Journal of Medical Humanities*, 21 (2): 71–84.

Marx, K. (1988) *Selected Writings*, ed. D. McLellan. Oxford: Oxford University Press.

May, R., Angel, E. and Ellenberger, H. (eds) (1958) *Existence: A New Dimension in Psychiatry and Psychology*. New York: Basic Books.

Miller, P. and Rose, N. (eds) (1986) *The Power of Psychiatry*. Cambridge: Polity.

Moncrieff, J. (2008) *The Myth of the Chemical Cure: A Critique of Psychiatric Drug Treatment*. Basingstoke: Palgrave Macmillan.

Muir Gray, J.A. (1999) 'Postmodern medicine', *The Lancet*, 354 (9189): 1550–3.

National Collaborating Centre for Mental Health (2010) *Schizophrenia: NICE Guidelines on Core Interventions in the Treatment and Management of Schizophrenia in Adults in Primary and Secondary Care – Updated Edition*. NCG: No. 82. London: British Psychological Society and Royal College of Psychiatrists.

Parker, I., Georgaca, E., Harper, D., McLaughlin, T. and Stowell-Smith, M. (eds) (1995) *Deconstructing Psychopathology*. London: Sage.

Porter, R. (2002) *Madness: A Brief History*. Oxford: Oxford University Press.

Ramon, S. and Giannicheda, M. (eds) (1989) *Psychiatry in Transition: The British and Italian Experiences*. London: Pluto Press.

Repper, J. (2012) 'Recovery: a journey of discovery', in S. Tee, J. Brown and D. Carpenter (eds), *Handbook of Mental Health Nursing*. London: Hodder Arnold.

Repper, J. and Perkins, R. (2003) *Social Inclusion and Recovery: A Model for Mental Health Practice*. London: Ballière Tindall.

Rose, N. (1986) 'Psychiatry: the discipline of mental health', in P. Miller and N. Rose (eds) *The Power of Psychiatry*. Cambridge: Polity.

Rosenhan, D. (1973) 'On being sane in insane places', *Science*, 179 (4070): 250–8.

Sabia, D. (2010) 'Defending immanent critique', *Political Theory*, 38 (5): 684–711.

Scheff, T. (ed.) (1975) *Labelling Madness*. Englewood Cliffs, NJ: Prentice Hall.

Scheff, T. (2009) *Being Mentally Ill: A Sociological Theory*. New Brunswick, NJ: Transaction Publishers.

Sedgwick, P. (1982) *Psycho Politics*. London: Pluto Press.

Speed, E. (2006) 'Patients, consumers and survivors: a case study of mental health service user discourses', *Social Science and Medicine*, 62 (1): 28–38.

Szasz, T. (1972) *The Myth of Mental Illness: Foundations of a Theory of Personal Conduct.* St Albans: Paladin.

Szasz, T. (1976) *Schizophrenia: The Sacred Symbol of Psychiatry.* New York: Basic Books.

Szasz, T. (2008) 'Debunking anti-psychiatry: Laing, law and largactil', *Current Psychology,* 27 (2): 79–101.

Szasz, T. (2010) 'Psychiatry, anti-psychiatry, critical psychiatry: What do these terms mean?', *Philosophy, Psychiatry, Psychology,* 17 (3): 229–32.

Torrey, E. and Yolken, R. (2010) 'Psychiatric genocide: Nazi attempts to eradicate schizophrenia', *Schizophrenia Bulletin,* 36 (10): 26–32.

Younge, G. (2011) *Who We Are and Why Should it Matter in the 21st Century?* London: Penguin.

# 7

# Biological Theories

## FIONA McCANDLESS-SUGG

### Learning Objectives

- Gain an overview of biological theories as ways to understand aetiology and treatment in mental health nursing.
- Identify some historical factors in the search for biological determinants of mental disorders.
- Appreciate that prominent researchers are aware of the limits of biological explanations.
- Acknowledge the limitations of genetic theories and one of the neurochemical theories of the causes of mental disorders.
- Appreciate psychopharmacology as an area of mental health practice where some knowledge of biology is important in helping to understand effects and side-effects of drug treatments.

## Introduction

If a group of new mental health students were asked why they had chosen this field of practice, it is highly unlikely that any of them would volunteer, as an initial thought, that they wanted to learn about the biology of mental disorders. Of all the chapters in this book, this is perhaps the one that some, maybe many, would argue does not have a place in contemporary mental health nursing practice. Looking back over the history of biological psychiatry, we see a chequered story. At times, advances in biological science seemed to offer wonderful prospects for changing the lives of people who experienced mental distress. There has also been a long history of eminent people in the mental health field rejecting this line of enquiry.

The person reading this chapter is amazing and unique. If we met and took the time to get to know each other, we would start to appreciate who we both are and 'what makes us tick'. If, during the course of our conversations, I started to display behaviours that you were not expecting, for example laughing and crying incongruently, or including someone in the conversation that you could not see, would you still want to talk to me? Would my behaviour lead to a degree of rejection, or would you want to know more about the possible reasons why I was not behaving as you would expect? We can fear things that we do not understand; however, dismissing biological explanations could limit our ability to care for people holistically.

This chapter is most definitely not a return to the nature–nurture debate, with emphasis on arguing that nature, or our biological makeup, can explain why people develop mental illness. Nor will it provide an extensive overview of all possible biological theories of mental disorders; to do so would involve many hundreds of thousands of words and also run the risk of this being the chapter that would most quickly become outdated. What this chapter aims to do is provide mental health students with a critically sympathetic overview of some of the biological theories that have influenced our understanding of the aetiology (possible causes) of mental disorders and of treatment in mental health care.

## Historical development

'Psychiatry is a continuously evolving concept that has, historically, conveyed widely varying meanings for patients, physicians, and the general public' (Yudofsky and Hales, 2002: 1261). Psychiatry is the area of medicine where doctors have chosen, after years of training to gain knowledge in the treatment of a wide range of medical conditions, to specialise in treating people with mental illness. Griesinger (1845, cited by Kendell, 2001) declared that mental illnesses are diseases of the brain and the discovery in the nineteenth century that infection with syphilis was associated with mental disorders seemed to demonstrate that searching for the biological determinants of mental illness could be fruitful. In 1906, Alois Alzheimer gave the first description of the neuropathology of a form of dementia that continues to bear his name, which demonstrated that changes in the brain were associated with mental illness (Small and Cappai, 2006).

Alzheimer studied under Emil Kraepelin, who is credited with developing the distinction between mental disorders with predominantly mood disturbance, which he called manic-depressive psychosis, and a 'different' group of disorders that he called dementia praecox, to distinguish them from the type of dementia that seemed to affect predominantly older people. Andreasen (2001: 169) credits Kraepelin with recognising 'the importance of neuroscience long before the word was invented'. Although modern psychiatrists would now diagnose bipolar disorder, instead of manic depression, and schizophrenia (a term introduced by Bleuler) instead of dementia praecox, Kraepelin's distinction between different categories of mental illness is still recognisable in modern psychiatry.

Leach (2009: 8) argues that medical approaches are the predominant approach in mental health care, yet 'despite the well-intentioned desire to relieve suffering through the application of medical science, there has been much disagreement about the role of biophysical and biochemical factors in mental health'. The term 'disagreement' seems to underestimate the degree of dissent; Kingdon and Young (2007) published a provocative debate entitled 'Research into putative biological mechanisms of mental disorders has been of no value to clinical psychiatry'. Van Praag (2010: 164) echoes this in his piece 'Biological psychiatry: still marching forward in a dead end', and argues that the 'pathophysiology of mental pathology is still largely unknown'. Within the popular nursing press, there have also been calls to reject biological explanations, for example, an article by Monro (1999) – 'There is sin in them there genes'. It is correct that searching for biological causes of mental distress is akin to searching for the proverbial needle in a haystack; despite the advances in technology since the time of Kraepelin, Alzheimer, their contemporaries, and subsequent people who wanted to investigate psychiatry from a biological perspective, identifying the 'cause' of major mental disorders has proven elusive.

One mental disorder that is biologically determined is the early-onset form of dementia known as Huntingdon's disease. This disease is an inherited form of dementia that is autosomal dominant, meaning that the offspring of an affected parent has a 50% chance of inheriting the gene that causes the disorder. If the gene is inherited, the disease will develop at some point in that person's life. The disorder was characterised by George Huntingdon in 1872 (Walker, 2007), but the actual gene responsible for the disorder was not identified until 1993 – some 121 years after the genetic pattern of transmission had been described! There are two important points to note here: first, Huntingdon's disease follows a variation of Mendelian inheritance so, compared to the vast majority of other mental disorders, researchers were looking for '*the* gene'; and, second, great technological leaps forward were needed before science had the means to identify '*the* gene'. Unfortunately, just knowing what is 'wrong' in Huntingdon's disease has, as yet, not led to a cure for this devastating disorder.

Psychopharmacology is an area of biological science that offers the potential to develop drug treatments for mental disorders. Even though biological science has not helped us greatly, at the moment, to understand the aetiology of mental illness, has it helped with treatment? The section dealing with theory and practice will examine this in more detail and provide an overview of some of the groups of drugs that are used in mental health practice.

In 1982, the English and Welsh National Boards (ENB and WNB) for Nursing, Midwifery and Health Visiting published a new syllabus for training in mental health nursing. There was a heavy emphasis on teaching the interpersonal skills required for mental health nursing practice. Care was meant to be humanistic and holistic; however, biological content was lacking in this syllabus. Nurse education underwent a radical change when Project 2000 (United Kingdom for Nursing, Midwifery and Health Visiting [UKCC], 1986) was implemented, and there was recognition that student nurses needed a core knowledge that incorporated biological science. *Fitness for Practice* (UKCC, 1999: 17), which is also known as the Peach Report, acknowledged that 'new genetic approaches' meant that 'nurses and midwives of the future will have to have a basic knowledge of genetics, at the very least'.

In 2000, Rinomhota and Marshall published a book on the *Biological Aspects of Mental Health Nursing*. In the preface, the authors acknowledge that 'over the past two decades the pendulum has swung away from the medical model towards psychosocial and humanistic models with an apparent rejection of anything biological. Thankfully, however, in recent years the pendulum seems to be settling more centrally with the development of biopsychosocial-spiritual models.' In his foreword to the book, Professor Kevin Gournay outlines the key areas for mental health nurses in the twenty-first century to consider: first, advances in genetics and neurochemistry and what these mean for our understanding of mental health and ill health; second, the importance of nurses understanding how new pharmacological treatments work; and, third, the prospect of mental health nurses being offered the opportunity to train as nurse prescribers. Gournay was writing at an exciting time in the history of our understanding of mental disorders; in 2000 the first draft of the human genome was mapped.

## The biological theories of mental disorders

This chapter is about biological theories of mental health; however, contemporary theory does not view these in isolation from other explanatory frameworks. Biology can potentially help mental health practitioners in two ways. First, it may offer a contribution to explanations about why some people develop mental health issues. Second, it can provide us with information about effective treatments for mental distress. It is vital to appreciate that the most prolific researchers in the field will be the first to acknowledge that biological psychiatry will not provide all of the answers we need in mental health care. Kendler (2008), one of the most prominent researchers in the field of biological psychiatry that is broadly known as psychiatric genetics, openly acknowledges that biological reductionistic models are not appropriate when looking for the 'causes' of mental illness. Engel (1977: 135) acknowledged the limitations of the prevailing biomedical model and proposed a biopsychosocial model that would provide 'a blueprint for research, a framework

**TABLE 7.1**  Observed or reported behaviours that are characteristic of manic and depressive episodes

|  | Manic episode | Major depressive episode |
|---|---|---|
| **Mood Emotional** | • Elevated or irritable<br>• Increased self-esteem<br>• Grandiosity | • Low[a]<br>• Emotional numbing<br>• Loss of pleasure<br>• Loss of confidence<br>• Low self-esteem |
| **Cognitive** | • Subjective experience of thoughts racing<br>• Distractibility<br>• Sharpened thinking | • Poor concentration |
| **Psychomotor behaviour** | • Increased activity<br>• Increased speech (content and/or rate) | • Psychomotor retardation or agitation |
| **Motivational/ behavioural** | • Increased energy<br>• Increased libido<br>• Decreased need for sleep<br>• Increased involvement in pleasurable activities with high risk of painful consequences, e.g. sexual indiscretions, excess spending | • Tearfulness<br>• Suicidal<br>• Anergia<br>• Insomnia or hypersomnia<br>• Decreased or increased appetite<br>• Decreased libido |
| **Perceptual** | • Heightened perception | • Depersonalisation<br>• Derealisation |
| **Mood-congruent psychotic behaviour** | • Grandiose delusions | • Delusions of guilt<br>• Nihilistic delusions |

[a]Low mood not required for DSM-IV-TR (APA, 2000) diagnosis of major depression.

**TABLE 7.2**   Biopsychosocial model of mental disorders

| Diathesis | + | Stress | ⟶ | Mental disorder |
|---|---|---|---|---|
| Biological | | Biological | | Biological |
| and/or | | and/or | | and/or |
| psychological | | psychological | | psychological |
| and/or | | and/or | | and/or |
| social | | social | | social |
| Factors | | Factors | | Expression of mental distress |
| Cultural and spiritual influences | | | | |

for teaching, and a design for action in the real world of healthcare'. Table 7.1 gives an overview of some of the behaviours that might be reported by, or observed in, someone experiencing mania or depression. It would be impossible to explain this purely in terms of biological mechanisms, or indeed treat people experiencing these levels of distress by biological treatments alone.

Table 7.2 provides an overview of a possible biopsychosocial model for understanding mental disorders. Note that it broadly follows a diathesis-stress conceptualisation, whereby people who develop mental disorders have a predisposition, or vulnerability, that is influenced by stress, resulting in expression of mental distress. Also see that underlying predisposition, stress and expression, are cultural and spiritual influences. In addition to factors that might be viewed as conferring vulnerability, this model could also include factors that protect someone who is exposed to stress. Kendler (2012: 380) gives an overview of some factors that have been associated with development of schizophrenia from a biological perspective; these include 'obstetric complication, season of birth, extensive exposure to cannabis, intrauterine viral exposure and famine'. Not everyone who experiences these biological 'stresses' will develop schizophrenia, so it seems that, yet to be determined, factors mediate in who is more at risk. Furthermore, individual differences mean that factors conferring vulnerability in one person might very possibly differ from those that elevate risk in another.

Kendler (2012) attempts to expand on the biological, psychological and 'higher-order' 'difference-makers' that have been associated with an increased risk of developing schizophrenia, depression or alcohol dependence An overview of these is given in Table 7.3. As Kendler's work has been in the field of psychiatric genetics, it is worth considering what this area of research has contributed to our understanding of mental disorders.

**TABLE 7.3**   Biopsychosocial 'difference-makers' (adapted from Kendler, 2012)

| | | |
|---|---|---|
| **Biological effects** | Molecular genetic | Are there any genes that have been shown to be associated with mental disorders? |
| | Molecular neuroscience | Which neurotransmitters might be associated with mental disorders? |
| | Systems neuroscience | Are there structural and functional differences between the brains of people with mental disorders, and those of people without mental disorders? |
| | Aggregate genetic effects | What clues do twin and adoption studies give us about heritability of mental disorders? |
| | Other biological risk factors | What other biological risk factors have been proposed/investigated? |
| **Psychological effects** | Neuropsychology | Any clues from psychology, for example in how people with mental disorders process information? |
| | Personality and cognitive/attitudinal patterns | Are there any traits that seem to be associated with mental disorders? |
| | Trauma exposure | What environmental risk factors/stressful life events seem to be associated with mental disorders? |
| **Higher-order** | Social | Covers a multitude of experiences that people have. |
| | Political | Kendler, here, highlights evidence indicating that the price of alcohol, for example, impacts on the risk of alcohol dependence. |
| | Cultural | Again, covers a multitude of attributes. |

Mental disorders are known to run in families, so does this mean that they are genetic? Not at all, the familiarity could be the result of shared environment rather than genetics. Rudin (1916, cited in Gejman et al., 2011) is credited with being the first person to conduct a family study of schizophrenia, and he noted that a Mendelian model of inheritance could not account for a model of transmission. Gejman et al. (2011) also point out that most people with schizophrenia do not have a parent, sibling or child (that is, a first-degree relative) with the diagnosis, which indicates that genetics of the disorder are complex. Twin and adoption studies are two other approaches to uncovering the contribution that genetic factors make in mental disorders (and indeed other complex conditions and traits).

Twin studies compare the rate of concordance for a characteristic in identical (monozygotic: MZ) and non-identical (fraternal; dizygotic: DZ) twins. MZ twins are 'genetically identical'; whereas DZ twins share approximately 50% of their genes, as they would with their other first-degree relatives. If MZ twins are found to be more alike compared to DZ twins on the characteristic of interest, for example, mental disorder or personality trait, this suggests that genes have an influence because twins are assumed to share comparable environmental experiences. Gejman et al. (2011) report that MZ twins are 40–50% concordant for schizophrenia and DZ twins are 6–10% concordant, which does indicate that genes are involved. Smoller and Finn (2003) demonstrate that concordance rates for bipolar disorder range from 38.5 to 62% for MZ twins and 4.5 to 9.1% for DZ twins. A difference in MZ/DZ concordance rate has also been reported for other mental disorders, including obsessive compulsive disorder, panic disorder, major depressive disorder and Alzheimer's disease (Shih et al., 2004), and alcohol dependence (Kendler, 2012).

Adoption studies can aid understanding of the genetics of characteristics by examining concordance between biological versus adoptive relations. Again, adoption studies have demonstrated genetic influences on schizophrenia (Gejman et al., 2011), bipolar disorder (Smoller and Finn, 2003) and major depressive disorder (Shih et al., 2004). So quantitative genetic studies, what Kendler (2012) calls aggregate genetic effects, all support genetics playing a role in the development of mental disorders.

The latter part of the twentieth century was an exciting time for researchers who were interested in finding the genes for mental disorders; technological advances, combined with the mapping of the human genome, offered opportunities to identify genes that conferred increased susceptibility towards mental disorders. Understanding what was happening at the molecular level could potentially also mean that rational treatments, based on understanding of the biological basis of a disorder, could also be developed.

What is clear from molecular genetic studies of mental disorders is that they are even more complex than had been imagined. With Huntingdon's disease, eventually the genotype for the phenotype was discovered, and people who are 'at risk' as a result of having a first-degree relative with the disorder can receive counselling and genetic testing to show if they will go on to develop the disorder too. Research has shown that the genes for a specified mental disorder, for example bipolar disorder or schizophrenia, will be many and have a small effect on vulnerability (Crow, 2011), which means that large samples are needed (Craddock et al., 2009). The effect of environmental factors is also influential (Craddock et al., 2009; Rutter, 2010; Wermter et al., 2010), thus one very important point that this area of research reinforces is that biological reductionist approaches will be unhelpful in understanding the aetiology of mental disorders.

Zuckerman (1999) developed a multi-factorial model of vulnerability to psychopathology; however, he is best known as a psychologist who devised the sensation-seeking scale for the study of personality. Kraepelin was looking at mental disorders as discrete entities that would differ in course and prognosis, whereas Zuckerman has extensively studied an aspect of human variation ('phenotype') that is viewed as dimensional rather than dichotomous. Molecular genetic research has challenged Kraepelin's conceptualisation of mental disorders (Craddock and Owen, 2005, 2010) being discrete, standalone, entities – could this mean the end for the diagnostic classification of schizophrenia? Very possibly, and genetic research is making a significant contribution to this.

Kendler (2012) included 'molecular neuroscience' and 'systems neuroscience' as biological 'difference-makers'. Technological advances in these fields have been influential in helping to understand what could be happening in mental disorders and also where contemporary theories are limited. Table 7.4 gives an overview of some neurotransmitters and the mental disorders that they have been associated with. It is vital to acknowledge that, as with genetic involvement in mental disorders, the relationship between neurotransmitters and mental disorders is extremely complex. The involvement of neurotransmitters will be revisited in the next section, where actions of drug treatments are discussed. To illustrate the complexity of the relationship between neurotransmitters and mental disorders, the dopaminergic hypothesis of schizophrenia will be briefly considered.

**TABLE 7.4**  Neurotransmitters and mental disorders

| Neurotransmitter | Possible association |
| --- | --- |
| Dopamine | Schizophrenia |
| Acetylcholine | Alzheimer's disease |
| Noradrenaline | Mood disorders |
| Serotonin | Mood disorders Schizophrenia |
| Gamma aminobutyric acid (GABA) | Anxiety |

Neurotransmitters are chemical messengers involved in passing signals from nerve cell to nerve cell. Dopamine is a neurotransmitter associated with pleasure/reward pathways, addiction thrills, memory and movement (Mutsatsa, 2011). Of all of the neurotransmitter theories in psychiatry, the dopaminergic hypothesis of schizophrenia has been the most dominant. Kendler and Schaffner (2011) presented an analysis of this theory and acknowledge that, despite it being the most influential biological theory of schizophrenia in the late 1970s, there was no direct evidence in support of it. Research continued, the theory was refined; however, Kendler and Schaffner (2011) conclude that it has not performed well as a scientific theory and suggest that 'As our science and field matures beyond ideologically driven controversy, it would be wise and mature for all of us, regardless of whether we see ourselves as biological, social or psychodynamic, to be more self-critical about the theories we adopt' (p. 59). As part of an aetiological theory, dopamine does not seem to help a great deal; nevertheless, dopamine will be considered again in the next section.

Technological advances mean that it is now possible to 'see' what is happening in the living human brain via neuroimaging. A range of techniques is available including Magnetic Resonance Imaging (MRI), functional MRI (fMRI), Positron Emission Tomography (PET) and Single Photon Emission Computed Tomography (SPECT). There has been suggestion that neuroimaging is, yet again, a biologically reductionistic approach (Lennox, 2009); however, it should also be acknowledged that the techniques are being used to investigate environmental influences on brain changes (Linden, 2012). Fusar-Poli et al. (2012) reviewed the available evidence on neuroimaging in people who were considered at high risk of bipolar disorder and concluded that there is evidence of neurological abnormalities in this group. The studies were all cross-sectional though, and there is a need for longitudinal studies. As is now the case with genetic research, it is important to aim for large samples and collaboration between researchers in order to identify robust biomarkers in psychiatry.

Many of the most influential people working in biological psychiatry readily acknowledge the limitations of the bio-reductionist approach. Biology cannot be viewed as separate from psychosocial, cultural and spiritual factors that influence vulnerability, stress and expression in mental disorders. People are amazing and unique; approaches to understanding and care need to acknowledge this and incorporate biopsychosocial-cultural-spiritual levels of understanding. It is essential to recognise that the people that we care for may have very different conceptualisations of why they are distressed, and this has implications for how we work together.

# Biological theory applied to practice

The ENB and WNB (1982) placed great emphasis on the interpersonal skills that mental health nurses needed to develop in order to have a therapeutic alliance with the people they care for. In the 30 years since this syllabus was implemented, biological science has continued to search for the basis of mental disorders in the hope that we can understand what is happening and develop rational treatments that are based on the underlying pathophysiology. In the preceding section it became clear that research in biology has demonstrated how complex mental disorders really are; they cannot be reduced to a few aberrant genes influencing structure and/or function of the central nervous system. What does this mean for the therapeutic relationship in mental health nursing?

In order to work effectively with the people in our care we need to develop a mutual understanding about their explanations for why they became unwell or mentally distressed. For someone who has relatives with mental health issues, genetic explanations might make a great deal of sense. Mental health nurses will meet people who are not the first person in their family to come into contact with mental health services. We may be asked questions such as 'Should I have children?', 'Will my children get this?', 'Have I passed this on to my children?', for example, which could be seen as questions that would be asked in genetic counselling. Pre-registration nurse education does not equip students with the skills of a genetic counsellor; however, the UKCC (1999) and Gournay (2000) acknowledged that nurses would need to appreciate the importance of genetic research in health care. Understanding the nature of the genetics of complex behaviours, such as mental disorders, is an important consideration. There are currently no genetic tests for mental disorders (apart from Huntingdon's disease) and, given our current understanding, it seems unlikely that there ever will be for the majority of the mental disorders that are currently identified in classifications systems such as the *Diagnostic and Statistical Manual of Mental Disorders* (DSM-IV-TR: APA, 2000), or subsequent revisions.

The 'power' of the internet is an important consideration too; rarely a week goes by without a 'breakthrough' being made in health care. So much information is available for people to try to make sense of their experiences of mental distress. Some of this will be empowering and meaningful, whilst other information could be misleading. As a student nurse you will be helped to develop your skills in critically analysing and evaluating evidence, and you will appreciate where 'evidence' has its limitations. Some of the people that we care for may not be as discerning, for any of a variety of reasons, so it is important to be sympathetic to their views and understand why the explanations they have could make perfect sense to them and their personal situation.

Some of the people that we care for may be recruited as participants into research projects and want to discuss this with you. Obviously the researchers themselves should be the first point of contact for questions about their studies; however, taking an interest in the person's experience can also enhance the therapeutic alliance. As a student nurse, it could alert you to new approaches in mental health research and help you to be aware of emerging evidence for understanding and treating mental disorders.

The remainder of this section will focus on another important aspect of mental health nursing practice – medication management. Although biology has not greatly enhanced our understanding of the causes of mental disorders it has helped us to understand the drugs that we use, how these work and why they are associated with certain side-effects. The drugs that are used in mental health care are very powerful preparations that act on the central nervous system. Section four of the British National Formulary (BNF – the formulary is updated each year in March and September) list 11 groups of drugs that act on the central nervous system. Five of these (4.1 Hypnotics and anxiolytics; 4.2 Drugs used in psychoses and related disorders; 4.3 Antidepressant drugs; 4.9 Drugs used in parkinsonism and related disorders; and 4.11 Drugs for dementia) will be considered. The guiding principles for medicines management can be found in the Nursing and Midwifery Council (NMC, 2008) publication *Standards for Medicine Management* (although you should be alert for any revisions to this). Guidelines on the management of mental disorders and various drugs groups can also be obtained from the National Institute for Health and Clinical Excellence (NICE: nice.org.uk). For a comprehensive overview of drugs that are used in mental health care, David Healy's (2009) *Psychiatric Drugs Explained*, which is now in its fifth edition, incorporates historical perspectives in addition to extensive information on biological mechanisms of action and side-effects.

According to Rinomhota and Marshall (2000) the drugs commonly used in mental health care exert their effects on one of three ways:

- Modifying re-uptake of a neurotransmitter into the presynaptic neuron
- Activating or inhibiting postsynaptic receptors
- Inhibiting enzyme activity.

## Benzodiazepines

Anxiolytics are drugs that reduce anxiety and hypnotics are drugs that induce sleep. The main drug group is the benzodiazepines, which includes diazepam and temazepam. Gamma aminobutyric acid (GABA) is an inhibitory neurotransmitter and, according to Mutsatsa (2011: 174), it is the body's own natural anti-anxiety medicine. GABA reduces activity of neurons in some areas of the brain by binding to GABA receptors. Benzodiazepines work by boosting the effect of GABA in the brain by binding to GABA receptors (Mehdi, 2012). These drugs should only be used for short-term (two to four weeks) treatment of severe anxiety or insomnia (see the BNF [2013] and NICE [2011] guidelines for anxiety).

Benzodiazepines became controversial in the 1980s when it became evident that significant numbers of people had been taking these on prescription for a number of years. It seemed that the medical profession had 'created' a group of 'addicts', which is an example of iatrogenesis (a condition induced by the medical profession). In addition to the problem of people developing a tolerance to and a dependence on this group of drugs, there is also an associated withdrawal syndrome. A later controversial association concerned one of this group of drugs known as flunitrazepam (no longer in the BNF), which is more commonly known as Rohypnol – the 'date-rape' drug. Despite the controversies that have been associated with this group of drugs, they still have a place in contemporary mental health care. First line interventions for anxiety and insomnia should involve psychosocial approaches and these should be incorporated as part of holistic care, even when short-term treatment with anxiolytics or hypnotics is indicated because the anxiety or insomnia is severely debilitating.

## Antipsychotics

In the previous section, we saw that the dopaminergic hypothesis has not made a major contribution to our understanding of the aetiological basis of schizophrenia despite a long history of research; however, evidence demonstrates that the effect that antipsychotic drugs have on psychosis is related to their ability to block dopamine receptors. According to Kendler and Schaffner (2011), this does not support dopamine as an aetiological theory and they cite the example of diuretic therapy (which acts on the kidneys) for congestive cardiac failure as one example where the action of a drug does not give us much information about the aetiology of a condition.

Antipsychotic drugs have been used since the 1950s to treat schizophrenia. There are several different groups of drugs, which are now classed as typical and atypical and some are available in a long-acting injectable form. Five types of dopaminergic receptors, $D_1$ to $D_5$, are currently known and antipsychotics exert their therapeutic effects by blocking the $D_2$ receptor. As noted previously, dopamine is associated with movement though, and blocking the receptors produces movement-related side-effects, or extrapyramidal side-effects (EPSE), that include:

- Stiffness (akinesia)
- Abnormal movements (dyskinesia)
- Abnormal muscle tone (dystonia)
- Restlessness (akathisia).

Dopaminergic side-effects (drug-induced parkinsonism) might lead to a person also being prescribed a drug from section 4.9 of the BNF (4.9.2 Antimuscarinic drugs used in parkinsonism), as there are three drugs – orphenadrine, procyclidine and trihexyphenidyl – that can help. Like all drugs though, there are side-effects associated with these preparations, including confusion, euphoria, hallucinations, anxiety and restlessness. Think about some of the ways that people might express mental distress; this could include feelings of confusion, elevated mood, hallucinatory experiences, anxiousness and restlessness. Antipsychotic medications might be used in treating someone with one or more of these, and it was noted above that restlessness is a recognised side-effect of these drugs. When working with people who are being treated with medication it is vital to be mindful of what is potentially a drug side-effect, what could be a result of drugs that are used to counteract the side-effects, and what might mean that the drugs are not having a therapeutic effect.

A very serious side-effect of antipsychotic medication is tardive dyskinesia, which is associated with abnormal movements of the face and mouth. However, tardive dyskinesia is not improved by drugs in section 4.9.2 of the BNF and, potentially, could be made worse. Hormonal side-effects of antipsychotic drugs could even result in lactation, i.e. production of breast milk, in females and males taking this medication. You might want to take some time to reflect on how these side-effects, and the others outlined below, might feel to the person who is experiencing them. Side-effects may result in people looking or acting differently to those around them – what impact could this have on social inclusion?

Other, non-dopaminergic, side-effects, include:

- Weight gain
- Diabetes
- Dry mouth
- Postural hypotension
- Seizures
- Constipation
- Photosensitivity
- Sexual problems.

This list is not exhaustive, but incomplete without mention of a rare but potentially fatal side-effect known as neuroleptic malignant syndrome (NMS). Many mental health nurses will have never seen this in practice, but if suspected it is essential that medical attention is sought urgently. Signs and symptoms include muscle rigidity, elevated temperature, pulse and blood pressure.

Clozapine was the original second generation, also known as atypical, antipsychotic drug. Initial reports had suggested that it was not associated with the range of EPSE observed with older antipsychotics and it did not cause tardive dyskinesia. However, it was found to affect production of white blood cells, resulting in a potentially fatal side-effect known as agranulocytosis, and withdrawn. Research studies continued to support its efficacy in treating schizophrenia, so it was introduced into the UK in 1990 with strict guidelines for prescribing and blood monitoring (Gray et al., 2009). Clozapine acts on $D_2$ receptors, and also on serotonergic ones, which is why it might appear to be more effective in some people compared to the first generation of antipsychotics. The range of drugs currently licensed as second generation antipsychotics, with their side-effect profiles, can be found in the most recent edition of the BNF. Although more recent developments in drug treatments are not associated with some of the troublesome side-effects of the earlier ones, they too present some adverse effects that can have significant implications for the health and well-being of people taking them.

When working with people who are taking medication, it is important to know what side-effects to look out for. It is also important to be mindful that people may develop side-effects that would not be expected. If this happens, it is important that these are reported – in the person's records, to other members of the multidisciplinary team, and to the Medicines and Healthcare Products Regulatory Authority (MHRA: www.mhra.gov.uk) through the yellow card scheme. When drugs are licensed for use they have been through rigorous testing before being considered 'safe'. The side-effect profile is known to an extent; however, the testing has been conducted in controlled environments. Once a drug is released for widespread use, we can start to get a much better idea of the side-effect profile, and it is vital that all suspected adverse drug reactions are reported.

## Lithium

Section 4.2 of the BNF also includes drugs used for the treatment of mania; one of these – lithium – is interesting because it came into widespread use following biological research that was based on a flawed hypothesis about the cause of mania. In the 1940s, John Cade was conducting animal experiments to investigate the theory that urea was a causal factor in mania, and noted that lithium had a calming effect. Quite how this happens is still poorly understood, but it remains a treatment for acute mania and for maintenance as a mood stabiliser. Prior to starting on lithium, people will have kidney and thyroid function assessed as the drug is known to affect this in some of the people who take it. Kidney and thyroid function will be assessed regularly – between three-monthly and yearly, unless presence of symptoms suggest sooner. The drug also has a very small therapeutic window, meaning that plasma levels need to be assessed every three months to determine that the person is receiving a therapeutic/non-toxic dose.

## Antidepressants

There are broadly four groups of antidepressant drugs, tricyclic antidepressants (TCAs), monoamine oxidase inhibitors (MAOIs), selective serotonin re-uptake inhibitors (SSRIs) and 'others', which do not fit into one of the other categories based on mode of action (see section 4.3 of the BNF). Dopamine, serotonin and noradrenaline are monoamine neurotransmitters, and classical theories of depression linked low concentrations of these with low mood. TCAs have been used in mental health practice for many years and their mode of action helped to develop theories about the causes of depression, as they prevent the reabsorption of noradrenaline and serotonin back into the presynaptic neuron. When monoamines are reabsorbed, they can be broken down by an enzyme called monoamine oxidase (MAO); MAOIs stop this process happening. However, these drugs are rarely used because of their potential interaction with foods that contain tyramine.

SSRIs were introduced in the 1980s, although the first one – zimeldine – had to be withdrawn due to serious side-effects; as the name suggests they act selectively on serotonin. The SSRIs have been subject to a great deal of attention from the MHRA and, of all the groups of drugs used in mental health care, are perhaps the ones that we know most about, in part because early on there were reports that they were associated with an increased risk of suicide. Like all drugs, they are associated with a range of side-effects and there is also a condition called serotonin syndrome that, like NMS, is rare but could be serious enough to warrant hospitalisation.

## Drugs for dementia

It was noted earlier that one of the breakthroughs in biological psychiatry came when Alzheimer described what happened in the brains of people with dementia. It took several decades before drug treatments were developed to address what was hypothesised to cause the neurological changes seen in the condition. Dementia affects memory and, although we don't have a complete understanding of the processes involved, it has been noted that the brains of people with Alzheimer's disease have significantly decreased numbers of acetylcholine neurons in the brain. Acetylcholine is a neurotransmitter associated with memory and is broken down by acetylcholinesterase. Three drugs – donepezil, galantamine and rivastigmine – are currently licensed as cholinesterase inhibitors for dementia. One other drug – memantine – is currently licensed for use in Alzheimer's disease, and this works by blocking the effect of another neurotransmitter – glutamate. Even though we don't currently know exactly what is happening in the brains of people who develop Alzheimer's disease and other forms of dementia, it is vital to appreciate that there are structural and chemical changes that mean the brain is not functioning as it should. Introducing pharmacological preparations into a complex system that is already 'imbalanced' could lead to further detrimental changes, and compound the difficulties that someone with dementia, and their carer, already experience.

Intuitively, it might seem, based on how medication works for mental disorders, that some chemical imbalance is responsible for the expression of mental distress. Research in psychopharmacology has demonstrated that it is much more complex than that. Nevertheless, drugs are part of a biological approach to treatment in mental health care and it is essential that nurses understand what effects they have on the person who is taking them.

CASE EXAMPLE

Sue is a woman in her early forties. Over a 20-year period she has experienced episodes of depression and been treated with antidepressants. These were usually prescribed by her GP, but twice she has been referred to a psychiatrist and treated as an outpatient.

Sue's most recent episode of depression caused her to re-evaluate her understanding of her own mental health. She had seen her GP with familiar symptoms and was prescribed an antidepressant that she had not tried before. Within six days she was back at her GP, extremely agitated and insisting that 'this is not right'. Her GP was sympathetic and started her on the SSRI that had worked well in the past, but this time it did nothing to make her feel any less depressed or agitated. Consulting her GP again, she was told that she was 'not responding' and to 'up the dose', but she eventually went back to the GP and said that she had stopped taking them, as she felt they were making her much worse than they should do. Sue's GP referred her to a psychiatrist, who prescribed an atypical antipsychotic to address her agitation, with a view to starting her on a different type of antidepressant when she was calmer. She was also referred to a community team for weekly support. Sue took the antipsychotic for a week, until the agitation had subsided, but – after discussion with her keyworker – she felt strong enough to tell the psychiatrist that she would not be trying any more medication.

Sue realised that episodes of depression usually happened after a prolonged period when she was 'pushing herself to the limit'. She had always accepted biological explanations for her moods and readily accepted medication, but on the last occasion she felt that this 'had back-fired' and the medication compounded her distressed state. As a result of this, Sue has attempted to get more of a balance in her life and know her limits. So far so good; she doesn't rule out taking medication again in the future if she ever feels as depressed as she has done previously, but she would rather not if possible for fear that she might experience a similar reaction to last time.

Sue's case illustrates how human experience cannot be reduced to biological levels of understanding and treatments; any more than purely psychological or sociological explanations can help us to comprehend why some people experience mental distress. Holistic, individualised, biopsychosocial-cultural-spiritual approaches are needed in order to understand and help the people that we care for.

## Summary

People who are 'different', who do not conform to the prevailing views or societal norms, can be subject to suspicion, discrimination, abuse and prejudice. We know this from the way that people with mental disorders have been treated historically and even in society today. In some cases, this will lead to rejection of the person. Given the lack of major advances in understanding the biological basis of mental disorders, it is easy to see

*(Continued)*

*(Continued)*

why some people are opposed to what they construe to be 'biological reductionism' of mental distress. Before rejecting biological explanations outright, it is important to acknowledge that current knowledge is based on research conducted to date. It took well over a decade before *the gene* responsible for Huntingdon's disease was identified, even though the mode of transmission had been described. Given the complexity of mental disorders and how mental distress is expressed, biological reductionist approaches will not provide the answers. However, they may make a contribution to our understanding of, and response to, mental distress if seen as a component in more complex formulations. Research from a biological perspective is also emphasising that environmental influences are significant in causes and treatment of mental distress.

Biological treatments are part of the 'toolkit' that helps mental health nurses to respond to the needs of the people for whom they care. It is vital that nurses understand the effects that biological treatments have, and the adverse effects that can be associated with them. The people we care for may look to biological explanations, such as genetics or 'chemical imbalances' when they try to make sense of their experiences, and they need nurses who can be sympathetic to their views. As Kendler and Schaffner (2011: 59) suggest, we need 'to be more self-critical about the theories we adopt', whilst keeping an open mind so we don't miss developments that could enhance the care that we are able to participate in.

# References

Andreasen, N.C. (2001) *Brave New Brain: Conquering Mental Illness in the Era of the Genome*. New York: Oxford University Press.

APA (American Psychiatric Association) (2000) *Diagnostic and Statistical Manual of Mental Disorders* (4th edn, text revision). Washington, DC: American Psychiatric Association.

BNF (British National Formulary) (2013) *British National Formulary (BNF) 65. The Authority on the Selection and Use of Medications*. London: BMJ Publishing Group Ltd and Royal Pharmaceutical Society.

Craddock, N. and Owen, M.J. (2005) 'The beginning of the end for the Kraepelinian dichotomy', *British Journal of Psychiatry*, 186 (5): 364–6.

Craddock, N. and Owen, M.J. (2010) 'The Kraepelinian dichotomy – going, going ... but still not gone', *British Journal of Psychiatry*, 196 (2): 92–5.

Craddock, N., Kendler, K., Neale, M., Nurnberger, J., Purcell, S., Rietschel, M., Perlis, R., Santangelo, S.L., Schulze, T., Smoller, J.W. and Thapar, A. (2009) 'Dissecting the phenotype in genome-wide association studies of psychiatric illness', *British Journal of Psychiatry*, 195 (2): 97–9.

Crow, T.J. (2011) 'The missing genes: what happened to the heritability of psychiatric disorders?', *Molecular Psychiatry*, 16 (4): 362–4.

ENB and WNB (English and Welsh National Boards for Nursing, Midwifery and Health Visiting) (1982) *Syllabus of Training: Professional Register – Part 3 Registered Mental Nurse.* London: English National Board.

Engel, G.L. (1977) 'The need for a new medical model: a challenge for biomedicine', *Science*, 196 (4286): 129–36.

Fusar-Poli, P., Howes, O., Bechdolf, A. and Borgwardt, S. (2012) 'Mapping vulnerability to bipolar disorder: a systematic review and meta-analysis of neuroimaging studies', *Journal of Psychiatry and Neuroscience*, 37 (3): 1170–84.

Gejman, P.V., Sanders, A.R. and Kendler, K.S. (2011) 'Genetics of schizophrenia: new findings and challenges', *British Journal of Psychiatry*, 12 (1): 121–44.

Gournay, K. (2000) 'Foreword', in A.S. Rinomhota and P. Marshall, *Biological Aspects of Mental Health Nursing.* London: Churchill Livingstone.

Gray, R., Bressington, D. and Chadwick, H. (2009) 'Psychopharmacology', in I. Norman and I. Ryrie (eds), *The Art and Science of Mental Health Nursing.* Maidenhead: Open University Press.

Healy, D. (2009) *Psychiatric Drugs Explained* (5th edn). London: Churchill Livingstone.

Kendell, R.E. (2001) 'The distinction between mental and physical illness', *British Journal of Psychiatry*, 178 (6): 490–3.

Kendler, K.S. (2008) 'Explanatory models for psychiatric illness', *American Journal of Psychiatry*, 165 (6): 695–702.

Kendler, K.S. (2012) 'The dappled nature of causes of psychiatric illness: replacing the organic–functional/hardware–software dichotomy with empirically based pluralism', *Molecular Psychiatry*, 17 (4): 377–88.

Kendler, K.S. and Schaffner, K.F. (2011) 'The dopamine hypothesis of schizophrenia: an historical and philosophical analysis', *Philosophy, Psychiatry, and Psychology*, 18 (1): 41–63.

Kingdon, D. and Young, A.H. (2007) 'Research into putative biological mechanisms of mental disorders has been of no value to clinical psychiatry', *British Journal of Psychiatry* 191 (4): 285–90.

Leach, J. (2009) 'Diverse approaches to mental health and distress', in J. Reynolds, R. Muston, T. Heller, J. Leach, M. McCormick, J. Wallcraft and M. Walsh (eds), *Mental Health Still Matters.* Basingstoke: Palgrave Macmillan.

Lennox, B.R. (2009) 'The clinical experience and potential of brain imaging in patients with mental illness', *Frontiers in Human Neuroscience*, 3 (12): 1–3.

Linden, D.E.J. (2012) 'The challenges and promise of neuroimaging in psychiatry', *Neuron* 73 (1): 9–22.

Mehdi, T. (2012) 'Benzodiazepines revisited', *British Journal of Medical Practitioners*, 5 (1): c501.

Monro, R. (1999) 'There is sin in them there genes', *Nursing Times*, 95 (33): 28–9.

Mutsatsa, S. (2011) *Medicines Management in Mental Health Nursing*. Exeter: Learning Matters.

NICE (National Institute for Health and Clinical Excellence) (2011) *Generalised Anxiety Disorder and Panic Disorder (with or without Agoraphobia) in Adults: Management in Primary, Secondary and Community Care*. London: NICE.

NMC (Nursing and Midwifery Council) (2008) *Standards for Medicines Management*. London: NMC.

Rinomhota, A.S. and Marshall, P. (2000) *Biological Aspects of Mental Health Nursing*. London: Churchill Livingstone.

Rutter, M. (2010) 'Gene–environment interplay', *Depression and Anxiety*, 27 (1): 1–4.

Shih, R.A., Belmonte, P.L. and Zandi, P.P. (2004) 'A review of the evidence from family, twin and adoption studies for a genetic contribution to adult psychiatric disorders', *International Review of Psychiatry*, 16 (4): 260–83.

Small, D.H. and Cappai, R. (2006) 'Alois Alzheimer and Alzheimer's disease: a centennial perspective', *Journal of Neurochemistry*, 99 (3): 708–710.

Smoller, J.W. and Finn, C.T. (2003) 'Family, twin, and adoption studies of bipolar disorder', *American Journal of Medical Genetics Part C (Seminars in Medical Genetics)*, 123C(1): 48–58.

UKCC (United Kingdom Central Council for Nursing, Midwifery and Health Visiting) (1986) *Project 2000: A New Preparation for Practice*. London: UKCC.

UKCC (United Kingdom Central Council for Nursing, Midwifery and Health Visiting) (1999) *Fitness for Practice: The UKCC Commission for Nursing and Midwifery Education*. London: UKCC.

Van Praag, H.M. (2010) 'Biological psychiatry: still marching forward in a dead end', *World Psychiatry*, 9 (3): 164–5.

Walker, F.O. (2007) 'Huntington's disease', *Lancet*, 369 (9557): 218–28.

Wermter, A.-K., Laucht, M., Schimmelmann, B.G., Banaschweski, T., Sonuga-Barke, E.J.S., Rietschel, M. and Becker, K. (2010) 'From nature versus nurture, via nature and nurture, to gene x environment interaction in mental disorders', *European Child and Adolescent Psychiatry*, 19 (3): 199–210.

Yudofsky, S.C. and Hales, R.E. (2002) 'Neuropsychiatry and the future of psychiatry and neurology', *American Journal of Psychiatry*, 159 (8): 1261–4.

Zuckerman, M. (1999) *Vulnerability to Psychopathology: A Biosocial Model*. Washington, DC: American Psychological Association.

# 8

# Ethical Theories

## NIGEL PLANT AND ARU NARAYANASAMY

### Learning Objectives

- Place current ethical thinking in an historical context.
- Develop an awareness of the contributions made by leading philosophers to ethical thinking that informs mental health practice.
- Develop an understanding of ethical frameworks and concepts that can be used to reflect and analyse mental health practice and inform clinical decision-making.
- Analyse how ethical thinking informs practice to promote care that is inclusive and anti-discriminatory.

## Introduction

Mental health practice contains a myriad of ethical issues, from those related to the purpose of mental health practice and the role of psychiatry in society to the ethics of providing treatment with or without consent and the ethics of particular interventions used by practitioners to promote mental well-being. As such, ethical mindedness is an instrumental component of clinical decision-making and therefore an understanding of ethical frameworks and perspectives is an important factor in promoting accountable practice which in turn should promote recovery.

This chapter will introduce a number of leading philosophers whose thinking informs approaches to the study of ethics, before outlining the major ethical theories. We place these in the practice context with a brief scenario that serves to illustrate the dilemmas practitioners face in working in a service user-centred way focusing on the issues of service user autonomy and decision-making before going on to highlight the importance of inclusivity and diversity and the need to ensure that mental health practice is both empowering and anti-discriminatory.

# The historical development of ethics in nursing

There has been an interest in ethics in nursing since the 1870s and North America led the way in its development. Since then, a body of knowledge based upon moral philosophy began to emerge with a steady output of moral-oriented literature. From these influences and including the works of Florence Nightingale, codes of ethics were developed to guide practice. Consequently, ethics featured in many nursing curricula mainly in the US and the American Nursing Association (ANA) took a prominent role in developing a focus of ethics in nursing. The ANA was instrumental in drafting the first code for professional nurses in 1950 and it went through several changes over the years.

In the United Kingdom and Europe, the influence of Florence Nightingale was prominent in the development of ethical thinking in nursing. She brought Christian influences and military discipline to nursing ethics as a consequence of her background and experiences. The Nightingale Pledge was adopted in nursing in the UK and Europe.

---

## Nightingale Pledge, 1893

I solemnly pledge myself before God and in the presence of this assembly, to pass my life in purity and to practice my profession faithfully. I will abstain from whatever is deleterious and mischievous, and will not take or knowingly administer any harmful drug. I will do all in my power to maintain and elevate the standard of my profession, and will hold in confidence all personal matters committed to my keeping, and all family affairs coming to my knowledge in the practice of my calling. With loyalty will I endeavour to aid the physician in his work, and devote myself to the welfare of those committed to my care. (*Source*: Davis et al., 2006: 24)

---

Much of Europe was influenced by moral ethics through religious orders in nursing such as the Deaconesses and Knights Hospitallers (Narayanasamy, 1999). Early literature in nursing puts much emphasis on morality and the moral position of nurses towards doctors and patients. It was then an ethical requirement that nurses should be of strong moral character, show unquestioning obedience and loyalty to doctors and devotion to their work and duty to patients. Nursing was seen as a vocation and selflessness was valued as a high moral quality in nurses. The book *Ethics for Nurses* (Wray, 1962) extolled the virtues of obedience, selflessness, duty and vocation, which was published as a series of articles in the *Nursing Times*. Indeed, under the heading 'Respect for the Doctor' the book stated:

> Ward routine has a certain pattern to encourage respect for the doctor; he is always accompanied by the sister, the ward is quiet, he is never contradicted; and by various means he is shown to be a person of pre-eminent skill and wisdom. (Wray, 1962: 22)

However, nursing began to move from the emphasis on vocation to a profession and with this ethics began to take shape with nurses questioning the supremacy of doctors which was partly reinforced and maintained by the literature such as *Ethics for Nurses* and the Nightingale Pledge. This change is reflected in development of the International Council of Nurses code of ethics in 1973, which offered a universal understanding and application of ethics to nursing practice.

With the advent of the United Kingdom Central Council for Nursing, Midwifery and Health Visiting (UKCC) in 1983, came the Code of Professional Conduct based on ethical concepts of deontology and utilitarianism to safeguard the patients within professional nursing. The Project 2000 nursing curriculum introduced by the UKCC placed greater emphasis on ethics in nursing and ethical concepts and principles and moral philosophy were addressed extensively in nurse education as a consequence of this initiative. Concepts and principles included topics such as deontology, utilitarianism, teleology, religious and moral thinking, personhood/value of life, freewill and determinism, justice and resource allocation, truth-telling and honesty, pre-conceptual issues and abortion, technology and ethics, to name a few.

However, the theoretical supremacy of ethics in nursing began to decline when nurse education based on Project 2000 was replaced by the Fitness for Practice curriculum. In our view this was a mistake as ethics and other theoretical subjects lost significant ground in nursing. Since then, ethics has not featured as a discrete subject but taught across the curriculum at best and at worst is barely mentioned. With the advent of the Graduate Nursing Curriculum, we are optimistic that ethics will regain ground as critical thinking students would be using greater levels of analysis as they examine questionable practices and transgressions of professional boundaries as part of their collaborative work in health care.

Having looked at the brief history of ethics in nursing we now provide a short history of some of the thinkers who influenced ethics in nursing through their grand narratives. Although there are a number of thinkers on moral philosophy and ethics, we give attention to Immanuel Kant, Jeremy Bentham and John Stuart Mill to provide a historical background to the exposition on ethical theories and principles that follow. Deontology (or duty ethics) is attributed to Immanuel Kant, and Jeremy Bentham set out the principles of utilitarianism, which was further developed and refined by John Stuart Mill.

## Immanuel Kant (1724–1804)

Kant was born in Konigsberg in East Prussia where he lived, worked and died. He produced several, influential philosophical works (Billington, 1993). He is well known in ethics for his work on deontology. He was interested in the question; 'What is a moral action?' (Warburton, 1992: 39). Kant emphasised that a moral action has to be executed out of a sense of duty rather than with an intention to gain something out of it. For example, if you are nursing someone to health to get fulfilment in life then you are not acting morally but if you are nursing this person out of sense of compassion then you *are* acting morally. His moral theory of deontology is considered to be absolute because he stressed the importance of telling the truth, sense of duty, rights, obligations and selflessness. Other moral philosophers such as William David Ross tried to modify deontology to make it workable.

## Jeremy Bentham (1748–1832)

Jeremy Bentham was born in Spitalfields, London, on 15 February 1748 (Thompson, 1999). Although his father intended that his very bright son become a lawyer, Bentham became disillusioned with law and instead he decided to write about it, mainly critically to bring about its improvement. Improved health and social conditions are attributed to the social reforms brought about by Bentham. His concerns over the social conditions in his day led him to be involved both with hospitals and prisons. His determination to improve people's lives motivated him to develop the moral theory of utility, which was based on the principle that what was done in a society would be judged right or wrong on the basis of its benefit to the majority of its citizens. The benefits of an action are judged good or bad according to its consequence or outcome. We further explore this theory later. Bentham genuinely believed that all members of society are entitled to maximum happiness and that everyone had an equal right to happiness irrespective of their circumstances. He believed that human beings were motivated by pleasure and pain and people pursued pleasure and sought to avoid pain (Bowie, 2011). Such a preoccupation with happiness is known as hedonism. According to Thompson (1999), Bentham advocated that happiness should be measurable in terms of the following:

- Its duration
- Its intensity
- How near, immediate and certain it is
- How free it is from pain, and whether or not it is likely to lead on to further pleasure.

## John Stuart Mill (1806-73)

John Stuart Mill was a child prodigy who became a philosopher, political economist and civil servant. Influenced by his father, Mill became an ardent follower of Bentham at a very young age. He further developed the ethical theory of utilitarianism mainly in response to criticism that it encouraged decadency and debauchery because of its emphasis on pleasure and happiness as the end. He introduced the idea of higher and lower pleasure to overcome the accusation that utilitarianism was evidence of a corrupt mind. He proposed that higher pleasure was to do with human intellect, while lower pleasure was associated with animals. Mill claimed that when faced between a pleasure of the body and a pleasure of the mind, the mind is preferred (Bowie, 2011). In summary, he gave utilitarianism real philosophical credibility by enriching the concept of happiness.

# Advances in nursing

The twenty-first century has brought numerous challenges to nursing in the form of globalisation, sustainability, economic entrenchment, technological advances, reducing world poverty, combating oppression, better nutrition, well-being, better health and social justice for all. Scientific advances such as nanotechnology and genetic engineering promise to bring great improvements to health but these privilege the wealthy who will always have enhanced access to health care facilities to keep ahead in terms of longevity and aesthetics while the rest are left behind. Ethics becomes a central issue in the context of these challenges. Nurses and students of nursing need a sound understanding and critical application of ethical principles and codes of professional practice to deal with problems and issues arising from moral and ethical dilemmas that patients and health care practice pose. In the next section we set out to explain the principles of deontology and utilitarianism.

Understanding moral theory will help us to determine the best or right course of action in making clinical decisions. This prompts us to consider what is right or wrong and how we determine the right thing to do. Here we will introduce you to some of the major ethical theories, before proceeding to consider how these theories may inform mental health practice and decision-making.

# Deontology

Deontological theory originates from the work of Immanuel Kant (1724–1804) a Prussian philosopher from the eighteenth century. The term deontology originates from the Greek word *deon* or duty, and it is on this notion of duty that deontological theories are based. So the person should always adhere to their duty or obligations. The focus here is therefore on the duty of the action rather than the consequence of what is done. Therefore acting ethically requires that one acts according to one's duty. Examples of deontology might be always telling the truth or always keeping one's promises.

These laws are seen as binding and universal in that they apply to everyone, therefore to the deontologist it is the very nature of the act that is seen as being important or 'categorical' rather than the consequences of the act, meaning that the moral obligation becomes one to act according to one's duty. The converse of this is that to act out of self-interest, for example to undertake an action so that others view you in a positive light, or to avoid being embarrassed or to fit in with a group of friends, is not seen as being morally praiseworthy regardless of the act itself. It is the very intention that underpins the act that becomes the defining characteristic in terms of the moral worth that can be attributed to the act. Therefore it is both the nature of the act and the intention or will of the person undertaking the act which become the defining properties in judging the moral nature of the act.

We can see then that morality to the deontologist is about categorical rules that we all should follow because that is the right thing to do rather than because it will make someone happy or prevent harm being caused. In making these rules we should will these to be binding and applicable to everyone, for example you should do unto others as you would have done unto you, or you should always treat people as an end in themselves rather than a means to an end.

While deontology gives us much to think about and is evident in our day-to-day thinking, for example 'each moment of life is precious', it provides absolutes and doesn't accommodate grey areas of thinking. Similarly, it may be that we find our duties conflict with each other thus creating moral dilemmas as to which action we should follow, and deontology does not provide us with an answer as to how we should resolve these conflicts.

## Utilitarianism

Utilitarianism or 'consequentialist ethics' derives in modern times from the thinking of two particular philosophers, Jeremy Bentham (1748–1832) and John Stuart Mill (1806–73). This approach to ethical decision-making focuses not on duty but on the consequences of the action; as such no moral act is intrinsically right or wrong. Rather the moral rightness is to be judged by the consequences, i.e. the non-moral good the action brings about, for example, the happiness it brings or the knowledge created. In adopting this approach utilitarianism considers the interests of others over the interest of the individual and in so doing opposes any ideas about acting on the basis of self-interest.

In deciding what one should do, the utilitarianist needs to consider the consequences of his or her actions and should act to bring about the best consequences possible. The issue becomes one of how the benefits are to be judged and therefore relies on a theory of intrinsic value. Here Jeremy Bentham and John Stuart Mill work on the principle of utility and guide us to make decisions on the basis of happiness and the balance between the amount of pleasure or pain derived, or to coin a phrase, the greatest good for the greatest number. While utilitarianism focuses on the act itself and the act that brings about the best results without giving particular attention to the context within which the decision is being made, it does recognise the wider world and its influence on decision-making by accounting for example for the law, professional accountability, public expectation, etc.

An advantage of this approach is that in making a decision all the options available should be weighed in the balance, as such the theory opens possibilities for decision-making that would not be open to the deontologist. However, critics of this philosophy point out that the theory may be used to view acts as morally appropriate when they are not, for example it may be argued that it is morally right for someone to steal from a very wealthy person on the basis of the pleasure or consequences the theft may bring about.

## Virtue ethics

Virtue ethics proposes a very different way of thinking about ethics; whereas utilitarianism and deontology focus on the act itself, virtue ethics points us towards the nature of the person, i.e. the virtuous person. We are therefore not concerned about the rules we should follow in making a decision between right or wrong, instead we are drawn towards the motives and intentions of what we wish to achieve and ask ourselves 'what the virtuous person in this situation would do'.

Virtue ethics is therefore about the development of personality traits that will enable us to make the right choices. Traits such as kindness can be developed and nurtured and translated into different situations so that acting through kindness becomes a way of being. While virtue ethics stems from the works of Aristotle and Plato, the relevance to current health care practice with the emphasis on compassionate care, dignity and recovery is easy to see with the focus being on the values that underpin the care received by the patient. Posing the question of what would the virtuous mental health professional do?

## Activity

Elliot is a newly appointed health care assistant in a mental health unit. He is charming and popular with patients. You overhear him using sexist remarks about staff and others when he is chatting with patients. Patients enjoy his company as he always has amusing stories to tell them, especially about his conquests, which are punctuated with sexist remarks. On occasions he tries to 'chat up' student nurses and younger members of the female staff with sexual innuendos. Some staff tolerate him because of his charming and appealing looks.

What are the ethical implications of Elliot's behaviour?

You may have indicated Elliot's behaviour is unethical and this needs to be pointed out to him. It is ethical that he needs to make conscious avoidance of sexist remarks and jokes, patronising sentiments towards women and men. It is important that all social and health care staff set and maintain personal standards in the way we use language that undermines sexual identities. In a civilised society, there is no place for people to use language which is offensive, patronising or excluding to anyone. Offensive language always devalues individuals. Such offensive behaviours sometimes make indelible imprints in individuals' minds with potentially serious consequences that may dent self-esteem and self-image.

In the next section we provide the rudiments of the ethical principles that you could apply in nursing practice to situations that may be ethically challenging.

# Ethical principles in practice

Over recent years there has been an emphasis on principle-based ethics in nursing largely due to the work of Beauchamp and Childress (2005) and their book *Principles of Biomedical Ethics*, which is now in its sixth edition.

The four principles proposed are: autonomy, beneficence, non-maleficence and justice. According to Beauchamp and Childress (2005) all the concepts are seen to have equal value, though over the years it has been said that the concept of autonomy weighs heaviest.

## Autonomy

Autonomy has become a fundamental principle underpinning health care practice and is founded on the notion of self-determination, i.e. the individual is best placed to make decisions about issues that affect him or her. The relevance to mental health practice is beyond doubt, as is the premise that individuals are best placed to make decisions about their care, treatment and lifestyle. It is this premise which underpins mental health practice that focuses on recovery, values the service user experience and empowers the service user to participate in decision-making. In doing so the practitioner promotes, creates and/or maximises the autonomy of the service user.

## Beneficence

Beneficence enshrines the principle of doing good for patients or clients. In everyday language this principle means to 'do the most positive good' (Seedhouse and Lovett, 1992: 10). All acts of nursing should be based on the principle of bringing good to patients or clients and their families. It is best to consider the patient's or client's best interest when dealing with all aspects of their care. However, it is not always easy to establish what is good and who decides what is good? Like the word yellow it is difficult to define what is good because it is a subjective term and open to varieties of definitions. It is best to be guided by the principle that any action that brings about great benefits to patients in terms of well-being constitute good.

## Non-maleficence

This is based on the absolute principle of never harming the patient or client. Every effort should be made in nursing to prevent harm to patients or clients but sometimes it is a difficult principle to achieve. Not all nursing actions avoid pain, for example an injection may hurt a patient or client but it is based on the principle of beneficence where overall it will alleviate distress by bringing about analgesic effect if given to control pain. Although the principle of non-maleficence may be difficult to apply in some situations, every effort should be made to minimise harm.

## Justice

Justice is the final principle, which is based on the ethical premise that all acts should be fair and equitable. All patients and clients have a right to good care and treatment based on their needs. It is about how to respect everyone and that the goodness of the act, in this case nursing care and treatment, is fairly distributed. No individuals should be subjected to discrimination or treated unjustly. The principles of anti-discriminatory practices ensure that justice prevails in nursing.

Abdul, a young Asian man, is admitted in to a mental health assessment unit having become withdrawn and apparently responding to auditory hallucinations. Abdul has been admitted informally and is content to be there though he doesn't understand why he has been admitted and is refusing medication. He looks apprehensive and is unable to respond to nurses' questions about his well-being and nursing needs. It is clear that Abdul is unable to respond because of communication difficulties. However, he constantly writes something in his diary and when you ask him what he has written he points out to a paragraph that he had written. In the diary he has written about Allah as his God who is going to look after him while he is in hospital and that nurses will be understanding and treat him well.

Consider the ethical issues that the clinical team need to consider in making decisions as to how to engage Abdul in his care.

**CASE EXAMPLE**

In respecting Abdul's autonomy the care team wish to engage Abdul in discussions about his treatment and be respectful of his expressed preferences. In doing so the practitioners would not only be respecting Abdul's autonomy but would be acting to promote it by sharing information with him, talking with him about the risks and benefits of the treatment proposed and engaging him in discussions about his values and beliefs regarding his illness and his preferred course of treatment.

A dilemma may occur if Abdul continues to refuse the treatment that the care team believe to be beneficial to him. While it is generally accepted that the individual is best placed to determine their 'best interests', the team may feel that Abdul's refusal of treatment in some way compromises their duty to promote beneficent care and in doing so fear that care may fall below the legal standard by failing to meet the standards expected in exercising their duty of care. Here we can see a dilemma arising between the patient's autonomy and the notion of beneficence. The danger is that for the nurse to practise from a position of beneficence risks care being paternalistic. This might be based on what the care team think is best for Abdul; on the other hand, the care team would want to know whether Abdul's decision to refuse treatment is a reflection of his wishes or whether the decision arises from his mental illness (see the Mental Capacity Act 2005). The care team aim to promote care that is just and is respectful of Abdul's beliefs and values and may advocate for him from this perspective. However Abdul's refusal of treatment may potentially lead to a worsening of his condition and this may be something the team are very aware of through their previous dealings with him. From an ethical viewpoint the team would wish to provide Abdul with care that meets his mental health needs, reduces distress and safeguards his autonomy at a time when Abdul is not able to exercise this himself. While we may share information with him and would encourage him to participate in treatment, there is a fine line to be drawn between practice which is supportive and practice that is coercive.

The dilemma may be more compounded by Abdul's informal status and while this is not a chapter on mental health law there may be calls for Abdul to be sectioned under the Mental Health Act (1983) as amended by the 2007 Act. We should remember that a principle of the Act is that care is provided in the least restrictive manner and that even if Abdul is sectionable under the Act, in providing him with treatment we would wish to work to preserve a therapeutic relationship and as far as is possible involve Abdul in decisions about his care. Nevertheless we cannot ignore the fact that under mental health law, treatment of convincing necessity can be provided without the patient's consent; in so doing the practitioner works to protect both the interests of the patient and society. It is through attention to ethical reasoning that these potentially competing interests are resolved.

We have to acknowledge that there is a potential for tension between the notion of patient autonomy and the interests of society as a whole and this is an issue that is common in mental health practice where the interests of society and the protection of others necessarily impact on the freedom of the individual and in so doing necessitate effective and comprehensive clinical assessment of risk.

In planning care for Abdul it is important that the care team respect his individuality by providing mental health care that is anti-discriminatory, accounting for and reflecting Abdul's values, beliefs and culture and work as far as possible to enable and empower Abdul (Dalrymple and Burke, 2006).

## Summary

By the very nature of mental health practice mental health practitioners work with people who find difficulty in exercising their autonomy and are considered to be vulnerable. The ethos of mental health practice is the promotion of recovery in which the service user is enabled and empowered by the mental health practitioner who not only respects their experience of their illness and their recovery but who also promotes, creates and supports the service user in decision-making. This chapter has introduced you to theories and concepts related to moral thinking and provided examples of how these can inform and promote care that not only promotes autonomy but is empowering, respectful of diversity and is anti-discriminatory.

# References

Billington, R. (1993) *Living Philosophy: An Introduction to Moral Thought*. London: Routledge.

Beauchamp, T.L. and Childress, J.G. (2005) *Principles of Biomedical Ethics* (6th edn). New York: Oxford University Press.

Bowie, R.A. (2011) *Ethical Studies*. Cheltenham: Nelson Thornes.

Dalrymple, J. and Burke, B. (2006) *Anti-oppressive Practice* (2nd edn). Maidenhead: Open University Press.

Davis, A.J., Tschudin, V. and de Raeve, L. (2006) *Essentials of Teaching and Learning in Nursing Ethics*. Edinburgh: Churchill Livingstone.

Narayanasamy, A. (1999) 'Learning spiritual dimensions of care from a historical perspective', *Nurse Education Today*, 19 (3): 386–95.

Seedhouse, D. and Lovett, L. (1992) *Practical Medical Ethics*. Chichester: John Wiley and Sons.

Thompson, M. (1999) *Ethical Theory*. London: Hodder and Stoughton.

Warburton, N. (1992) *Philosophy: The Basics*. London: Routledge.

Wray, H. (1962) *Ethics for Nurses*. London: Macmillan.

# 9

# Compassion and Mental Health Nursing

## THEO STICKLEY AND HELEN SPANDLER

### Learning Objectives

- Understand what is meant by compassion.
- Appreciate the need for compassion in mental health nursing practice.
- Weigh up the tensions for mental health nurses practising compassion in today's consumer-driven culture.

## Introduction

The concept of compassion in nursing is well established. Usually this has been associated with the need for nurses to demonstrate empathy towards people who are suffering. In mental health care, however, people's distress is often experienced internally and can be manifested in external behaviour. The underlying distress is much less obvious than the suffering and pain associated with cancer or heart failure. For mental health nurses, compassion may mean being able to empathise with people's life experiences and demonstrate understanding of how these experiences may cause psychological problems. The concept of compassion therefore in mental health nursing may be more complicated than in physical nursing. This chapter will describe compassion and identify some key theories related to the topic, identify what compassionate caring might look like in practice and consider the barriers to compassionate mental health nursing.

# Historical development

The concept of compassion is found in all cultures and whilst we may feel that we instinctively understand what it means, it is quite difficult to explain. One way of understanding the concept is by thinking about 'empathy'. This means the ability to understand another person's experience without necessarily having those experiences oneself. Empathy and compassion involve more than intellectual understanding, but require a kind of emotional understanding. Compassion 'in action' may be interpreted as an act of human kindness. In this chapter, we consider how it can be developed and encouraged in mental health nursing practice, not just by individuals, but by developing cultures of compassion within services (Spandler and Stickley, 2011).

When we think of the old 'lunatic asylums' of the eighteenth century we may easily conjure up images of care that was appalling (Porter, 2004; Scull, 1993), however the subsequent 'moral treatment' of the insane brought with it humane approaches that were positively therapeutic. The York Retreat, founded in 1796 under the leadership of William Tuke, has become the best known example of providing moral treatment (Kennard, 1983). In the York Retreat, patients were encouraged to engage with certain activities that were deemed to be good for them. Although as Digby (1985) observes, it was not so much the activities that were provided that were considered curative, but the provision of such by people who genuinely cared and provided good therapeutic relationships. Thus the effectiveness of compassionate care in mental health has a long tradition.

After the Second World War, there emerged a new way of thinking about human relationships and this later became known as humanistic psychology (see Chapter 4). At the time, thinkers such as Carl Rogers and Abraham Maslow were hugely influential in the world of psychotherapy. This approach was much less about the knowledge and skill of the therapist and more about providing healthy, positive relationships that may help a person to change and grow. They believed that we are all individual and as such have unique and different views not only of the world we live in, but of each experience that we encounter. Rogers became known as the father of client-centred or person-centred counselling. Rogers was particularly interested in how a person made sense of their life experiences. He believed that each one of us has the capacity to change and solve our own problems given the right conditions. Thus, people are the experts in their own lives. The conditions he refers to include: genuineness, empathy, unconditional positive regard, honesty and transparency. He believed that if the therapist can provide these conditions, the person with whom the therapist is working will feel valued and good about themselves. This focus upon the human qualities of the therapist was a new idea in considering what it meant to develop and maintain therapeutic relationships. The act of using empathic understanding is in itself an act of compassion.

Humanistic psychology has had an enormous influence upon health care and educational theory and practice for decades. However, more recently, as health care has become more technical and target-driven, it could be argued that there has been less emphasis on creating humane and compassionate approaches to health care. In mental health care, the need for compassion has become even more marginalised. Some have observed that compassion is no longer the focus of nursing practice (Chamber and Ryder, 2009). One recent study has suggested that whilst compassion has not exactly been completely lost, there may now be fewer opportunities for professionals to express it (Youngson et al., 2009).

There has, however, been a recent interest in reasserting the significance of compassion within health care relationships. When the Nursing and Midwifery Council (NMC) published their new standards for nurse education, they were keen to emphasise that the need for compassion was as important as scientific knowledge:

> Care that is competent as well as compassionate is grounded in scientific knowledge and appropriate use of technology as well as in humanitarian professional values. All nurses must keep abreast not only of scientific developments … but also advances in understanding how to provide compassionate care. (NMC, 2010: 4)

The King's Fund in the UK have been very active in encouraging the development of compassionate care in nursing and it is becoming recognised as fundamentally important to the delivery of nursing care, especially in hospital settings (Maben et al., 2009; NHS Confederation, 2008).

In mental health care specifically, there has also emerged what might be referred to as 'compassion-focused' therapies that incorporate practices of self-compassion, through meditation and mindfulness exercises (Gilbert, 2005, 2010; Williams et al., 2007). Furthermore, the literature shows that there are a number of specific compassionate approaches being introduced for particular client groups, such as people with dementia (Scott et al., 2012), survivors of child sexual abuse (Gilbert, 2005), those experiencing anxiety and depression (Segal et al., 2002) and hearing voices groups (Mayhew and Gilbert, 2008).

## Policy

In the UK, the call for compassionate care has featured in NHS policy for a long time (DH, 2008). The NHS recognises the importance of compassionate care and places its significance at the heart of NHS philosophy. The NHS Constitution defines what compassion means in practice:

> We respond with humanity and kindness to each person's pain, distress, anxiety or need. We search for the things we can do, however small, to give comfort and relieve suffering. We find time for those we serve and work alongside. (DH, 2009a: 12)

About 60% of the mental health workforce comprises mental health nurses. The commitment to compassionate care is evident within the NMC. In 2007 the NMC published a paper entitled *Essential Skills Clusters (ESCs) for Pre-registration Nursing Programmes* (NMC, 2007). This identifies the skills needed for nursing practice that are thought to underpin the necessary knowledge and values for nursing. The ability to deliver compassionate care is rooted within these skills. The need, therefore, for compassionate care within NHS delivery is seen as a necessary skill or quality for nurses to provide. Compassionate care is also called for by the King's Fund in the UK (King's Fund, 2009) and the British Medical Association (BMA, 2011).

It is worth noting, however, that this ethos has not been translated into specific mental health policies. At the time of writing, the overarching framework for mental health policy is *No Health Without Mental Health* (DH, 2011). Similar to its predecessor (*New Horizons: A Shared Vision for Mental Health*, DH, 2009b), it makes no mention of compassion. Both documents are replete with references to recovery and the concept of hope, but the absence of any discussion about compassion leaves the reader of these policies wondering what hope looks like in practice. A compassionate and understanding system is one that will breed hope; compassionate mental health nurses are the ones that radiate optimism (Spandler and Stickley, 2011).

Compassion therefore should be at the heart of the therapeutic relationship between nurses and clients. These ideas are not new and have their origins in humanism and compassion, rooted in a well-established philosophy of care.

# Theories of compassion

## Compassion and love

There is a rich and well-established literature about the centrality of compassion to healthy human development. This can be found across a number of disciplines including spiritual traditions (especially Buddhism), neuroscience, developmental psychology, humanism, etc. These support the idea that compassion is necessary and essential to being human. It is difficult to separate the concept of 'compassion' from the concept of love, especially in a more ancient understanding of the word, where love has a number of meanings. In today's language we tend to restrict the word love to intimate relationships and family, but in years gone by, it was normal to refer to loving one's neighbours. Fromm (1957) argues that one of the problems of our language is that we make one word express an entire range of emotions. Hence love for example could refer to the affection we might feel for a pet kitten to the deepest kind of relationship. Whilst we have only one word for love, classical Greek has a number of words such as eros and agape. Erotic love is associated with sexual feelings, but agape can be understood as altruistic love in which an individual can experience compassion for a complete stranger, as if that stranger were related to the person.

We discussed earlier the contribution of Carl Rogers to this topic. His emphasis upon 'unconditional positive regard' has been regarded by some as the need for love in the therapeutic relationship (Stickley and Freshwater, 2002). Referring to counselling, Petruska Clarkson recognises the closeness of the love dilemma to the therapist's work commenting that:

> We are required to act constantly in the arena of love, yet renounce all personal gratification; we work in one of the most potent cauldrons of intimacy, yet we are prohibited to drink from it. (Clarkson, 1995: 25)

Stickley and Freshwater (2002) also go on to suggest that the notion of Rogers' concept of unconditional positive regard actually equals love. It could be argued that because Rogers replaced the word 'love' with 'unconditional positive regard' he helped to remove the concept of love from the vocabulary of the therapy world. Unconditional positive regard may easily be viewed as a skill or technique, which diminishes the potency of love in its original form.

## Cultivating compassion

Gilbert (2005) asserts that human beings are a social species who depend on encouragement, care, support, safety and affection of others to survive and thrive. He identifies that compassion means being able to be moved by the distress of others and to become able to tolerate and understand it. These qualities motivate us to care for and be sensitive to others' feelings. To help cultivate compassion it is often helpful to visualise the other person's life. Patience is also a key quality of compassion. In that act of compassionate caring, the carer may also develop a sense of purpose, meaning and hope. It is by exercising compassion that nurses may feel a deep sense of satisfaction and fulfilment in their work.

However, theorists of compassion regularly point out that it is hard to be compassionate to others when we ourselves do not feel cared for. It is for this reason that nurses need to be well supported and supervised in their work, so that they themselves feel valued. Just as important is the ability of nurses to be able practise self-compassion, in other words to find ways to care and look after themselves; only then are they genuinely able to offer support to others (Gilbert, 2005). In order to be helpful to others, we must not neglect ourselves:

> Many doctors, nurses, social workers psychotherapists and teachers are suffering and do not know how to recognise and transform their pain. They want to help relieve other people's suffering, but they do not know how yet to take care of their own pain and suffering … [helping professionals] should learn the practice of mindfulness and self-care as part of the curriculum, not only as an intellectual pursuit, but as part of daily life. (Titch Nhat Hahn, 2003: 41–2)

Whilst compassion may be deeply human, it doesn't come 'naturally'. It has to be consciously cultivated and nurtured by individuals, groups and communities. Supportive environments are necessary for compassionate care to flourish.

## Challenges to compassion in practice

In mental health practice, many people become service users reluctantly. Whilst this might also be the case for people with physical health problems, there is an important difference. People with physical health problems are usually keen to receive the physical treatments available to them. They are therefore usually compliant with the wish of the medical team to bring the person into hospital and to give the person the required treatment for their illness. In mental health, however, things can be very different. Many people enter hospital against their will (this is what is referred to as 'being sectioned'). People often do not wish to take prescribed medication as it is often associated with unwanted side-effects. Some people are taken to hospital because of their seemingly dangerous or inexplicable behaviour. Whilst the treatment that is offered in these acute circumstances may temporarily help, the problems that often cause such distress are usually still there when the person is discharged. Whilst hospital admission may offer respite, it cannot normally solve problems such as experiences of abuse, domestic violence, the effects of alcohol or illegal substances and so on. This is a crucially important point to understand in relation to the nurse–patient relationship in mental health. People with physical health problems may demand care and understanding from their nurses while they are in hospital, but people in psychiatric wards may be angry at being there in the first place. The power battles that may result from this may be one reason why compassionate care is difficult to give in such environments.

Some people might argue that it is impossible to be compassionate when people are being coerced into treatments or detained in hospital and that any coercion is therefore unethical (see, for example, Thomas Szasz, 2013). Others might argue that this is actually one of the reasons why compassion is *even more important*, precisely because these situations may be potentially traumatic. Whatever we think of compulsion, compassion is always important, in any context. In acute mental health crises, people's own support networks, usually their families and friends, have often broken down. It can sometimes be even harder for families and friends to be compassionate as they are 'too close' to the situation.

As well as challenges such as these, qualities of compassion are often squeezed out in health care systems (Maben et al., 2009; Youngson, 2008). On top of this, nurses often feel frustrated about their inability to provide the kind of care and support that they would want to deliver (Koekkoek et al., 2009). Sadly, for these kinds of reasons, some nurses leave the profession all together.

In recent years in the UK, cognitive behavioural therapy (CBT) has been considered the best psychological treatment for people with a range of mental health problems. This has been associated with an initiative called Improving Access to Psychological Therapies (IAPT). Whilst not wanting to criticise this initiative, nor the work done by nurses and psychologists, it is interesting to see the focus upon technical strategies rather than upon the qualities of therapeutic relationships. This can be seen in the increasing popularity of manualised or computerised therapies. Whilst IAPT and CBT offer one framework for developing therapeutic care, we would argue that what is needed is an investment in understanding and developing compassionate caring relationships rather than investments in technical 'fixing'.

There are even bigger challenges to compassion in wider society. Unfortunately, in the last 20 or 30 years in the UK, capitalism has demanded an ever increasing focus upon personal achievement, individualism, independence, choice and competition. This focus has also bred selfishness and the pursuit of profit, status and power (Bunting, 2004; James, 2008). In today's health services there is an increased emphasis on value-for-money and it has now become routine that services are privatised. It seems that the dominant values in mainstream society (and recently in the NHS) that we are supposed to aspire to are diametrically opposed to qualities associated with compassion. It could be argued that society is more interested in consumerism than compassion. However, there is much recent research that highlights the damaging psychological effects of a capitalist system. One major observation is the impact of economic inequality that leads to high crime, major mental health problems, poor physical health, anxiety, depression, addictions and so on (Wilkinson and Pickett, 2009). Materialism and individualism are also said to cause mental health problems and a breakdown of trust (Trzesniewski and Donnellan, 2010; Twenge and Campbell, 2010).

This is one of the many reasons why society needs to find ways of providing genuinely therapeutic environments for people who suffer mental distress. It would be even better if our society was based more on compassionate and caring values towards one another.

## Compassion as accepting service users' views

When we think about what service users might want from mental health services, we could well ask ourselves: 'If I were using mental health services, what would I want?' People that use services are ordinary people just like us, although they are often facing difficult, extraordinary, or unusual situations or experiences. If you or I were to experience extreme emotional or psychological distress, we would both presumably want to be shown understanding and warmth from our fellow human beings. One problem is that people who experience mental distress may sometimes behave in certain ways that might make others feel judgemental, scared or uncomfortable.

A good example of this is health care professionals' attitudes to people who self-harm. People who self-harm have often been regarded as manipulative, a nuisance or labelled as 'attention-seeking' (Pembroke, 1994; Spandler, 1996). Nurses may not always use these words, but often people who harm themselves are regarded as less deserving of compassion than other patients (e.g. those who are physically ill).

A compassionate nurse will not judge the person's actions but instead, seek to understand the person, try to accept how they are coping with their distress and perhaps try to minimise the harm they are causing themselves, or indeed others (Spandler and Warner, 2007). This is important even if we find such behaviour upsetting, irrational or disagreeable. A compassionate approach in mental health nursing therefore means that the nurse needs to be aware of and then try to 'bracket off' judgemental feelings about a person's actions. They need to find ways of appreciating the person's life and their situation and understand that the person is coping with their situation in the best way they know how.

In a similar way, organisations like the Hearing Voices Network have pioneered the idea and practice of 'accepting voices'. Many people hear or see things that other people cannot hear. Only some of these are distressed by this experience. Distressing voices often relate to difficult or abusive early life experiences. Rather than trying to get rid of people's unusual experiences, some practitioners and voice hearers have found ways to live with and accept their voices and understand their meaning (Knight, 2009; Romme et al., 2009).

Finally, some practitioners are working more creatively and compassionately with service users who do not want to take psychiatric medication. Usually the approach to mental health care, especially when people are experiencing what is known as 'psychosis', is to convince people to take medication (usually antipsychotics). This happens, despite their dubious and unknown long-term effectiveness, as well as their often unwanted effects or side-effects (Moncrieff, 2009). Instead, some practitioners have started to adopt a 'harm reduction' approach which accepts that people often do not want to take medication. Rather than entering a futile battle about taking medication (and service users will often find ingenious ways of not taking them anyway), nurses can work alongside service users. For example, they may provide realistic information to enable them to make informed decisions and to reduce any harm that might result from not taking medication (Aldridge, 2012).

These examples can be seen as compassionate ways of working because they are about being with a person in crisis by accepting and working with his/her current coping strategies, gradually building up resilience and understanding.

CASE EXAMPLE

Pete is 34 years of age. He is unsure what came first, the drug use or the psychosis. Whichever it was, as a teenager, he left home and lived with friends in an empty house. He 'squatted' for 10 years, but he was occasionally arrested and detained in mental health units. He has always felt rejected by society. He thinks people consider him a scrounger and a worthless human being. He seems distrustful and angry towards everyone he meets and is quickly rejected by them. Having experienced periods of homelessness, Pete was transferred to a residential rehabilitation unit. The manager of the unit is Mary. She is in her late fifties and has had four sons of her own; they are now grown up. From when Mary first met Pete, she felt a sense of connection to him. Despite Pete's angry outbursts and the fact that Mary felt pushed away and rejected by Pete, she continued to make herself available if he needed her. In other words, she was very patient. She recognised and accepted her own feelings about this (for example, her own fear of rejection). She did not take out her feelings on Pete, for example by retaliating or rejecting him. However, she made sure she found ways to look after herself so she didn't feel resentful or guilty. Mary imagined what it must have felt like being a teenager and feeling rejected by his family (and how she would feel if her children rejected her). She also imagined that if she was in that situation at that age, she too may have resorted to using drugs and alcohol. Mary saw beyond Pete's dishevelled appearance and looked into Pete's eyes and saw his humanity.

Over time, as they got to know one another, Mary discovered that Pete was interested in learning about digital photography; he had never owned a camera, but had seen others using them. Mary had a spare camera at home and brought this into work for Pete to use (she probably bent the rules doing this). Mary also showed Pete how to save the images on the office computer and over a period of months, Pete learned Photoshop and enjoyed producing stunning photographs of the cityscape. Eventually Pete gained access to a college course on digital photography. He began to think about doing a degree and for the first time in many years, dared to create a personal ambition for his life.

## Summary

The concept of compassion in general nursing is well established and prominent in NHS policy for physical illness. This is much less so in mental health policy. People who use mental health services have often been judged according to their behaviour and there remain strong negative stereotypes associated with psychiatric labels. Mental health nursing has been greatly influenced by humanistic principles and the need for empathic understanding is central to the therapeutic relationship. Mental health nurses need to demonstrate understanding of how negative life experiences may cause psychological problems and learn to become non-judgemental about people's behaviours. Compassion is also rooted in ordinary human love, a neglected area of study. There are many barriers to compassionate nursing practice not least of which, understanding at a policy and practice level. Furthermore, health care systems are becoming more orientated towards business models and the target-driven culture. Although we have argued that compassion is central to mental health nursing practice, it may not be as valued by managers as quantifiable results. We can be certain, that compassionate practice is greatly valued by the people that matter the most: our clients and patients.

# References

Aldridge, M.A. (2012) 'Addressing non-adherence to antipsychotic medication: a harm-reduction approach', *Journal of Psychiatric and Mental Health Nursing*, 19 (1): 85–96.

BMA (British Medical Association) (2011) *The Psychological and Social Needs of Patients.* London: British Medical Association.

Bunting, M. (2004) *Willing Slaves: How the Overwork is Ruling our Lives.* London: Harper Collins.

Chamber, C. and Ryder, E. (2009) *Compassion and Caring in Nursing.* Oxford: Radcliffe Publishing.

Clarkson, P. (1995) *The Therapeutic Relationship.* London: Whurr.

Department of Health (2008) *High Quality Care for All: NHS Next Stage Review Final Report.* London: The Stationery Office.

Department of Health (2009a) *The NHS Constitution.* Norwich: The Stationery Office.

Department of Health (2009b) *New Horizons: A Shared Vision for Mental Health.* London: The Stationery Office.

Department of Health (2011) *No Health Without Mental Health: A Cross-government Mental Health Outcomes Strategy for People of All Ages.* London: The Stationery Office.

Digby, A. (1985) *Madness, Morality, and Medicine: A Study of the York Retreat, 1796–1914.* New York: Cambridge University Press.

Fromm, E. (1957) *The Art of Loving.* London: HarperCollins.

Gilbert, P. (ed.) (2005) *Compassion: Conceptualisations, Research and Use in Psychotherapy.* London: Routledge.

Gilbert, P. (2010) *The Compassionate Mind.* London: Constable.

James, O. (2008) *The Selfish Capitalist: Origins of Affluenza.* London: Vermillion.

Kennard, D. (1983) *An Introduction to Therapeutic Communities.* London: Routledge and Kegan.

King's Fund (2009) *The Point of Care.* Available at: www.kingsfund.org.uk/research/projects/the_point_of_care/index.html (accessed on: 13/1/2011).

Knight, T. (2009) *Beyond Belief: Alternative Ways of Working with Delusions, Obsessions and Unusual Experiences.* Berlin: Peter Lehman Publishing.

Koekkoek, B., Van Meijel, B., Schene, A. and Hutschemaekers, G. (2009) 'A delphi study of problems in providing community care to patients with non-psychotic chronic mental illness', *Psychiatric Services*, 60 (5): 693–7.

Maben, J., Cornwell, J. and Sweeney, K. (2009) 'In praise of compassion', *Journal of Research in Nursing*, 15 (1): 9–13.

Mayhew, S. and Gilbert, P. (2008) 'Compassionate mind training with people who hear malevolent voices: a case series report', *Clinical Psychology and Psychotherapy*, 15: 113–38.

Moncrieff, J. (2009) *The Myth of the Chemical Cure: A Critique of Psychiatric Drug Treatment.* Basingstoke: Palgrave.

NHS Confederation (2008) 'Compassion in health care: the missing dimension of healthcare reform?', *Futures Debate*. Available at: www.nhsconfed.org/Publications/Documents/compassion_healthcare_future08.pdf (accessed on: 5/7/2013).

NMC (Nursing and Midwifery Council) (2007) *Essential Skills Clusters (ESCs) for Pre-registration Nursing Programmes*. London: Nursing and Midwifery Council.

NMC (Nursing and Midwifery Council) (2010) *Pre-registration Nurse Education in the UK*. London: Nursing and Midwifery Council.

Pembroke, L. (ed.) (1994) *Self-harm: Perspectives from Personal Experience*. London: Survivors Speak Out.

Porter, R. (2004) 'Is mental illness inevitably stigmatising?', in A. Crisp (ed.), *Every Family in the Land*. London: The Royal Society of Medicine Press.

Romme, M., Escher, S., Dillon, J., Corstens, D. and Morris, M. (2009) *Living with Voices: 50 Stories of Recovery*. Ross-on-Wye: PCCS Books.

Scott, S., Sampson, E.L. and Jones, L. (2012) 'The compassion programme: looking at improving end-of-life care for people with advanced dementia', *International Journal of Palliative Nursing*, 18 (5): 212–16.

Scull, A. (1993) *The Most Solitary of Afflictions: Madness and Society in Britain, 1700–1900*. New Haven, CT: Yale University Press.

Segal, Z., Williams, J.M.G. and Teasdale, J. (2002) *Mindfulness-based Cognitive Therapy for Depression: A New Approach to Preventing Relapse*. New York: Guilford Press.

Spandler, H. (1996) *Who's Hurting Who? Young People, Self-harm and Suicide*. Manchester: 42nd Street.

Spandler, H. and Stickley, T. (2011) 'No hope without compassion: the importance of compassion in recovery-focused mental health services', *Journal of Mental Health*, 20 (6): 555–66.

Spandler, H. and Warner, S. (eds) (2007) *Beyond Fear and Control: Working with Young People who Self-harm*. Ross-on-Wye: PCCS Books.

Stickley, T. and Freshwater, D. (2002) 'The art of loving and the therapeutic relationship', *Nursing Inquiry*, 9 (4): 250–6.

Szasz, T. (2013) 'Thomas Szasz 1920–2012', *Asylum*, 20 (1).

Titch Nhat Hahn (2003) *Creating True Peace*, New York: Free Press.

Trzesniewski, K.H. and Donnellan, M.B. (2010) 'Rethinking "Generation Me": a study of cohort effects from 1976–2006', *Perspectives on Psychological Science Journal*, 5 (1): 58–75.

Twenge, J.M. and Campbell, W.K. (2010) 'Birth cohort differences in monitoring the future dataset and elsewhere: further evidence for Generation Me: Commentary on Trzesniewski and Donnellan', *Perspectives on Psychological Science Journal*, 5 (1): 81–8.

Wilkinson, R. and Pickett, K. (2009) *The Spirit Level: Why More Equal Societies Almost Always do Better*. London: Allen Lane.

Williams, M., Teasdale, J., Segal, Z. and Kabat-Zinn, J. (2007) *The Mindful Way Through Depression*. London: Guilford Press.

Youngson, R. (2008) *Compassion in Health Care: The Missing Dimension of Health Care Reform?* NHS Confederation Futures debate paper 2. London: NHS Confederation.

Youngson, R., Dickson, N., Sweeney, K. and Gallagher, U. (2009) *NHS Policy Salon: Discussion Summary: Has Compassion Got Lost?* London: King's Fund/NHS Confederation.

# 10

# Theories for Public Mental Health and Mental Health Promotion

## SALLY BINLEY AND THEO STICKLEY

### Learning Objectives

- Appreciate the historical origins of mental health promotion.
- Recognise the contested nature of 'mental health'.
- Understand of the contribution of Aaron Antonovsky to the topic.
- Acknowledge the role of communities in mental health promotion.

## Introduction

In this chapter we argue that for public mental health (and therefore mental health promotion) to be effective, it needs to be wholly engaged with communities of people. A salutogenic approach is recommended that harmonises with an individual's world view and own 'sense of coherence'. People do not become mentally ill without a context for such problems to exist. Any attempt to promote mental health needs to understand and acknowledge the personal and social contexts. Mental health nurses both individually and collectively need to grasp these complexities and take responsibility for effective public mental health.

## Historical perspective

In order to fully appreciate the concept of mental health promotion it is helpful to understand how general health promotion theory and practice have emerged over time. This section therefore gives an overview of the history of how modern approaches to promoting health came about; we will then consider mental health promotion specifically.

In the mid-nineteenth century, the prevailing 'Miasma theory' stated that diseases such as cholera or the Black Death were caused by pollution or a noxious form of 'bad air'. In 1854, John Snow, a physician in London, carefully observed the incidence of a devastating cholera outbreak and controversially concluded that it was, in fact, contaminated water from a particular public water pump that was responsible for the infection. It was later discovered that the pump had been built close to an old cesspit.

In doing so, Snow contributed to the founding principles of epidemiology and the eventual understanding of how infectious diseases are spread. This understanding led to improvements in water quality and sanitation which contributed significantly to a reduction in infectious diseases and an increase in life expectancy in the late nineteenth and early twentieth centuries. Tackling these environmental factors was, according to McKeown (1979), significantly more important than medical interventions in achieving these essential improvements in the health of the population.

This understanding of how environmental factors impact the health of the wider population is a fundamental element of public health and health promotion. As infectious diseases declined, chronic diseases such as heart disease and cancer became the leading causes of death in developed countries and highlighted the fact that individuals' lifestyles were also significant in the development of ill health.

This focused attention on people's behaviour and their lifestyle choices such as smoking and exercise, and consequently, health promotion activity concentrated on preventing disease by encouraging people to reduce or stop their risky health behaviours. This approach, though, was accused of 'victim-blaming' in that it focused too much attention on the responsibility of individuals for their own health with little or no regard for the role that government and other institutions have in determining the health of the population. An example of how this approach has continued to this day can be seen in the current debate about minimum pricing per unit of alcohol. The debate argues that government policy will have the greater impact on alcohol-related ill health rather than relying on individuals to reduce their drinking.

The 1980s saw a significant increase in the development of health promotion theory and practice, with health considered to be the 'extent to which an individual or group is able to realise aspirations and satisfy needs, and to change or cope with the environment' rather than purely the absence of disease (WHO, 1986).

Health promotion was defined by the World Health Organization in the Ottawa Charter (WHO, 1986). The Charter outlined strategies to achieve 'health for all' by the year 2000 and defined health promotion as:

> ... the process of enabling people to increase control over, and to improve, their health. To reach a state of complete physical, mental and social well-being, an individual or group must be able to identify and to realise aspirations, to satisfy needs, and to change or cope with the environment.

The Charter also described health as 'a resource for life' and 'not the object of everyday living' and discusses fundamental prerequisites for health which include: peace, education and social justice. So in this context, the responsibility for promoting health is clearly much wider than the remit of the individual or indeed the health sector alone.

It is therefore suggested that sectors such as education, law enforcement and private business have just as much responsibility for promoting health as health services themselves. For example, schools may well teach children about healthy eating but if they only provide unhealthy school meals and sell snacks such as crisps and chocolate from vending machines then the ability of the students to implement the messages they receive in the classroom is limited.

The Ottawa Charter listed key activities for the practice of health promotion as follows:

- Building public health policy
- Creating supportive services
- Strengthening community action
- Reorienting health services
- Developing personal skills.

There are a number models of health promotion which offer different perspectives on the type of activities involved, and these can be explored through wider reading. However, key examples of health promoting activities can be grouped under certain headings:

- Legislative measures – e.g. laws that enforce 'healthy' behaviours such as wearing a seat belt or not using your mobile phone when driving.
- Behaviour change methods – e.g. a variety of approaches are available to support people to reduce or stop their unhealthy behaviours, such as stopping smoking.

- Population-wide prevention measures – e.g. vaccinating children against communicable diseases such as measles or screening for early signs of ill health, such as breast screening.
- Empowerment approaches which support individuals and groups to take control over their health and environment through the development of knowledge and skills.


## Mental health promotion

Having outlined a brief history of health promotion, we now go on to give an overview of how the concept became applied to mental health. Early developments in health promotion tended to focus on physical health and so the WHO definition could simply be used to describe mental health promotion as: 'the process of enabling people to take control over and to increase their mental health' (Tilford, 2006). However, this definition became regarded by many as woefully inadequate and a more detailed definition is offered by the Canadian Public Health Association in 1996:

> Mental health promotion is the process of enhancing the capacity of individuals and communities to take control over their lives and improve their mental health. It uses strategies that foster supportive environments and individual resilience, while showing respect for equity, social justice, interconnections and personal dignity.

Tilford (2006: 41) questioned whether it was necessary to define mental health promotion as a separate activity at all:

> Since health promotion adopts an holistic definition of health logically its actions are directed towards mental as well as physical health and mental health promotion is an integral part of general health promotion.

However, she also acknowledges that this approach of including mental health in general health promotion can lead to it being overlooked altogether. In terms of general health promotion policy development, mental health has featured more significantly as thinking has progressed. Moreover, there has been a gradual shift in emphasis from reducing mental illness to the promotion of mental well-being.

Targets to reduce mental illness were specified in policies such as the *Health of the Nation* in 1992. This strategy was the central health policy in England from 1992 to 1997; however the emphasis here was on reducing deaths from suicide rather than on positive approaches to enhancing mental well-being.

In 1997 a change in government signalled a move towards a more population-wide approach to promoting health and a significant report on inequalities in health was published in 1998 (the Acheson Report). This highlighted the link between health and social class and the impact of deprivation on life expectancy and general health outcomes. This in turn led to a rapid succession of documents which aimed to tackle inequalities and improve the health of the most deprived populations. One such series of policies in the UK were the National Service Frameworks (NSFs); NSFs were published around a range of issues such as coronary heart disease, cancer, diabetes and, in 1999, mental health. These frameworks set out to eradicate the discrepancies in services that patients suffering from these conditions were experiencing, depending on where they lived; this was known as the 'postcode lottery'. They sought to establish a national set of standards that any patient could expect if they accessed services for their condition, regardless of where they lived.

In terms of mental health, this included standards on primary care services for people with common mental health problems through to standards on inpatient care for people with severe and enduring mental illness. Of particular significance, however, was the inclusion of a standard (Standard 1) on mental health promotion. The stated aim of this national standard (DH, 1999: 14) was:

> To ensure health and social services promote mental health and reduce the discrimination and social exclusion associated with mental health problems.
>
> Health and social services should:
>
> - promote mental health for all, working with individuals and communities
>
> - combat discrimination against individuals and groups with mental health problems, and promote their social inclusion.

This was a significant step forward for the development of mental health promotion and the first time it had been recognised in national policy. The significant difference was the emphasis on society and local communities and the recognition of social inclusion as fundamental elements of promoting mental health:

> Mental health promotion is most effective when interventions build on social networks, intervene at crucial points in people's lives, and use a combination of methods to strengthen:
>
> - individuals to enhance their psychological well-being
>
> - communities in tackling local factors which undermine mental health. (DH, 1999: 14)

Thus, the focus was no longer just upon individuals and their behaviour, but it also looked at greater social forces at work that are responsible for people's mental ill health. This was later developed in government policy when, in 2004, the Social Exclusion Unit published the report: *Mental Health and Social Exclusion* (SEU, 2004).

# Theories for public mental health

Before we introduce key theories for mental health promotion, we need to think about a key question: 'What is mental health?' We need some kind of idea as to what it is, before we can promote it. There is a problem though, because the idea of mental health is a contested concept (the following ideas have been further developed in Stickley and Timmons, 2007).

In the western world, the medical model of mental illness prevails and dominates statutory mental health services. It has defined official policy since the 1858 General Medical Act, which recognised that insanity was a disease of the brain and ordained doctors as keepers of the mad and the authority in their treatment (Rogers and Pilgrim, 2001).

## The medical model

The medical model asserts that mental illness is a pathology and in the same way that any physical disease can be assessed by signs and symptoms, so can mental illness. A diagnosis can be duly ascribed and treatment can be offered, a process that is verified by a body of empirical science. People who experience this form of illness seek help from the medical profession who are trained to recognise the symptoms and are able to diagnose according to the classification of diagnostic manuals such as the DSM-IV and the ICD-10. An accepted psychopharmacology enables doctors to prescribe drugs that affect the central nervous system and the brain's chemistry. Because the science of biopsychiatry is considered universal, there is little scope for subjective and cultural variations. If somebody is deemed to have symptoms of schizophrenia for example, they will be diagnosed irrespective of whether they are from Surbiton or Senegal, whether they are an Iranian refugee or a white merchant banker. For people who are considered sufficiently ill, they may be required to stay in hospital until they are considered well enough to resume their role in society. (For more about the philosophical problems of the medical model, see Chapter 1.)

## Lay beliefs

Closely aligned to the medical model are lay beliefs about mental illness, which are strongly affected by the images of mental illness as portrayed by the media and which are usually relating to stories of violence and crime committed by people with mental health problems. There are a variety of conceptualisations of mental health; whilst we do not intend to offer expositions of all the theoretical positions, it is important to acknowledge alternative understandings to medical and lay beliefs. These theoretical views overlap and at times contradict each other.

## Social theories

Sociology offers a number of alternatives to lay and medical beliefs. People are understood in their social context and the role of people considered 'mentally ill' has evolved with society. Parsons (1951) proposed the 'sick-role' identity which ensures that the incapacity which people may experience does not interfere with the smooth running of society. There are circumstances where people prefer to be ill than to be unemployed as the benefits of illness outweigh the disadvantages. For example, some people may feel protected from being made to feel that they 'should' work by others and 'illness' provides a good reason not to work. Furthermore, some people may receive high rates of state benefits that exceed unemployment benefits and enjoy not having to bear the responsibility to work. Some believe that capitalism is largely to blame for what is categorised as disease. Factors such as workplace stress and pollution are examples of this. People's environments are more significant in determining mental health rather than their biology.

In his book *Madness and Civilization* Foucault (1965) shows how madness (the term he preferred) is not a biological phenomenon, and can only be understood in the context of the society in which it exists. He believed that society 'constructs' its own version of madness. Aaron Goffman (1961) analysed psychiatric hospitals and regarded them as social rather than therapeutic institutions. He saw the asylums as 'total' institutions that controlled every aspect of inmates' lives. This separation from society and the controlled existence effectively stigmatises people contained in asylums and prevents them from not only functioning but also reintegrating into society and forces a 'sick' identity on to them. Goffman shows how the total institution creates more problems than it solves.

## Anthropology

Some anthropologists would argue that any understanding of mental illness cannot be separated from the culture of the person. As a concept, mental health can only be understood by seeing it in the context of the beliefs, values, systems and institutions of that culture (Helman, 2000). Mental illness is not universally accepted across cultures and it is therefore suggested as only ever culturally determined (Jaynes, 1990).

## Humanistic theory

A humanistic view of human experience will offer another conceptualisation of mental health. From this perspective, life is seen as a journey with its ups and downs and mental distress may be regarded as a process of self-discovery (Rogers, 1951). Rather than 'breakdown', it may be better to consider the possibility of 'breakthrough'. Under stress we may all suffer emotionally and psychologically. Furthermore, expressions of distress no matter how apparently garbled can be understood to those who have ears to hear. This position was demonstrated in action by the psychiatrist R.D. Laing (1960). He believed that no matter how bizarre or apparently unintelligible the individual presented, there was always meaning. It is far easier to diagnose as mad and prescribe medication than to spend time with a distressed person and work hard at listening and committing to an empathic relationship. This approach has informed the Hearing Voices Network, largely based upon the seminal work of Romme and Escher (1993). (For more about humanistic theory see Chapter 4.)

## Alternative beliefs

There are many alternative beliefs to the notion of mental health and mental illness. In recent years, for example, the nursing literature has seen a growth in interest towards concepts of holism and alternative (or complementary) therapies. Most of these complementary practices have their origins in eastern religion, thought and medicine. Concepts of mental illness in eastern thinking are seen in the context of balances of body energy. For example, traditional Chinese medicine, which has underpinned a majority of alternative therapies, considers the body to be a microcosm of the universe and any notion of illness is directly related to the individual's relationship with his/her own life force. Mental illness is seen in the context of blockages of energy pathways in the body (Miller, 2006). If these pathways can be unblocked, then equilibrium can be restored and the individual's life force can be restored. These vital forces maintain physical and mental well-being. In some cultures, a spiritual explanation of mental illness is offered, where irrational and incoherent behaviour may be caused by demonic possession. The spiritual leader (whether it be a shaman or Church of England vicar) is called to exorcise the offending spirits.

There are therefore many theories of mental health that are not always reconcilable. These competing discourses may inform the development of mental health promotion initiatives according to their particular beliefs. To date, most national mental health promotion initiatives seek to combat stigma and attempt to 'normalise' experiences of mental distress. However, given the high proportion of people experiencing mental health problems from lower social classes, there is a need for mental health promotion initiatives that acknowledge this fact and that promote social answers to social problems.

## Total health promotion

As we have seen there are many conceptualisations of what mental health is. The problem however is that the medical model continues to dominate in mental health services. The medical model continues to see mental ill health as an abnormality and some psychiatrists have acknowledged how their own profession may be a contributing factor to maintaining stigma because of diagnostic categories (Crisp, 2004; Kendall, 2004). Crisp (2004) calls for doctors to take responsibility for the labels they use that cause 'discriminatory identification (that produce) potentially negative generic characteristics at the expense of individuality' (Crisp, 2004: xv). Kendall accuses his own profession of using 'stigmatising, derogatory terms to refer to patients with various kinds of mental illness (Kendall, 2004: xxiii). Porter (2004) blames the diagnostic labelling as much for the stigma surrounding mental illness and likens the process of determining diagnoses through the committees of the Diagnostic Statistical Manual to pantomime. This concern has been echoed by Seedhouse (2003: 7), who argues that 'as soon as we come to believe our classifications are real like rock ... we are trapped'. It is argued that the label puts people in a position in society that is inferior and stigmatised.

Historically, there have been campaigns that seek to normalise 'mental illness' by referring to 'it' as similar to any other illness, such as diabetes. However, some have argued that that such destigmatising campaigns actually reinforce rather than alleviate stigma as the 'problem' is located within the individual and the social injustices are not addressed (Repper and Perkins, 2003; Sayce, 2000). Although mental and physical health is often separated for convenience of service provision, they should be considered jointly. Any division is created largely for the benefit of professionals and that mental health underpins and is inseparable from all health should therefore underpin all health strategies (Seedhouse, 2003).

## Salutogenesis

Antonovsky (1996) criticises mental health promotion for its stagnant theory base and its tendency to compartmentalise the human condition. During his life (he died in 1994) he developed a theory he called 'salutogenesis' that focuses on factors that support human health and well-being rather than on factors that cause disease. Antonovsky studied the influence of a variety of sources of stress on health and was able to show that relatively unstressed people had much more resistance to illness than more stressed people. This he referred to as a 'sense of coherence'. Although contemporary medicine increasingly speculates about the origin of illnesses, Antonovsky suggested that the question of the origin of good health was of greater significance, especially to health promotion. Sense of coherence is defined by Antonovsky as:

> A global orientation that expresses the extent to which one has a pervasive, enduring though dynamic feeling of confidence that one's internal and external environments are predictable and that there is a high probability that things will work out as well as can reasonably be expected. (Antonovsky, 1987: 19)

This sense of coherence is the result of the collective effect of resources and processes that are conducive to health. Within the salutogenic orientation the view is held that there is a direct relationship between the strength of the sense of coherence and the person's ability to employ cognitive, affective (emotional) and instrumental strategies likely to improve coping and thereby well-being.

Salutogenesis requires a decisive change in attitude, one that recognises the influence of a person's relationship with others and the social environment on the maintenance of that person's mental health. As a person-centred approach to health promotion, salutogenesis supports an understanding of how the loss of meaningful interactions with others contributes to social isolation, and therefore social interaction is essential in attaining an improved sense of well-being. Health promotion initiatives can help contribute to a positive sense of identity and health 'resourcefulness' by encouraging individuals to participate in community activities. These initiatives have also been found to promote a sense of control over their illness in individuals receiving care. Individuals are encouraged to develop coping skills and a *sense of coherence* independently, the latter of which is key to mental health according to Antonovsky. This model also advocates that health resources are both individual and personal, echoing others' views that a *sense of coherence* is aided by an understanding of how an individual's cultural background affects their life experiences of valued participation.

The twentieth century witnessed advances in health care in the western world of unforeseen dimensions. It is curious to observe at the beginning of the present century, what little progress has been made in considering human beings as whole entities. The existing distinction in statutory research and practice between mental and physical health is an example of dualistic thinking. Seedhouse and Antonovsky are two amongst a very few that have intellectually addressed the problem of dualistic thinking in health promotion.

## Application to practice

In the UK, Standard 1 of the National Service Framework (NSF) for mental health (DH, 1999) first spelt out the requirement for mental health promotion. Additionally, with the introduction of the Department of Health's (2001) *Making it Happen*, mental health workers were given a guide for the implementation of mental health promotion in the UK. At a local level, Standard 1 of the NSF was instrumental in the development of a raft of projects aimed at raising awareness of mental health issues, attempting to reduce the stigma around mental illness and improving access to services. Local strategies were developed which set targets for mental health promotion across a range of settings including schools, workplaces and prisons. Activities included partnership working between the local authorities and health services to tackle domestic violence and provide training for health visitors to enable them to detect early signs of post-natal depression.

Putting Standard 1 into practice was not without its challenges and it could be argued that it was ahead of its time. However, it was an important step in progressing the thinking around mental health promotion and formed the basis for subsequent policy development. Current policy around mental health continues to drive the importance of working with communities to promote mental health and underlines the significant impact that poor mental health can have on overall health. Similarly, there is continued acknowledgement of the relationship between poor mental health and social factors such as poverty and poor education.

In 2011, a new policy framework for mental health was introduced, called *No Health Without Mental Health* (DH, 2011). The aims of the strategy are:

> As well as improving the mental health and wellbeing of the population, and services for people with mental health problems, this strategy will also help to deliver the best value for our society from the resources committed to mental health. (p.13)

The framework however was introduced at a time of severe economic difficulties in the western world. These difficulties have come at a time when studies of epidemiology suggest that inequality is a major cause of mental health problems (Wilkinson and Pickett, 2010). Furthermore, economic inequality is the most significant indicator for ill health and social disorganisation and psychosocial factors, such as the following, are indicators of poor health outcomes:

- Low social status affecting dignity and self-worth
- Poor social affiliations resulting in feelings of loneliness
- Early childhood experience that impacts upon psychological well-being in later life (Wilkinson, 2005).

The implementation of policies therefore that might 'improve the mental health and well-being of the nation' against a backdrop of an unequal society with tremendous problems of poverty and unemployment does not bode well without a strong political will from those in government to address economic inequality.

Returning however to Seedhouse and Antonovsky, what might a programme of work look like based upon their ideas? In the following section we give a brief overview of a community-based arts project that was developed in about 2003; the project is ongoing.

**CASE EXAMPLE**

Increasingly, mental health promotion has become associated with 'ordinary' type community-based activities such as sports or the arts. The following case study is arts-based and is reported more fully in Stickley (2012).

The Lost Artists Club (LAC) was the idea of two people who we shall refer to as Wendy and Rupert. They both lived in the poorest area of a Midlands city and were both on benefits. Both considered themselves artists, but felt they were outside the mainstream of society. Rupert played the saxophone, he also painted and wrote poetry. Wendy had done a creative arts degree years previously, but had to take time out because of her mental ill health. She used to perform her poetry in the 1980s, but she concentrated more on painting in recent years.

They both found the arts helped emotionally, and wanted a community of artists to relate to. They felt that what was lacking in their lives was not lack of artistic ability, nor fear of creating – both being quite prolific with their art – but difficulty finding like-minded people.

A small group of people including a mental health nurse and a few local artists met together to discuss how Wendy and Rupert could be helped in their ideas for developing a community-based arts initiative. It was through discussing these ideas together that the Lost Artists Club was born.

Through word of mouth people started coming along, at first to Rupert's living room. Wendy produced a leaflet and slowly the momentum grew. More and more people attended what they referred to as 'creative gatherings'. There were no inclusion/exclusion criteria, neither were there any referral procedures or risk assessments! The LAC was run by the people, for the people.

Over time, the group became constituted and received small amounts of funding. The group decided to meet monthly. After about one year, the LAC held an exhibition at a local gallery. Fourteen artists exhibited their work, and over 300 people saw the exhibition and gig at the end of the exhibition. The exhibition was an enormous success. The group also produced two CDs and a poetry/art booklet for the exhibition. In the years that followed over a hundred people became members of the LAC.

The group always believed that anyone can produce art. These highly talented, creative people could benefit from connecting with like-minded people. From its experience, art became a bridge for people to socially connect. Because of the LAC, new friendships were created and people had opportunities to create, perform and exhibit and find fulfilment in their creative expression.

# Summary

This chapter has described the origins of mental health promotion and attempted to identify some of the complexities of promoting mental health. Mental health itself is a contested concept, so in order to promote it nurses need to acknowledge the debates that surround its conceptualisation. We have emphasised the theoretical contribution of both David Seedhouse and Aaron Antonovsky. We have chosen these particular thinkers because their work acknowledges the complexities described and both emphasise the need to regard people holistically and in their social context. Mental health promotion needs to be holistic and focused upon people's life situations and involve people in their communities. For mental health promotion to be effective, initiatives need to make sense to the people on the receiving end. A short example has been given to help illustrate the main principles included in this chapter.

# References

Antonovsky, A. (1987) *Unraveling the Mystery of Health: How People Manage Stress and Stay Well*. San Francisco: Jossey-Bass.

Antonovsky, A. (1996) 'The salutogenic model as a theory to guide health promotion', *Health Promotion International*, 11 (1): 11–18.

Canadian Public Health Association (1996) *Action Statement for Health Promotion in Canada*. Available at: www.cpha.ca/en/programs/policy/action.aspx (accessed on 25/6/2013).

Crisp, A. (ed.) (2004) *Every Family in the Land*. London: The Royal Society of Medicine Press.

Department of Health (1992) *The Health of the Nation*. London: The Stationery Office.

Department of Health (1998) *Independent Enquiry into Inequalities in Health (the Acheson Report)*. London: The Stationery Office.

Department of Health (1999) *National Service Framework for Mental Health*. London: DH.

Department of Health (2001) *Making it Happen*. London: DH. Available at: www.dh.gov.uk

Department of Health (2011) *No Health Without Mental Health*. London: HM Government.

Foucault, M. (1965) *Madness and Civilization*. New York: Vintage.

Goffman, E. (1961) *Asylums*. New York: Anchor Books.

Helman, G. (2000) *Culture, Health and Illness* (4th edn). London: Arnold.

Jaynes, J. (1990) *The Origin of Consciousness in the Breakdown of the Bicameral Mind*. London: Penguin.

Kendall, R.E. (2004) 'Why stigma matters', in A. Crisp (ed.), *Every Family in the Land*. London: The Royal Society of Medicine Press.

Laing, R.D. (1960) *The Divided Self*. Harmondsworth: Penguin Books.

McKeown, T. (1979) *The Role of Medicine: Dream, Mirage or Nemesis*. Oxford: Basil Blackwell.

Miller, G. (2006) 'China: healing the metaphorical heart', *Science*, 311 (5760): 462–3.

Parsons, T. (1951) *The Social System*. London: Routledge and Kegan Paul.

Porter, R. (2004) 'Is mental illness inevitably stigmatising?', in A. Crisp (ed.), *Every Family in the Land*. London: The Royal Society of Medicine Press.

Repper, J. and Perkins, P. (2003) *Social Inclusion and Recovery*. Edinburgh: Ballière Tindall.

Rogers, C.R. (1951) *Client-centered Therapy: Its Current Practice, Implications and Theory.* Boston: Houghton Mifflin.

Rogers, A. and Pilgrim, D. (2001) *Mental Health Policy in Britain: A Critical Introduction* (2nd edn). Basingstoke: Palgrave.

Romme, M. and Escher, S. (1993) *Accepting Voices.* London: Mind.

Sayce, L. (2000) *From Psychiatric Patient to Citizen: Overcoming Discrimination and Social Exclusion.* London: Macmillan.

Seedhouse, D. (2003) *Total Health Promotion: Mental Health, Rational Fields, and the Quest for Autonomy.* Chichester: John Wiley.

SEU (Social Exclusion Unit) (2004) *Mental Health and Social Exclusion.* London: Social Exclusion Unit.

Stickley, T. (2012*) Qualitative Research in Arts and Mental Health.* Ross-on-Wye: PCCS Books.

Stickley, T. and Timmons, S. (2007) 'Considering alternatives: student nurses slipping directly from lay beliefs to the medical model of mental illness', *Nurse Education Today,* 27 (2): 155–61.

Tilford, S. (2006) 'Mental health promotion', in M. Cattan and S. Tilford (eds), *Mental Health Promotion: A Lifespan Approach.* Maidenhead: Open University Press.

Wilkinson, R. (2005) *The Impact of Inequality.* New York: The New Press.

Wilkinson, R. and Pickett, K. (2010) *The Spirit Level: Why Equality is Better for Everyone.* London: Penguin.

WHO (World Health Organization) (1986) International Conference on Health Promotion, Ottawa, Canada.

# 11

# Mindfulness and Mental Health Care

## TIM SWEENEY

### Learning Objectives

- Identify the origins of mindfulness.
- Define mindfulness.
- Understand the theoretical underpinnings of mindfulness.
- Identify key studies highlighting benefits arising from mindfulness practices.
- Understand how mindfulness works with depression.

## Introduction

Experiences of mental health problems have been reported throughout history and within all cultures and historic periods. One early record dates as far back as 10,000 BC in the form of 'trepanation', an act involving cutting small holes in the skull, possibly in an attempt to resolve mental health problems (Brothwell, 1963). References to mental disorders are apparent in Ancient Greece, in the hallucinations of Pythagoras (Pilgrim, 2007), through to contemporary accounts of a 'Prozac Nation' (Wurtzel, 1994).

Whilst the last century witnessed significant economic and social advances leading to improvements in physical health, standards of living and increased life expectancy for populations, there has been a substantial rise in the number of mental health problems including anxiety disorders, alcoholism, drug abuse, dementia and depression (WHO, 2001).

Mental health problems have recently been estimated to affect approximately 18% of the population in the UK at any one time (DH, 2009). The most common single disorder is depression, which presents a significant cause of disability across the world and affects up to 15% of the UK within their lifetime (National Collaborating Centre for Mental Health, 2010).

In recent years an ancient and traditionally eastern approach to managing suffering has been imported by the west to tackle this rising problem in the western world – mindfulness. Originating within Buddhist philosophy, mindfulness is a form of conscious awareness that is characterised by the capacity to be fully aware of the totality of momentary experience. One of the most widely quoted definitions of mindfulness is by Jon Kabat-Zinn, who describes mindfulness as:

> Paying attention on purpose, in the present moment, and non-judgementally to things as they are. (1990: 4)

Within the UK the last decade has seen a dramatic escalation of interest in mindfulness as benefits arising from this approach are increasingly recognised. In particular, its inclusion in National Institute for Health and Clinical Excellence Guidelines for Depression (NICE, 2004a, 2009) has generated increased enthusiasm for mindfulness in the form of mindfulness-based cognitive therapy (MBCT). MBCT is a therapeutic intervention which combines mindfulness with cognitive therapy to form a structured programme for the treatment of a wide range of physical and mental health problems.

The origins, theoretical underpinnings and applications of MBCT within modern health care are described in the following sections of this chapter. This begins with its Buddhist origins, starting over 2500 years ago.

## Historical development of MBCT

Buddhism was founded in the sixth century BC in North India by Siddharta Gautama. Born a prince, his early life of wealth and privilege had sheltered him from the harsh existence experienced by the vast majority of the population, and on leaving his castle one day he was struck by the scale and ubiquity of death and suffering. He subsequently resolved to more fully understand the human condition through the attainment of spiritual enlightenment (Kumar, 2002). This is synonymous with a state of nirvana: the end of suffering as all things are seen with total insight and clarity, aided by compassion towards the self and all beings (Goldstein, 2002).

To this end, he left his home and family and initially engaged in contemporary religious practices believed to bring about enlightenment, consisting of self-induced austerities such as near starvation (Goldstein, 2002). However, despite a determined effort to cultivate enlightenment utilising these methods over several years, he decided that this approach was inadequate. He consequently adopted a new approach to the development of insight, involving mindfulness meditation as a core component (Goldstein and Kornfield, 1987).

Having gained enlightenment through a process of mindfully experiencing a variety of urges and depravations, Siddharta Gautama became known as the Buddha, or Awakened One (Kumar, 2002). He subsequently spent the next 45 years teaching his philosophy – the Dharma (Kumar, 2002), which are written as discourses.

The aim of mindfulness meditation is therefore nothing less than final liberation from suffering (Thera, 1962). It is commonly referred to as *satipatthana* from the Pali language. The word *sati* refers to 'attention' or 'awareness' that is skilful, or good. *Patthana* refers to 'presence of'. Combined, this makes 'presence of skilful attentiveness' (Thera, 1962). It is also referred to as 'insight' or *vipassana* meditation. *Vipassana* is the Pali word for insight, or clear sightedness. It is found in all the Buddhist traditions and is the fundamental practice of paying attention (Goldstein, 2002).

The application of mindfulness to a range of health problems is suggested by its Buddhist roots, which incorporate the fundamental aims of developing compassion and reducing suffering (Ludwig and Kabat-Zinn, 2008). To this end, Jon Kabat-Zinn, an American biologist, started a Stress Reduction Clinic in Massachusetts in 1979 in an attempt to make mindfulness meditation accessible to people suffering from a wide range of physiological and psychological disorders (Saxe et al., 2001). This began as a department within a medical hospital offering people an alternative approach to managing chronic pain and stress conditions. It was intended to provide a complementary service to people receiving treatment for health problems only partially addressed through the medical model (Kabat-Zinn, 2002).

Building on assertions made by Walsh (1980) and Jung (1969) amongst others (e.g. Deikman, 1982) about the potential value of engaging in eastern spiritual meditative practices, Kabat-Zinn combined this approach with the western psychological and behavioural science paradigms and research methodology (Kabat-Zinn et al., 1985). The subsequent introduction of mindfulness meditation to the western world during the establishment of the Stress Reduction Clinic in the late 1970s and onwards represents what appears to be the first concerted attempt to deliver mindfulness to a population outside a purely Buddhist framework.

Intensive mindfulness training is taught to participants experiencing a broad spectrum of physical and mental health problems (Kabat-Zinn et al., 1992). Kabat-Zinn's treatment programme, mindfulness-based stress reduction (MBSR), is an eight-week group training and believed to be especially useful in helping patients with chronic disorders develop skills to better manage these difficulties (Majumdar et al., 2002), due to the heightening of mindful awareness positively altering the patients' perception of their symptoms. This facilitates a change in relationship with symptoms as these are observed with non-judgemental attention, allowing alternative, more helpful strategies to emerge, rather than the continuation of self-defeating attempts to resolve them (Ludwig and Kabat-Zinn, 2008).

As the fundamental unifying element across all facets of the MBSR programme (Davidson and Kabat-Zinn, 2004), it is argued that purposeful engagement in mindfulness meditation results in greater levels of mindful awareness (Kabat-Zinn, 2003), and that this is the mechanism mediating improvements in the functioning and well-being of participants (Kabat-Zinn, 1982, 2005a; Kabat-Zinn et al., 1998).

Within the MBSR programme mindfulness is regarded as a universal and intrinsic human facet independent of a religious framework, relating to the innate capacity to pay attention. This capacity is deepened and refined through repetition and practice (Kabat-Zinn, 2003; Meili et al., 2004). It is therefore taught not as a Buddhist practice but as a method for developing awareness (Kabat-Zinn, 2002). This context changes the precise focus of the intervention from attainment of enlightenment to management of stress and pain.

During the 1990s, three eminent clinical psychologists working in the field of cognitive science and depression were in the process of attempting to develop a form of cognitive therapy that prolonged the relapse-preventing properties of this intervention (Segal et al., 2002). On discovering the work of Jon Kabat-Zinn and colleagues they were struck by the way this programme attempts to help people develop a different relationship to emotional pain, and realised its potential applicability to depression. They subsequently went on to develop mindfulness-based cognitive therapy (MBCT).

MBCT is a group treatment combining mindfulness meditation and cognitive therapy. It was developed for use in recurrent depressive disorder as a means of attempting to reduce risk of recurrence in susceptible individuals (Segal et al., 2002). Borrowing heavily from the MBSR programme, MBCT more precisely focuses on targeting processes believed central to depressive vulnerability: rumination and self-critical thinking patterns triggered by a mild drop in mood (Teasdale et al., 2000). MBCT involves attentional training through mindfulness meditation. Through this teaching, participants become more aware of momentary changes in mood, allowing them to intervene at precisely the point at which low mood typically escalates into depressive relapse (Williams et al., 2007).

In summary, mindfulness has moved from inhabiting an eastern religious and philosophical framework focusing on the pursuit of spiritual enlightenment, to residence within a secular training programme focusing on the relief of a specific form of emotional pain – depression.

Within both Buddhism and cognitive therapy, becoming more aware of mental processes is regarded as a key component of reducing suffering and attaining emotional well-being. The following section will outline the basic theory of each approach in relation to MBCT, which has led to their combination in this form of treatment for depression.

# Theories underpinning mindfulness and MBCT

## Buddhism

Buddhist teachings describe the development of a detached relationship with internal experiences, including thoughts, as a central feature of its approach to reducing suffering. This approach teaches that suffering is an integral part of human existence and is only increased by attempts to contain it. For example, within a Buddhist philosophy rumination may be conceptualised as a well-meaning, but self-defeating attempt to escape from distress through identifying its causes by engaging in analytical thinking. However, this increased preoccupation with the causes of unhappiness may unwittingly only create further suffering. In this respect, the deliberate effort to resolve difficulty actually becomes the principal factor maintaining it. Alternatively, attempts to avoid suffering through suppressing negative thoughts, memories and feelings, whilst potentially helpful in the short term, curtail opportunities to resolve these more comprehensively in the longer term, and are likely to result only in further rumination in an attempt to overcome the problem. This pattern is highlighted in diagrammatic form in Figure 11.1.

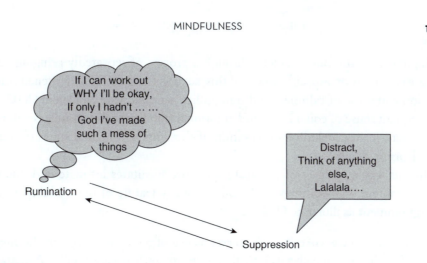

**FIGURE 11.1**   Key processes accounting for vulnerability and maintenance for depression

In summary, attempts to avoid suffering through either *thinking about* its causes in order to overcome it, or through alternative methods of trying *not* to think about it, only unwittingly perpetuate the suffering these strategies are designed to resolve. Developing a different approach to managing emotional pain and difficulty is instead offered within Buddhism through the process of mindfulness. Rather than approaching experience with the intention of making this 'better' or 'right' in some way, Buddhist teachings instead assert that increased contentment arises from an increased detachment from urges to fulfil particular desires with a correspond-ing ability to fully engage with the actuality of moment-to-moment experience (Kumar, 2002). In this way, the tension between desired and actual states dimin-ishes and suffering is reduced. It is the act of letting go of things, whether material, conceptual or emotional, which leads to freedom (Goldstein, 2002). Mindfulness facilitates this process.

Within Buddhism, mindful awareness is developed through meditation exercises which systematically direct attentional focus on to aspects of experience, such as sounds and bodily sensations. Buddhist teachings, or *Sutras*, provide comprehensive instructions for the cultivation of mindfulness, as in the *Satipatthana Sutra*:

> Experiencing the whole body I shall breathe in … breathe out, thinking thus, he trains himself. (Soma and Pereira, 1949: 46)

In practising this, the individual is directly and mindfully experiencing the body (Hanh, 1975). Furthermore, mindfulness of the body is regarded as a method for bringing the mind into balance. Through a process of repeatedly bringing awareness to the body or a specific aspect of this, such as the breath, a heightened concentration and sense of calmness and tranquillity is developed (Goldstein, 2002). The subsequent sense of equanimity and emotional stability enables a fuller exploration of present reality, including observation of thoughts and mental states (Goldstein and Kornfield, 1987).

In this way, awareness of physical experience facilitates intimate understanding of the content and workings of the mind – a key feature of the Buddhist route to enlightenment as illustrated below:

> Whatsoever there is of evil … whatsoever there is of good – all issues from the mind. If the mind is comprehended, all things are comprehended. (Buddha, Anguttara Nikaya vol. I, in Thera, 1962: 22)

This systematic observation of the mind in Buddhist meditation practices helps us to notice the tendency to categorise phenomena as pleasant or unpleasant and react accordingly. This can gradually reduce the preoccupation with reacting to avert pain or cling on to pleasure. The act of simply resting in awareness in this way engenders understanding that attempting to endlessly meet preconditions for contentment results only in further dissatisfaction and disappointment (Thera, 1962). Mindfulness therefore provides an opportunity to instead experience events fully and respond skilfully without being swept along by automatic and habitual reactions. It is the heightened awareness arising from mindfulness meditation that allows this to occur (Goldstein and Kornfield, 1987).

As highlighted above, mindfulness is developed through focusing on everyday activities such as breathing, the body, feelings and the mind. Beginning with formal meditation practices and then bringing mindfulness to these activities continuously throughout the day is necessary to generate levels of awareness consistent with the attainment of enlightenment. This involves awareness of every thought, feeling and sensation that arises without instantly reacting to them, but simply acknowledging their existence (Hanh, 1975). This provides an opportunity to then choose how best to respond to these events.

Having repeatedly practised bringing awareness to specific facets of experience, such as the breath, attention is expanded to include any observable phenomena. This meditation technique is called 'bare attention' and is regarded as a key form of mindfulness directing individuals towards enlightenment (Thera, 1962).

Bare attention is a form of relating to internal and external events without reacting, but rather observing them fully (Thera, 2005). It is the clarity of understanding about the true nature of experience that this brings that is sought. Bare attention involves focusing on any and all phenomena such as thoughts, feelings, sights and sounds that arise within the field of awareness. It is described as bare as it attends only to the initial facts of perception, without engaging in usual reactions to these events, such as reflecting on them. As described above, such reactions are automatic and often characterised by aversion or clinging to experience. The exacerbating effects of automatically reacting to suppress or eradicate unwanted internal events are countered by calmly facing and naming such difficulties within the meditation practice. Labelling this internal material enables a clearer recognition of its nature (Thera, 2005), allowing it to more readily become an object of mindful awareness (Thera, 1962).

The ability to recognise and step back from such phenomena in this way is a key aim of mindfulness meditation (Thera, 2005). This requires the individual to focus only on the present moment, counteracting the tendency to dwell in the past or fantasise about the future. This is regarded as a pointless waste of energy and potential source of suffering (Thera, 1962). In contrast, mindfulness meditation promotes full contact with the reality of what is actually present, rather than being lost in memories, imaginings and projections about the future.

In this way, bare attention encourages objective observation of present moment experience, rather than the more usual filtering of phenomena through idiosyncratic and often biased interpretations with corresponding reactions. An accurate recognition of what is present allows clarification of the constituent parts of experience so that it can be more fully understood and experienced. This reduces the risk of being unwittingly swept into reactions to events that cause unhappiness and distress (Thera, 2005).

Meditation techniques within Buddhism also involve meditations specifically aiming to generate compassion, such as 'loving kindness' meditation or *metta* where the individual encourages thoughts of compassion towards him/herself and others. This involves incorporating words into a meditation practice such as 'may you be free from suffering' (Goldstein and Kornfield, 1987).

Such compassion is considered a necessary component of mindfulness as distractions are managed within this with equanimity and acceptance. Therefore, a compassionate attitude is regarded as a necessary prerequisite for the development of mindfulness, whilst at the same time being a core feature of it (Kumar, 2002).

In summary, mindfulness is conceptualised within Buddhism as a necessary component of the path to contentment and spiritual enlightenment. It involves observing internal and external phenomena without reaction in an effort to fully comprehend the true nature of experience. Bare attention tempered with a compassionate attitude is a primary method for achieving this.

Cognitive therapy is the other facet of MBCT alongside mindfulness. Its theoretical background is now summarised in the section below.

## Cognitive therapy

Chapter 5 in this book provides a more in-depth explanation of cognitive therapy, but for the sake of this chapter, I will outline this approach and its relevance to mindfulness. The Beckian cognitive model was developed principally in the 1970s as a new form of psychological therapy for the treatment of mood disorders. Based fundamentally on the assertion that 'men are disturbed not by things but the views which they take of them' (Epictetus, in Ellis, 1979: 190), it applied this concept to mental health problems in a way that was revolutionary.

Cognitive therapy differs from alternative previous treatments for emotional disorders by emphasising the crucial role that thoughts play in determining how a person feels and acts. In essence, conscious thoughts are used as a window into the individual's internal experience. These thoughts are tangible evidence of the meaning that the person gives to events, which in turn accounts for how he or she feels about it. These factors influence the person's behaviour. These features of an individual's experience can form what is termed a vicious circle, as thoughts, emotions and behaviour unwittingly conspire to perpetuate distress, as highlighted in Figure 11.2 (you will find a similar example in Figure 5.1).

Within cognitive therapy, individuals are taught to identify problem situations in terms of their constituent parts, as highlighted above. Through this process they become increasingly aware of the direct influence of their thoughts and actions on their emotions, and how these can maintain distress.

Central to the cognitive model is the proposition that it is the *content* of thoughts and beliefs that is principally responsible for depression, typically involving themes of loss, worthlessness and failure (Segal et al., 2002), as highlighted in the example above. It is this content that interventions seek to positively alter and to which the success of therapy is attributed. Consequently individuals learn to identify and challenge the negative content of their thoughts during therapy. However, studies focusing on mechanisms accounting for the success of cognitive therapy suggest instead that the *process* of thinking may actually be more important than the specific *content* of thoughts. For example, a study carried out by John Teasdale et al. (2001) suggested that the efficacy of cognitive therapy results from its success in

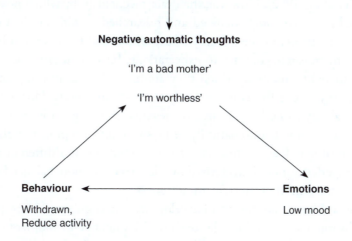

**Critical situation**

A mother is physically unwell and is temporarily unable to look after her children

**Negative automatic thoughts**

'I'm a bad mother'

'I'm worthless'

**Behaviour**

Withdrawn,
Reduce activity

**Emotions**

Low mood

**FIGURE 11.2** Vicious circle highlighting maintenance factors

assisting reductions in an absolute, black and white thinking style, rather than simply through decreasing the negative content of thinking as proposed by Beck's cognitive model.

Recent theories also proposed that it is our relationship with, and response to negative experiences and thoughts that determine whether these intensify or abate (Teasdale, 1998), in keeping with theories espoused in Buddhist teachings above. For example, the differential activation hypothesis (Teasdale and Barnard, 1993) argues that it is an individual's reaction to a drop in mood that determines whether or not this escalates into a full blown episode of depression. Those vulnerable to depression can quickly become entangled in a self-maintaining vicious circle as described in Figures 11.1 and 11.2, in the face of only slight reductions in mood due to their tendency to react by dwelling on the problem in a misguided effort to resolve this. However, this response typically only entraps them further within their depression as they become increasingly absorbed in their difficulty, and consequently more distressed by it.

As a result of these recent theoretical and research developments, the emphasis within cognitive therapy for depression has moved from specifically targeting the content of negative thoughts to instead helping people to change the way they relate to them.

Cognitive therapy for depression as developed and implemented by Beck et al. (1979) assists many people in recovering from what can be a life-threatening problem (Keller et al., 1992). However, the exact mechanism by which positive change is achieved has been widely debated and researched within the field of cognitive therapy. Beck's theory of the primacy of cognitions and their content has not been borne out by research, contrary to expectations. Instead, altering our relationship with our thoughts to one in which they are recognised as passing mental events, not necessarily fact or the 'truth', is likely to be advantageous. This involves developing the ability to be less reactive to negative thinking, to learn to stand back from thoughts, without automatically being swept into attempts to fight, argue and ruminate on them. Central to this is the development of a different relationship with our experience, one characterised by a less reactive, more balanced approach to this: one characterised in short, by mindfulness.

In summary, both Buddhism and developments in cognitive therapy propose that the establishment of a mindful relationship with moment-to-moment experience is likely to be helpful for those susceptible to depression. This has led to the combination of these approaches through the development of MBCT.

The use of MBCT is supported by findings from several recent randomised controlled trials which demonstrate its effectiveness in reducing the risk of future depressive episodes by approximately 50% for those with a history of multiple episodes of depression, and therefore particularly susceptible to future relapse (e.g. Kuyken et al., 2008; Ma and Teasdale, 2004; Teasdale et al., 2000). It has consequently become a recommended treatment for recurrent depression within the UK for this population (DH, 2009; NICE, 2004b).

Whilst these trials have consistently supported the value of MBCT in reducing the risk of depressive relapse in a vulnerable population, the mechanisms by which it achieves its effects remain relatively unexplored. These studies nevertheless appear to support the hypothesis that (for those with multiple episodes) depression is triggered by the gradual development of autonomous processes that involve the reactivation of depressive thinking patterns by a mild drop in mood (Teasdale and Barnard, 1993). MBCT is hypothesised to achieve its effects by disrupting these processes though the development of a mindful perspective.

## Theory applied to practice

In addition to approaches which seek to capitalise on the therapeutic effects of mindfulness directly, such as MBCT, a number of authors have proposed that mindfulness is an implicit component of a range of psychological therapies, pre-dating mindfulness-based interventions. For example, Martin (1997) asserts that mindfulness has always been a component of western psychotherapies, including both psychodynamic psychotherapies and cognitive therapy, due to their observational stance and aim to develop self-awareness in recipients. Development of an ability to 'step back' allowing individuals to see the difference between reality and their interpretation of this is clearly a common factor in many psychotherapies and is a phenomenon closely related, if not identical, to mindfulness.

The observation that an accurate view of reality is regarded as a fundamental component of healthy psychological adjustment within virtually all theories of mental health has been made (Martin, 1997), and other authors have commented on similarities between specific psychological therapies and mindfulness-based interventions. These have included existential phenomenological therapy (Claessens, 2010), Gestalt therapy (Dryden and Still, 2006; Tonnesvang et al., 2010), humanistic psychotherapy (Dryden and Still, 2006; Ellis, 2006), Adlerian concepts (Waller et al., 2006) and rational emotive behaviour therapy (Ellis, 2006). It is the basic aim of many such psychological therapies to increase levels of self-awareness and self-acceptance. As noted above, this is a fundamental intention of mindfulness and mindfulness-based interventions. It can therefore be argued that the differences in these approaches exist not in their aims, but in their methods for achieving these (Dryden and Still, 2006; Ellis, 2006).

Similarities between cognitive behaviour therapies and mindfulness are particularly noted in the literature (Dryden and Still, 2006; Ellis, 2006; Kang and Whittingham, 2010; Singh et al., 2008; Tonnesvang et al., 2010) and this view is further supported by the combination of these approaches in numerous mindfulness-based interventions. Despite this, some authors regard CBT and mindfulness as incompatible, citing different philosophies and underpinning theories as representing fundamental obstacles to their combination. For example, Harrington and Pickles (2009) argue that CBT is rooted in scientific method in an attempt to clarify the nature of reality, whereas mindfulness is conceptualised as an attempt to transcend reality, and that this approach is more aligned with mysticism. Therefore, CBT and mindfulness belong to different paradigms that cannot be combined with any validity. The focus in traditional cognitive therapy on content of thinking, rather than the processes involved in this, is a further distinction between these approaches (Hofmann et al., 2010). Nevertheless, as the health benefits of mindfulness have become more recognised, additional mindfulness-based interventions targeting numerous health disorders have emerged, including dialectical behaviour therapy (Linehan, 1993), mindfulness-based cognitive therapy (MBCT; Segal et al., 2002), relapse prevention (Marlatt, 2002) and acceptance and commitment therapy (Hayes et al., 1999). All of these approaches are derived from cognitive behavioural theories of change but also incorporate mindfulness as a central aspect. The application of MBCT is outlined below.

## Mindfulness-based cognitive therapy in practice

Mindfulness-based cognitive therapy (MBCT) is a group treatment combining mindfulness meditation and cognitive therapy. It was developed for use in recurrent depressive disorder as a means of attempting to reduce risk of recurrence in susceptible individuals (Segal et al., 2002).

The approach is specifically recommended for people who are currently in remission from a depressive episode but nevertheless vulnerable to future depression due to the recurrent nature of their disorder. Those with three or more episodes have been found to gain particular benefit from MBCT, whilst those with fewer episodes have not been found to benefit (Kuyken et al., 2008; Ma and Teasdale, 2004; Teasdale et al., 2000).

MBCT involves attentional training through mindfulness meditation. Through this teaching, participants become more aware of momentary changes in mood, allowing them to intervene at precisely the point at which low mood typically escalates into depressive relapse (Williams et al., 2007). These steps are hypothesised to reduce the risk of depressive relapse (Segal et al., 2002).

*The National Institute for Health and Clinical Excellence Guidelines for Depression* (NICE, 2004a, 2009) recommend that MBCT should normally be delivered in groups of 8–15 participants and consist of weekly two-hour meetings over eight weeks and four follow-up sessions in the 12 months after the end of treatment. The MBCT programme is delineated in Segal et al.'s *Mindfulness-based Cognitive Therapy for Recurrent Depression: A New Approach to Preventing Relapse* (2002).

The programme attempts to increase participants' levels of mindful awareness through repeatedly practising mindfulness and cognitive therapy exercises. During weekly two-hour classes participants engage in mindfulness meditation practices, followed by a short discussion about their experiences to highlight teaching points. Exercises from cognitive therapy for depression are also included. MBCT teachers lead participants through the exercises and ensuing discussion, in the form of an educational class. As in cognitive therapy, participants are also required to undertake in-between session tasks which aim to increase and consolidate learning from within sessions. It is expected that participants carry out approximately 45 minutes of meditation and other awareness training exercises per day for the duration of the course. Examples of some of the key MBCT exercises are outlined below.

## The raisin exercise

This exercise is designed to illustrate the automatic tendency of the mind to wander away from direct contact of moment-to-moment experience. It involves participants being led through the process of eating a raisin, whilst paying particular attention to the immediate sensations and internal experiences accompanying this seemingly mundane event. Slowing down the day-to-day process of eating allows the experience to be truly savoured. Within this participants invariably notice aspects of the experience that otherwise are typically ignored. This exercise highlights our habitual tendency to exist on automatic pilot, whereby potentially rich and life-enhancing experiences pass unnoticed. It also demonstrates the qualitatively different experience of paying close attention to our experience as it is unfolding.

## The body scan

The body scan involves systematically moving attention around the body over a period of 40 minutes. This exercise aims to assist participants in developing increased awareness of bodily experiences, in particular those associated with depressed mood such as tension, restlessness and lethargy. Increasing awareness of physical sensations may assist people to more readily spot signs of deterioration in mood and take evasive action.

## Mindfulness of breathing

In this practice attention is repeatedly brought to the sensations of breathing. Training awareness to adhere to one particular focus, mindfulness of the breath also highlights the tendency of the mind to wander and that this comprises its natural state. The exercise allows participants to notice typical patterns of thinking and reacting that occur for them, increasing awareness of internal experiences that otherwise drive behaviours and rumination.

## Walking down the street

This exercise from cognitive therapy teaches participants the role of thinking in influencing emotions. Participants imagine walking down a street and being ignored by someone they know, noticing typical thoughts and feelings that arise in response to this. The aim is again to increase awareness of thoughts and other significant internal experiences that can trigger a downward mood spiral if passing unnoticed and unchallenged.

## Bringing a difficulty

This practice occurs within the second half of the programme and involves gradual exposure to unpleasant and often avoided thoughts, memories and feelings in an effort to counteract the instinctive and often self-defeating tendency to suppress unwanted internal experiences. Participants focus on a stressful situation, bringing this to the forefront of their mind, gently inviting themselves to feel how the difficulty is experienced within their body. This can allow participants to develop an alternative and acceptance-based strategy to experiencing difficulty, rather than usual attempts to avoid and suppress unpleasant difficulties which only tend to rebound back into consciousness, leading into protracted periods of rumination in an effort to resolve this.

All the above exercises underline the importance of increasing awareness for those vulnerable to depression, highlighting that attention, instead of adhering to the present moment, has a tendency to focus on negative and unsatisfactory aspects of experience. Repeatedly bringing awareness back to the here-and-now begins to undermine this potentially dangerous tendency, limiting the possibility that depression can creep up whilst the mind is otherwise occupied.

Within all mindfulness practices, instructions are given with exhortations to be gentle in carrying these out. At all times an emphasis is given to directing attention with a tone of kindness and self-compassion. This is designed to counteract the usual tendency of those with recurrent depression to experience a more punitive and harsh internal dialogue, in itself presenting a factor likely to maintain depression.

A case example highlighting a participant's experiences of engaging with MBCT is outlined below.

Edward was a 62-year-old man who had experienced recurrent depression for the preceding 17 years. At assessment he described at least one episode per year of moderate to severe depression lasting several months, despite ongoing use of antidepressant medication. These problems had led to him retiring early from his job as an electrical engineer, employment he had always enjoyed. Edward described finding it difficult to exert any sense of control over his mood and mental health, feeling entirely at the mercy of these, and simply waiting for episodes to pass. Episodes of depression were characterised by increased self-criticism and guilt, a lack of motivation and a tendency to become socially withdrawn.

During the pre-class interview, Edward initially expressed feeling sceptical that MBCT would be of any benefit. During this meeting, his tendency to respond to low mood and events by ruminating on these or alternatively attempting to ignore them was identified. The potential advantages of increasing capacity for mindful attention to offset these tendencies were discussed. Going through the rationale for MBCT, including the potential benefits of training awareness, Edward was willing to attempt the approach.

Edward's scepticism continued through the first half of the programme, during which time he noted his difficulty in maintaining awareness on aspects of experience, such as the breath. However, hearing that this was also the experience of others within the group gradually began to reassure Edward that the behaviour of his mind was not unique or a symptom of his 'defectiveness' as he had assumed. This further undermined his usual tendency to criticise himself for 'getting things wrong'. Having naturally high standards, Edward usually responded to problem situations by making unrealistic demands of himself. Demands that would become more self-defeating as his depression progressed. Becoming aware through mindfulness meditation of this tendency highlighted to him that an increased capacity to take a break, rather than drive himself harder, was likely to be more helpful and less damaging to his health than previous strategies.

Exploring typical behavioural reactions to a drop in mood, including his tendency to isolate himself socially, allowed Edward to experiment with alternative strategies and in doing so recognise more helpful alternatives. Becoming more compassionate towards himself and less self-critical as a consequence also clearly assisted him in more effectively managing the fluctuations of his mood.

Immediately following the group and throughout the two-year follow-up period, Edward described an absence of depressive episodes, attributing this to an increased ability to notice early signs of low mood and to react to these with skill and kindness.

# Summary

The ancient and eastern tradition of Buddhist mindfulness meditation has been creatively combined with a western and modern psychological therapy to form mindfulness-based cognitive therapy. Whilst originating within apparently such different traditions, the approach is theoretically coherent, using methods at the heart of both approaches to work with one of the biggest health problems on the planet: depression.

Through the MBCT programme the unconscious use of strategies to contain suffering, such as rumination, distraction and avoidance, is observed and their unwitting role in aggravating suffering is clarified. Mindfulness meditation highlights our fundamental lack of control over internal phenomena such as thoughts, feelings and sensations. Energy is therefore directed not towards altering or controlling the content of experience, but in reorienting ourselves towards it, thereby altering the trajectory of distress associated with this.

Throughout the MBCT programme participants gradually engage in practices that aim to initially help them develop a more stable capacity for attention, and then to gently bring this to avoided and painful aspects of experience, the suppression of which may inadvertently be maintaining distress. Throughout this, increasing awareness of internal experiences, particularly those associated with depression, enables participants to spot early warning signs of relapse more quickly, enabling them to take skilful action to avoid this. Mindfulness meditation and cognitive therapy exercises combine to form an approach to working with depression that increases people's capacity to be present for each moment that they are alive, radically increasing opportunities for happiness and pleasure, as well as potentially reducing the risk of profound episodes of suffering.

# References

Beck, A., Rush, A., Shaw, B. and Emery, G. (1979) *Cognitive Therapy of Depression.* New York: Guilford Press.

Brothwell, D.R. (1963) *Digging up Bones: The Excavation, Treatment and Study of Human Skeletal Remains.* New York: Cornell University Press.

Claessens, M. (2010) 'Mindfulness-based third wave CBT therapies and existential-phenomenology. Friends or foes?', *Existential Analysis*, 21 (2): 295–307.

Davidson, R.J. and Kabat-Zinn, J. (2004) 'Response', *Psychosomatic Medicine*, 66 (1): 149–52.

Deikman, A. (1982) *The Observing Self.* Boston: Beacon Press.

Department of Health (2009) *New Horizons: A Shared Vision for Mental Health.* London: Department of Health.

Dryden, W. and Still, A. (2006) 'Historical aspects of mindfulness and self acceptance in psychotherapy', *Journal of Rational-Emotive and Cognitive Behaviour Therapy*, 24 (1): 3–27.

Ellis, A. (1979) *Reason and Emotion in Psychotherapy*. New York: Citadel Press.

Ellis, A. (2006) 'Rational emotive therapy and the mindfulness-based stress reduction training of Jon Kabat-Zinn', *Journal of Rational-Emotive and Cognitive Behaviour Therapy*, 24 (1): 63–78.

Goldstein, J. (2002) *The Emerging Western Buddhism: One Dharma*. New York: HarperCollins.

Goldstein, J. and Kornfield, J. (1987) *Seeking the Heart of Wisdom*. Boston: Shambhala Publications.

Hanh, T.N. (1975) *The Miracle of Mindfulness*. Boston: Beacon Press.

Harrington, N. and Pickles, C. (2009) 'Mindfulness and cognitive behavioural therapy: are they compatible concepts?', *Journal of Cognitive Psychotherapy: An International Quarterly*, 23 (4): 315–23.

Hayes, K.C., Strosahl, K.D. and Wilson, K.G. (1999) *Acceptance and Commitment Therapy: An Experimental Approach to Behaviour Change*. New York: Guilford Press.

Hofman, S., Sawyer, A. and Fang, A. (2010) 'The empirical status of the "new wave" of cognitive behavioural therapy', *Psychiatric Clinics of North America*, 33 (4): 701–10.

Jung, C.D. (1969) 'Forward to introduction to Zen Buddhism', in C.D. Jung (ed.), *Psychology and Religion*. Princeton, NJ: Princeton University Press.

Kabat-Zinn, J. (1982) 'An outpatient program in behavioural medicine for chronic pain patients based on the practice of mindfulness meditation: theoretical considerations and preliminary results', *General Hospital Psychiatry*, 4 (1): 33–47.

Kabat-Zinn, J. (1990) *Full Catastrophe Living: How to Cope with Pain, Stress and Illness Using Mindfulness Meditation*. New York: Dell Publishing.

Kabat-Zinn, J. (2002) 'Commentary on Majumdar et al: mindfulness meditation for health', *The Journal of Alternative and Complementary Medicine*, 8 (6): 731–5.

Kabat-Zinn, J. (2003) 'Mindfulness-based interventions in context: past, present and future', *Clinical Psychology Science and Practice*, 10 (2): 144–56.

Kabat-Zinn, J. (2005a) 'Bringing mindfulness to medicine', *Alternative Therapies*, 11 (3): 57–64.

Kabat-Zinn, J. (2005b) *Coming to our Senses: Healing Ourselves and the World Through Mindfulness*. London: Piatkus.

Kabat-Zinn, J., Lipworth, L. and Barney, R. (1985) 'The clinical use of mindfulness meditation for the self-regulation of chronic pain', *Journal of Behavioural Medicine*, 8 (2): 163–90.

Kabat-Zinn, J., Massion, M.D., Kristeller, J., Peterson, L.G., Fletcher, K.E., Pbert, L., Lenderking, W.R. and Santorelli, S.F. (1992) 'Effectiveness of a meditation-based stress reduction program in the treatment of anxiety disorders', *American Journal of Psychiatry*, 149 (7): 936–43.

Kabat-Zinn, J., Wheeler, E., Light, T., Skillings, A., Scharf, M.J., Cropley, T.G., Hosmer, D. and Bernhard, J.D. (1998) 'Influence of a mindfulness meditation-based stress reduction intervention on rates of skin clearing in patients with moderate to severe psoriasis undergoing phototherapy (UVB) and photochemo-therapy (PUVA)', *Psychosomatic Medicine*, 60: 625–32.

Kang, C. and Whittingham, K. (2010) 'Mindfulness: a dialogue between Buddhism and clinical psychology', *Mindfulness*, 1 (3): 161–73.

Keller, M., Lavori, P., Mueller, T., Coryell, W., Hirschfeld, R. and Shea, M. (1992) 'Time to recovery, chronicity and levels of psychotherapy in major depression', *Archives of General Psychiatry*, 49 (2): 809–16.

Kumar, S.M. (2002) 'An introduction to Buddhism for the CBT therapist', *Cognitive and Behavioural Practice*, 9: 40–3.

Kuyken, W., Byford, S., Taylor, R.S., Watkins, E., Holden, E., White, K., Barrett, B., Byng, R., Evans, A., Mullan, E. and Teasdale, J.D. (2008) 'Mindfulness-based cognitive therapy to prevent relapse in recurrent depression', *Journal of Consulting and Clinical Psychology*, 76 (6): 966–78.

Linehan, M.M. (1993) *CBT of Borderline Personality Disorder*. New York: Guilford Press.

Ludwig, D.S. and Kabat-Zinn, J. (2008) 'Mindfulness in medicine', *Journal of American Medical Association*, 300 (11): 1350–2.

Ma, S. and Teasdale, J. D. (2004) 'Mindfulness-based cognitive therapy for depression: replication and exploration of differential relapse prevention effects', *Journal of Consulting and Clinical Psychology*, 72 (1): 31–40.

Majumdar, M., Grossman, P., Dietz-Waschowski, B., Kersig, S. and Walach, H. (2002) 'Does mindfulness meditation contribute to health? Outcome evaluation of a German sample', *The Journal of Alternative and Complementary Medicine*, 8 (6): 719–30.

Marlatt, A.G. (2002) 'Buddhist philosophy and the treatment of addictive behavior', *Cognitive and Behavioral Practice*, 9 (2): 44–50.

Martin, J. (1997) 'Mindfulness: a proposed common factor', *Journal of Psychotherapy Integration*, 7 (4): 291–312.

Meili, T., Kabat-Zinn, J. and Leskowitz, E. (2004) 'The power of the human heart: a story of trauma and recovery and its implications for rehabilitation and healing', *Advances*, 20 (1): 6–16.

National Collaborating Centre for Mental Health (2010) *Depression: The Treatment and Management of Depression in Adults (Updated Edition)*. National Clinical Practice Guideline 90. London: National Collaborating Centre for Mental Health.

NICE (National Institute for Clinical Excellence) (2004a) *National Institute for Clinical Excellence Guidelines for Depression*. London: Department of Health.

NICE (National Institute for Clinical Excellence) (2004b) *Depression: Management of Depression in Primary and Secondary Care*. Clinical Guideline 23. London: NICE.

NICE (National Institute for Clinical Excellence) (2009) *National Institute for Clinical Excellence Guidelines for Depression*. London: Department of Health.

Pilgrim, D. (2007) 'The survival of psychiatric diagnosis', *Social Science and Medicine*, 65 (3): 536–47.

Saxe, G.A., Herbert, J.R., Carmody, J.F., Kabat-Zinn, J., Rosenzweig, P.H., Jarzobski, D., Reed, G.W. and Blute, R.D. (2001) 'Can diet in conjunction with stress reduction affect the rate of increase in prostrate specific antigen after biochemical recurrence of prostate cancer?', *The Journal of Urology*, 166: 2202–7.

Segal, Z., Williams, J.M.G. and Teasdale, J. (2002) *Mindfulness-based Cognitive Therapy: A New Approach to Preventing Relapse*. New York: Guilford Press.

Singh, N., Lancioni, G., Wahler, R., Winton, A. and Singh, J. (2008) 'Mindfulness approaches in cognitive behaviour therapy', *Behavioural and Cognitive Psychotherapy*, 36 (5): 659–66.

Soma, B. and Pereira, C.A. (1949) *The Way of Mindfulness: The Satipatthana Sutta 1949*. Colombo: Ceylon Printing Press.

Teasdale, J. (1998) 'Cognitive vulnerability to persistent depression', *Cognition and Emotion*, 2 (3): 247–74.

Teasdale, J. and Barnard, P. (1993) *Affect, Cognition and Change*. Trowbridge, UK: Lawrence Erlbaum Associates.

Teasdale, J., Segal, Z., Williams, J.M.G., Ridgeway, V.A., Soulsby, J.M. and Lau, M.A. (2000) 'Prevention of relapse/recurrence in major depression by mindfulness-based cognitive therapy', *Journal of Consulting and Clinical Psychology*, 68 (4): 615–23.

Teasdale, J., Scott, J., Moore, R., Hayhurst, H., Pope, M. and Paykel, E. (2001) 'How does cognitive therapy prevent relapse in residual depression? Evidence from a controlled trial', *Journal of Consulting and Clinical Psychology*, 69 (3): 347–57.

Thera, N. (1962) *The Heart of Buddhist Meditation*. London: New Century Hutchinson.

Thera, N. (2005) *The Power of Mindfulness*. Sri Lanka: Buddhist Publication Society.

Tonnesvang, J., Sommer, U., Hammink, J. and Sonne, M. (2010) 'Gestalt therapy and cognitive therapy – contrasts or complementarities?', *Psychotherapy Therapy, Research, Practice, Training*, 47 (4): 586–602.

Waller, B., Carlson, J. and Englar-Carson, M. (2006) 'Treatment and relapse prevention of depression using mindfulness-based cognitive therapy and Adlerian concepts', *The Journal of Individual Psychology*, 62 (4): 443–54.

Walsh, R.N. (1980) 'The consciousness disciplines and behavioral sciences: questions of comparison and assessment', *American Journal of Psychiatry*, 137 (2): 663–73.

WHO (World Health Organization) (2001) *The World Health Report: Mental Health: New Understanding, New Hope*. Geneva: World Health Organization.

Williams, J.M.G., Teasdale, J., Segal, Z. and Kabat-Zinn, J. (2007) *The Mindful Way Through Depression: Freeing Yourself from Chronic Unhappiness*. New York: Guilford Press.

Wurtzel, E. (1994) *Prozac Nation: Young and Depressed in America: A Memoir*. New York: Riverhead Trade.

# 12

# Why Recovery?

JULIE REPPER AND RACHEL PERKINS

## Learning Objectives

- Appreciate the origins of the recovery movement.
- Understand the fundamental principles of recovery.
- Understand the relationship between recovery and policy and the complexities of implementation.
- Acknowledge the challenge of the recovery approach to mental health workers.

## Introduction

In many English-speaking countries in recent years, 'recovery' has become the informing approach in mental health policy. In this chapter, we explain how this has come about. We trace the origins of the concept to the US civil rights movement and describe how and why recovery has become so important to people's lives. Historically, psychiatric services have been seen by many to have become oppressive institutions, spreading pessimistic messages of despair. People have been given hopeless messages such as being told they will never work or form normal relationships, need to take strong medication for the rest of their lives and so on. The recovery movement has offered something entirely different; people are respected for their individuality, their strengths, wishes and abilities. Mental health professionals who embrace a recovery philosophy therefore have a much more optimistic approach to their work. In this chapter we will describe the policy context and some of the key ways in which the concept of recovery has been understood and misunderstood as it has been adopted by a powerful, professionally led, system. We will then explore some of the conditions necessary for its transformative potential to be realised. For mental health nurses working in a recovery-orientated way, we call for them to seek to develop 'hope-inspiring relationships' (see Repper and Perkins, 2003).

## Historical developments

Unlike most concepts within the mental health arena, ideas about 'recovery' do not have their origins in the writings of learned professionals and researchers. Instead they emerged within the US civil rights movement and the work of people with personal experience of surviving and thriving with a diagnosis of mental health problems (Chamberlin, 1977; Deegan, 1988). In the UK, Coleman (1999), in *Recovery: An Alien Concept*, said that reference to recovery could and would not be found in professional texts. However, by the end of the first decade of the twenty-first century the concept had been enthusiastically embraced, some would say 'taken over', by professionals, academics and policy-makers.

As mental health services have claimed ownership of recovery, so its origins have been sought in the development of psychiatry and services rather than the journeys of those individuals whom they serve. For example, Davidson et al. (2010) trace the origins of the 'recovery movement' in psychiatry to the work of pioneering reformers like Pinel and services like the York Retreat, established in 1796 to replace the chains, shackles, intimidation and neglect of the traditional 'mad house' with respect, friendship and kindness. However, such 'humanitarian psychiatry' continues to place treatment at centre stage and the focus remains on what professional services can do to put right that which has 'gone wrong'.

As Mary O'Hagan (2009: 16) points out, 'recovery can be seen through different lenses'. Even a cursory look at the burgeoning recovery literature shows that the concept has mutated over time and moved away from its roots within the mental health user/survivor movement. From the 'personal journey' described in earlier texts, it has too often taken on the status of a new professional 'model'. Given the ensuing confusion over its meaning, some have argued that the concept of recovery should be abandoned (see, for example, Beresford and Bryant, 2008; Pilgrim, 2008).

## Why recovery?

Recovery is not something that services or professionals do but a personal journey of discovery: making sense of, and finding meaning in, what has happened;

discovering your own resources, resourcefulness and possibilities; building a new sense of self, meaning and purpose in life; growing within and beyond what has happened to you; and pursuing your dreams and ambitions. Although everyone's journey is individual and uniquely personal, the writing of those with lived experience of recovery suggests that three things are critical in supporting recovery (see Repper and Perkins, 2003, 2012):

- Hope. It is not possible to rebuild your life unless you believe that a decent life is possible and you need people around who believe in your possibilities.
- Control. Taking back control over your destiny, the challenges you face and the help you receive to overcome them.
- Opportunity. The chance to do the things that you value, to access those opportunities that all citizens should expect and to participate in society as an equal citizen.

To date, recovery ideas have often been distorted to fit in with existing professional frameworks and practices. If professionals and services are to be valuable travelling companions in the recovery journeys of those whom they serve then far more fundamental changes are required.

First, instead of prescribing treatment and support and planning care for people, professionals and services must essentially form part of the self-management plans of those whom they serve. Thus they become part of the resources available for people to use in order to alleviate their distress, manage the challenges they face and achieve their ambitions. As Mary O'Hagan (2007: 4–5) has said, people with mental health challenges should view mental health services as 'carriers of technologies that we may want to use at times, just like architects, plumbers and hairdressers'. The development of 'personal health budgets' that allow people to purchase the supports, treatment and services they find helpful has the potential to really change the balance of power (see Alakeson and Perkins, 2012; Forder et al., 2012).

Second, we need to move beyond 'user involvement' to genuine co-production at all levels: from individual support and treatment planning to the design, delivery and development of services. The language and practice of services is firmly rooted in a 'them' and 'us' culture. Professionals speak of 'my patients/clients/caseload' and define 'their' needs in terms of what 'we' have to offer. 'User involvement' typically means involving 'them' in 'our' services. Recovery-focused practice requires moving from 'them' and 'us' to 'we'. If services are to be of assistance to people in managing the challenges they face then they must be designed around the preferences and convenience of those whom they serve. This requires a partnership between the 'carriers of technologies' and those who may wish to use them.

Third, we need a different kind of workforce. If services are to help people to rebuild their lives we must ask what sort of expertise is required. Technical treatment may be one component of this, but just how many mental health professionals do you need to run a mental health service? Are there not other sorts of expertise that may be useful? Maybe we need more welfare benefit experts, personal trainers, employment specialists, life coaches and most especially peer workers. There is a wealth of evidence that peer support (provided by people with their own experience of mental health problems and explicitly drawing on this experience) is central to recovery (Repper and Carter, 2011). This provides a different sort of relationship for people using services. Traditional relationships between professionals (even those who also have lived experience) and those whom they serve is hierarchical. There is the 'helper' and the 'helped' – there is the expert with special knowledge and there is the patient. Peer support is a reciprocal relationship, based on mutuality and a shared journey. It is a way of offering help and support as an equal in a relationship that empowers people to recover.

Fourth, relationships between services and the communities they serve need to change. Traditionally, it is assumed that the resolution of mental health problems is a task for the professional experts. People are taken out of their communities and relieved of their roles and responsibilities while experts try to resolve their difficulties. The idea is that, once their problems are resolved, they can return to whence they came and resume their ordinary social roles. For many people the reality is very different. Even though they may live in their community, they are not a part of it, and the identity of 'mental patient' eclipses all others.

O'Hagan (2007) has described how mental health professionals and services can, albeit unwittingly, serve to perpetuate marginalisation and exclusion in a kind of vicious circle. Those of us with mental health problems have come to believe that experts hold the key to our difficulties. Our nearest and dearest believe we are unsafe in their untrained hands and so they leave it to the experts. So we all become less and less used to finding our own solutions and less comfortable with embracing distress as a part of ordinary life.

## The policy context

'Recovery' as the stated aim of government policy in England first emerged in 2001 in *The Journey to Recovery: The Government's Vision for Mental Health Care* (DH, 2001). Whilst this document acknowledged the importance of service users' wishes and goals, it emphasised recovery as a desired outcome. The *Mental Health National Service Framework* (DH, 1999) described how services were to foster this via the creation of 'safe', 'sound' and 'supportive' services. This National Service Framework (NSF) used the term 'recovery' only three times, all in an exclusively 'cure'-based clinical context; however it did acknowledge that services should be based on 'service user and carer aspirations', that 'a place to live, meaningful occupation, further education and training' were important and that stigma and discrimination too often prevented people achieving these. Within nursing, the *Chief Nursing Officer's Review of Mental Health Nursing* (DH, 2006) described a recovery approach as the underpinning of all nursing practice: 'Mental health nursing should incorporate the principles of the Recovery Approach into every aspect of their practice.'

Following the *Mental Health National Service Framework, New Horizons: A Shared Vision for Mental Health* (DH, 2009) described the government's mental health strategy. This shifted the focus from the treatment of mental illness to the promotion of mental health and improving the lives of people with mental health problems and recognised that this required action not simply within health and social services but across government departments. *New Horizons* went beyond traditional treatment approaches in describing its underpinning principles as 'equality, justice and human rights; reaching our full potential; being in control of our lives; valuing relationships' (DH, 2009: 9). It stated that mental health services should be recovery-focused, defining this in the terms used by Anthony (1993: 17):

> … a deeply personal, unique process of changing one's attitudes, values, feelings, goals, skills and roles. It is a way of living a satisfying, hopeful and contributing life, even with the limitations caused by illness, recovery involves the development of a new meaning and purpose in life as one grows beyond the catastrophic effects of mental illness.

The focus on recovery and improving the lives of those with mental health problems is shared across the major political parties. The demise of the Labour government in 2010, resulted in a new Conservative/Liberal Democrat coalition government strategy, *No Health Without Mental Health* (DH, 2011). The focus and direction of this policy's 'seven key outcomes' remained the promotion of the mental health of the population and the improvement of life chances for those with mental health problems. It is noteworthy that none of these refers to the eradication of symptoms or cure, but recognise recovery as a means to an end rather than an end in itself. The second outcome makes recovery, defined in social terms, an explicit aspiration:

> More people with mental health problems will recover. More people who develop mental health problems will have a good quality of life – greater ability to manage their own lives, stronger social relationships, a greater sense of purpose, the skills they need for living and working, improved chances in education, better employment rates and a suitable and stable place to live. (DH, 2011: 6)

The other five focus on better physical health, improving people's experience of services, reducing avoidable harm, decreasing stigma and discrimination and improving the well-being of the population as a whole. This places an emphasis on the development of public services that empower those whom they serve, increasing choice and control – including the development of personal budgets so people can make their own decision about what support they want and who will provide it. Social action and human rights, as well as greater diversity of support/service providers, are all seen as key to achieving these outcomes.

## Understandings, misunderstandings and mutations

### From individual journey to service intervention

The process of recovery described by those with lived experience of mental health problems is essentially one of an individual journey of discovery (Coleman, 1999; Deegan, 1988; Reeves, 1998; Repper and Perkins, 2003, 2012):

> … the lived or real life experience of people as they accept and overcome the challenge of disability. They experience themselves as recovering a new sense of self and of purpose within and beyond the limits of the disability. (Deegan, 1988: 11)

This is a journey in which professionals, and the services they inhabit, are not at centre stage, but may (or may not) have a marginal, supporting, role:

> The most challenging decisions ahead are not how to increase access to professional services but how to maximise life chances and enable people with mental health conditions to make the most of their lives. The real challenge is how to do things differently and use resources differently: recognise the limitations of traditional professional expertise, the value of the expertise of lived experience and rekindle the belief that citizens hold most of the solutions to human problems. (Perkins, 2010: 36)

However, in the UK, ideas about recovery in mental health services have too often been taken forward not by those with lived experience, but by professionals and policy-makers (DH, 2001, 2009, 2011; NIMHE, 2005). In this process of adoption, the concept of recovery has metamorphosed from the journey of an individual to a model of service provision. This can be seen in the introduction of special 'Support, Time and Recovery Workers' (DH, 2003) and 'Recovery Teams', and 'Recovery Interventions' like the 'Recovery Star' (McKeith et al., 2010) with its prescribed dimensions of recovery (living skills, addictive behaviour, managing mental health, etc.) and progression on a 10-step ladder from 'stuck' to 'self-reliance'. All a long way from 'the lived or real life experience' and 'deeply personal, unique process' of which Deegan (1988: 11) and Anthony (1993: 17) wrote.

Professional services have typically focused on how to 'put right' that which is assumed to have 'gone wrong', whether by pharmacological, psychological, social or occupational means. As mental health services have taken ownership, ideas about recovery have become encompassed within this 'cure'-based paradigm.

## Recovering 'from an illness' versus 'recovering a life'

In its origins among those with lived experience, recovery was seen to mean 'recovery of a life': 'recovering a new sense of self and of purpose' (Deegan, 1988: 11), 'a way of living a satisfying, hopeful and contributing life' (Anthony, 1993: 17). With the adoption of 'recovery' as a professional intervention, the cure-based paradigm prevailing within services has seen its meaning transformed into 'recovery from an illness'. Longitudinal studies of 'recovery rates' are cited as evidence that more people with a diagnosis of, for example, schizophrenia, 'recover' – are free of symptoms, medication and services – than has historically been assumed (see Warner, 2009).

Such arguments may be useful in counteracting the 'therapeutic pessimism' that abounds in many mental health services and to remind us that the small section of the population whom professionals see in services do not offer a representative picture of life following a diagnosis of mental health problems. However, such a perspective places recovery within the paradigms of traditional psychiatry. The goal of 'recovery interventions' and 'recovery teams' becomes 'symptom reduction' and 'discharge'. The assumption is that the purpose of mental health services is to 'cure people' and to contain and care for them unless and until this is achieved (Perkins, 2012).

Clearly, attempts to reduce and eliminate distressing symptoms are desirable, but as Deegan (1993: 10) observes, 'One of the biggest lessons I have had to accept is that recovery is not the same thing as being cured. After 21 years of living with this thing it still hasn't gone away.' While symptom reduction may assist in the process of 'recovering a life', it is not the 'end point': how many people are discharged from services when their symptoms have reduced, simply to sit and stare at the four walls of their flat with few/no social contacts and participation in the life of their communities? Whereas many people have shown that it is possible to recover 'a new sense of self and of purpose' (Deegan, 1988: 11) and 'a satisfying, hopeful and contributing life' (Anthony, 1993: 17) in the presence of ongoing or fluctuating cognitive and emotional challenges:

> Recovery is a process, not an end point or destination. Recovery is an attitude, a way of approaching the day and the challenges I face. (Deegan, 1993: 9)

The transformation of recovery from a 'process' – or continuing journey – to an 'outcome' or end point is, of course, rather convenient for services in an era of limited (and diminishing) resources. It can be used to justify economic imperatives to reduce reliance on services as a means to reduce costs (see, for example, Beresford and Bryant, 2008). A cynic might argue that it is this, rather than a desire to improve the lives of people with a diagnosis of mental health problems, that underpins the current popularity of ideas about recovery in current mental health policy. Whether or not this is the case, the tide of therapeutic optimism when combined with a view of 'recovery as outcome' has sometimes resulted in a failure to recognise the enormity of the challenge of recovering a life and all that this involves in a society where discrimination and exclusion remain rife.

## 'Everything is possible in the best of all possible worlds'?

In this tide of therapeutic optimism and belief in 'cure' it is easy to underestimate 'the catastrophic effects of mental illness' (Anthony, 1993: 17) and the 'limits of the disability' (Deegan, 1988: 11). The real challenge is growing within and beyond what has happened, and this takes enormous courage and tenacity. For mental health workers, people coming into services is an ordinary, everyday occurrence, it is easy to forget that, for each individual, it is a devastating and life-changing event, not only because of the problems that led to their diagnosis, but for all that becoming a 'mental patient' means in our society. The symptoms themselves can be terrifying, but often more disabling are the prejudice, discrimination and exclusion that accompany them. For many these challenges are magnified by other devastating experiences (abuse, loss of relationships, etc.) and the additional discrimination they may face as a consequence of their race, culture, age, gender, sexual orientation, disability, faith.

Being diagnosed with mental health problems might best be seen as a bereavement involving loss of status (the 'privileges of sanity'), self, meaning and purpose in life, and loss of the future you expected to have (Repper and Perkins, 2003, 2012). As with any loss, reluctance to accept what has happened, denial, despair, giving up and anger are ordinary and rational human reactions:

> We didn't believe our doctors … we adamantly denied and raged against their bleak prophecies for our lives. We felt it was just all a mistake, a bad dream … in a week or two things would be back to normal again. … Our denial was an important stage in our recovery. It was a normal reaction to an overwhelming situation. It was our way of surviving those first awful months. (Deegan, 1988: 12)

> We both gave up. Giving up was a solution for us. It numbed the pain of our despair. All of us who have experienced catastrophic illness and disability know the experience. (Deegan, 1988: 13)

> Anger follows in the footsteps of despair. Anger at the illness which has so devastated us. Anger at the helping system that may have failed. … Anger at society and its attitudes. Anger at God for not taking better care of us. Anger at parents and friends for not being more helpful. Anger at our self for not being able to manage. Our anger is a necessary and important part of the process. Anger is a stimulus to recovery. It is normal and natural. (Spaniol and Koehler, 1994: 12)

Yet, within mental health services, these ordinary responses to loss are typically seen as the 'lack of insight' and 'aggression' that are inherent in the person's 'disorder' – indicating that he or she is not 'ready' or 'suitable' for 'recovery'. When a person fails to 'make progress' services too often locate the 'problem' in the person's 'lack of motivation for recovery'.

Failure to recognise the enormity of the task of recovering a life and the meaning that a diagnosis has for the person has 'left many people with mental illness feeling devalued and ignored and has resulted in mistrust and alienation' (Spaniol et al., 1997: 14).

The process of recovering does not involve 'putting the past behind you' or 'getting back to normal', it involves the 'development of a new meaning and purpose in life as one grows beyond the catastrophic effects of mental illness' (Anthony, 1993: 17), 'recovering a new sense of self and of purpose within and beyond the limits of the disability' (Deegan, 1988: 11). It involves accommodating what has happened and facing the challenge of moving forwards, and the amount of courage and tenacity this requires should never be underestimated:

> You have the wondrously terrifying task of becoming who you are called to be. … Your life and dreams may have been shattered – but from such ruins you can build a new life full of value and purpose. (Deegan, 1993: 9)

> I know I have certain limitations and things I can't do. But rather than letting these limitations be occasions for despair and giving up, I have learned that in knowing what I can't do, I also open up the possibilities of all I can do. (Deegan, 1993: 11)

Even when the enormity of the task is recognised, the process of change must not be seen as a purely individual process and responsibility. Mental health problems occur within a social context and that context can either facilitate recovery and participation or impede it. The barriers imposed by an oppressive and discriminatory world must be recognised and challenged.

## Changing the individual or changing the world? Understanding recovery in a social and political context

Many ideas about recovery are highly individualised in nature, born of the culture of individualism in the USA. Explorations of discrimination, exclusion and rights have been separated from ideas about recovery. 'Recovery' and 'social inclusion' were quite separate work streams within both the Royal College of Psychiatrists (Boardman et al., 2010; Roberts et al., 2006) and the National Institute for Mental Health in England (NIMHE), who described recovery as improvement in the person's condition and/or experience and the importance of the person assuming an active and responsible life (NIMHE, 2005). The underlying assumption is that recovery is essentially an individual, rather than collective process for which the individual must take personal responsibility. This fails to acknowledge the political and social reality of prejudice, discrimination and exclusion (see Beresford and Bryant, 2008; O'Hagan, 2009; Perkins, 2012; Repper and Perkins, 2003, 2012).

Within mental health services, the route to social inclusion is typically seen in changing the individual to fit in to society via treatment and rehabilitation:

reducing symptoms and developing the person's skills. However, this is not the only route to participation and 'a satisfying, hopeful and contributing life' (Anthony, 1993: 17). It is also possible to change the world so that it can accommodate the individual (Perkins, 2012; Repper and Perkins, 2003, 2012). If a person faces ongoing mental health challenges then we must look to removing the environmental barriers that stop them participating in the life of their communities.

In *From Psychiatric Patient to Citizen* Sayce (2000) talked not about treatment and rehabilitation as routes to inclusion and citizenship but of breaking down the barriers to participation. It is argued that the social model adopted in the broader disability rights arena has much to offer in relation to the opportunities and life chances of people with mental health problems (Beresford et al., 2010; Perkins, 2012; Repper and Perkins, 2003, 2012; Sayce, 2000):

> It is society that disables people. It is attitudes, actions, assumptions – social, cultural and physical structures which disable by erecting barriers and imposing restrictions and options. ... The social model of disability is about nothing more complicated than a clear focus on the economic, environmental and cultural barriers encountered by people who are viewed by others as having some form of impairment – whether physical, sensory or intellectual. (Oliver, 2004: 6)

As early as 1992, Deegan recognised the parallels between ongoing or recurring mental health conditions and physical impairments, and the importance of considering barriers not only in the physical world but also in the social world:

> For most of us, mental health problems are a given ... the real problems exist in the form of barriers in the environment that prevent us from living, working and learning in environments of our choice [the task is] to confront, challenge and change those barriers and to make environments accessible ... environments are not just physical places but also social and interpersonal environments ... those of us with psychiatric disabilities face many environmental barriers that impede and thwart our efforts to live independently and gain control over our lives. (Deegan, 1992: 3)

Examples of this sort of disability rights perspective in relation to mental health can be seen in the work of the Mental Health Action Group at the Disability Rights Commission (Mental Health Action Group, 2003). An increasing amount of work around the broader disability rights agenda explicitly includes those with mental health conditions and the UK's cross-government advisory group on disability issues is now chaired by a mental health service user/survivor. Following the work of US authors (Chamberlin, 1993, 1995; Deegan, 1988, 1992), some UK authors have argued that considerations of recovery should be framed within this broader rights-based context (Beresford et al., 2002, 2010; Perkins, 2012; Repper and Perkins, 2003, 2012; Sayce, 2000).

A social model and rights-based approach requires us to think differently about the way we understand the challenges people face and the way we organise services – not what is wrong with the person, but what are the barriers (attitudes, actions, assumptions – social, cultural and physical structures) that prevent participation and how these might be eroded via the provision of support and adjustments, breaking down prejudice and creating inclusive communities that can accommodate mental distress. It provides a different way of thinking about 'living independently': not doing things unaided but having the support you need to do the things you want to do and control over that support (Office for Disability Issues, 2008).

## The struggle for power

If professionals and services are genuinely to promote the recovery of those whom they serve then a change in the balance of power within services is required. A recovery-focused service recognises the expertise of lived experience on a par with professional expertise and requires that professionals use their expertise in a different way. Services and professionals:

> … should be 'on tap' rather than 'on top': putting their expertise at the disposal of those who may need it; easily accessible when it is needed, in the background when it is not; recognising and augmenting the expertise of lived experience; supporting individual and community resources and resourcefulness and helping people to find their own solutions. (Perkins, 2010: 5)

Recovery involves becoming an expert in your own self-care – using your own resources and those available to you to manage the challenges you face and pursue your ambitions. Some people find professional help valuable but this forms but one part of an often rich tapestry:

> Over the years I have worked hard to become an expert in my own self-care. … Over the years I have learned different ways of helping myself. Sometimes I use medications, therapy, self-help and mutual support groups, friends, my relationship with God, work, exercise, spending time in nature – all of these measures help me remain whole and healthy, even though I have a disability. (Deegan, 1993: 10)

However, mental health professionals of all hues have a great deal invested in existing structures. There is an entrenched assumption that, because of their specialist understanding, professional 'experts' know best, and must prescribe what is good for people and ensure compliance. It is this struggle of professionals to maintain power that underpins the mutation of 'recovery' in the hands of mental health services. In order to retain their power, services have accommodated ideas of recovery within their existing paradigms and practices: recovery becomes cure, a process becomes an outcome, the focus of change is the individual rather than society. A 'community mental health team' may be re-christened a 'recovery team', but its relationship with those it serves remains the same.

Far from a change in the balance of power, if anything, professional power is increasing. Alongside the increased focus on 'recovery' within mental health policy there has been an increase in the exercise of the ultimate use of power in services, that is, to detain and compel via use of the Mental Health Act (Figure 12.1). In England and Wales, use of compulsion has increased alarmingly: in 2011–2012 the Mental Health Act was used on a record 52,851 occasions and since 2008 the power to compel has been extended beyond the hospital door in the form of 'Supervised Community Treatment Orders'.

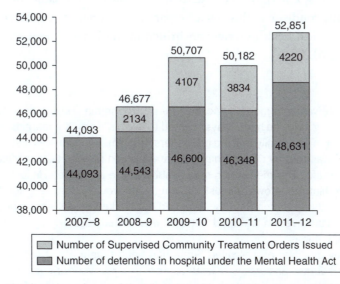

**FIGURE 12.1**  Total number of uses of the Mental Health Act 1983 in England (2007-12)

*Source*: NHS Information Centre for Health and Social Care (2012).

Mental health legislation is intrinsically discriminatory. It affords powers to detain and treat people deemed to have 'mental disorders' in a manner that would be inconceivable among those with physical health conditions (Szmukler, 2010) and contravenes the requirements of the United Nations Convention on the Rights of Persons with Disabilities (UNCRPD – ratified by the UK): 'respect for inherent human dignity and individual autonomy including the freedom to make one's own choices' (article 3), 'legal capacity on an equal basis with others in all aspects of life' (article 12) and the requirement that 'the existence of disability shall in no case justify a deprivation of liberty' (article 14). Mental health legislation is incompatible with the choice and control that are central to recovery. At the very least, we need to make every effort to reduce our use of compulsory detention and treatment, by, for example, increasing choice over support in crisis via using personal budgets, ensuring easy access to support when a crisis is looming rather than when it has already arrived and developing joint crisis plans (Henderson et al., 2004). Longer term, equal citizenship requires equality under the law and repeal of laws that apply to only one group of people. There may be times when any one of us lacks the capacity to make decisions for ourselves, and we may decide that at such times others (of our choosing) need to make decisions for us based, where possible, on our previously expressed wishes in crisis plans and advance directives. The right to refuse treatment must be the same for mental and physical health conditions: this must be part of the 'equality of esteem' between mental and physical health services enshrined in the Government mental health strategy (DH, 2011).

## CASE EXAMPLE

Paul was a 42-year-old man diagnosed with schizophrenia. Having been bullied at school for being 'odd', he had always seemed to live his life on the margins of society with no friends and a family that did not understand him. When he was first sectioned aged 20, he was told by the psychiatrist that he would have to take medication for the rest of his life. This medication made Paul 'feel like a zombie'. He lost his libido, and it made him feel drowsy almost constantly; he would often sleep for 12 hours each night and nap during the day. Paul had not worked consistently since he had left school. Paul lived in a rented flat and was visited regularly by a community mental health nurse.

A recently qualified nurse called Sonia had been taught about recovery during her nursing course. She was very keen to work in a recovery-orientated way when she qualified. When she joined the community team, the experienced nurses were encouraging of her, but she could tell that they were cynical about recovery. For them, it was another 'top-down' policy directive with little relevance to what they considered to be the 'real world' of mental health nursing. Sonia would not be put off though. She could see that Paul was an intelligent man, but also very lonely. Although quite socially isolated, Paul had no obvious way to make new friends; besides which, he never felt as though he had enough energy to make the effort. Sonia felt hopeful though, that she could help to bring about meaningful change in Paul's life. She knew, however, that any permanent change for the good would take time. First she concentrated on developing a therapeutic relationship with Paul; one that was built upon trust and respect. In the first six months of working with Paul, she began to share with him something of her philosophy of life: that all people are equal and have equal rights to education, employment, leisure facilities and access to good health care services. As Sonia got to know Paul, she noticed that he was quite artistic. She talked about art with him. Knowing that the local art gallery had an education department, she asked Paul one day if he would like her to visit with him. He said he would, though he was very aware of his lack of energy. In the following months, Sonia discussed with the team about reducing Paul's medication. A staged reduction was agreed with a positive effect. Paul found that he was becoming more alert and didn't need to sleep as much as he had been doing. He visited the gallery with Sonia four times over the next few months. Eventually he agreed to try out one of the groups in the education department. He enjoyed the group and discovered that they had a programme of groups and events over the next year. Within three years, Paul not only continued to enjoy the groups and events, he also began to volunteer at the gallery. For the first time in 20 years, Paul felt a sense of purpose in his life. He also felt a sense of belonging because he had made new friends and explored new opportunities as they arose. Sonia left the team after five years, but Paul had a sense that he didn't need to depend on her any more. Sonia had become quite attached to Paul and it was hard for her to eventually say goodbye. She remembered the cynicism of her team when she started, but she quietly knew beyond a shadow of doubt, that her belief in the recovery approach had made a life-changing difference to one lonely and sad man.

## Conclusion

Drawing this chapter to a close, we have decided to conclude with a strong message for mental health services and society. Mental health services must move from centre stage to the margins of people's lives. It must become as absurd for someone's primary identity to be that of 'mental health service user' as it would be for someone to define him/herself as a 'general practice service user' (Perkins, 2010). Mental health professionals should be there in the background providing easy access to a range of treatments when needed to assist people to thrive in those roles that are important to them: as partners, parents, workers, footballers …

People with mental health problems, as well as communities, need to start believing they hold most of the solutions to human problems, instead of professionals and services. (O'Hagan, 2007: 4)

The biggest challenge that we face is not creating better access to bigger and better professional services, it is maximising the life chances of people with mental health conditions by creating communities that can accommodate all of us. Recovery might best be framed within a social and rights-based model similar to that on which the broader disability rights movement is founded. We could usefully focus attention on those rights to which we are entitled within the United Nations Convention on the Rights of Persons with Disabilities – the rights to independent living on which broader disability policy is predicated.

All disabled people having the same choice, control and freedom as any other citizen – at home, at work and as members of the community. This does not necessarily mean disabled people 'doing everything for themselves' but it does mean that any practical assistance people need should be based on their own choices and aspirations. (Office for Disability Issues, 2008: 29)

## Summary

In this chapter, we described the origins of the recovery movement and traced the development of recovery becoming enshrined in policy in many countries. We have noted that recovery is primarily concerned with human values and beliefs. Recovery is more about people's individual journeys than it is about models or interventions. However, mental health nurses who work in a recovery-orientated way may help to bring about meaningful change in the lives of others. Nurses who adopt a recovery philosophy in their practice will invariably work in a way that inspires hope. The focus of the work should be to see the person beyond his or her role of using mental health services and to help to enable people to lead meaningful lives and enjoy their full rights of citizenship.

# References

Alakeson, V. and Perkins, R. (2012) *Personalisation and Recovery*. London: Centre for Mental Health/ImROC.

Anthony, W.A. (1993) 'Recovery from mental illness: the guiding vision of the mental health system in the 1990s', *Psychosocial Rehabilitation Journal*, 16 (4): 11–23.

Beresford, P. and Bryant, W. (2008) 'Saving the day centre', *The Guardian*, 11 June.

Beresford, P., Harrison, C. and Wilson, A. (2002) 'Mental health service users and disability: implications for future strategies', *Policy and Politics*, 30 (3): 387–96.

Beresford, P., Nettle, M. and Perring, R. (2010) *Towards a Social Model of Madness and Distress?* York: Joseph Rowntree Foundation.

Boardman, J., Currie, A., Killaspy, H. and Mezey, G. (2010) *Social Inclusion and Mental Health*. London: RCPSYCH Publications.

Chamberlin, J. (1977 [1988]) *On Our Own*. London: Mind.

Chamberlin, J. (1993) 'Psychiatric disabilities and the ADA: an advocates's perspective', in L.O. Gostin and H.A. Bayer (eds), *Implementing the Americans with Disabilities Act*. Baltimore: Brookes.

Chamberlin, J. (1995) 'Psychiatric survivors: are we part of the disability movement?', *Disability Rag and ReSource*, March/April: 4–7.

Coleman, R. (1999) *Recovery: An Alien Concept*. Gloucester: Handsell Publishing.

Davidson, L., Rakfeldt, J. and Strauss, J. (2010) *The Roots of the Recovery Movement in Psychiatry: Lessons Learnt*. Chichester: Wiley-Blackwell.

Deegan, P. (1988) 'Recovery: the lived experience of rehabilitation', *Psychosocial Rehabilitation Journal*, 11 (4): 11–19.

Deegan, P. (1992) 'The independent living movement and people with psychiatric disabilities: taking back control over our lives', *Psychosocial Rehabilitation Journal*, 15 (3): 3–19.

Deegan, P. (1993) 'Recovering our sense of value after being labelled mentally ill', *Journal of Psychosocial Nursing and Mental Health Services*, 31 (4): 7–11.

Department of Health (1999) *Mental Health National Service Framework*. London: Department of Health.

Department of Health (2001) *The Journey to Recovery: The Government's Vision for Mental Health Care*. London: Department of Health.

Department of Health (2003) *Mental Health Policy Implementation Guide: Support, Time and Recovery (STR) Workers*. London: Department of Health.

Department of Health (2006) *From Values to Action: Chief Nursing Officer's Review of Mental Health Nursing*. London: Department of Health.

Department of Health (2009) *New Horizons: A Shared Vision for Mental Health*. London: Department of Health.

Department of Health (2011) *No Health Without Mental Health*. London: Department of Health.

Forder, J., Jones, K., Glendinning, C., Caiels, J. et al. (2012) *Evaluation of the Personal Health Budget Pilot Programme*, Discussion Paper No. 2840_2. Kent: PSSRU.

Henderson, C., Flood, C., Leese, M., Thornicroft, G. et al. (2004) 'Effect of joint crisis plans on use of compulsory treatment in psychiatry: single blind randomised controlled trial', *British Medical Journal*, 329: 136–8.

McKeith, J., Burns, S., Onyemaechi, I. and Okonkwo, N. (2010) *The Recovery Star: User Guide* (2nd edn). London: Mental Health Providers Forum.

Mental Health Action Group (2003) *Coming Together: Mental Health Service Users and Disability Rights*. London: Disability Rights Commission.

NHS Information Centre for Health and Social Care (2012) *Inpatients Formally Detained in Hospitals under the Mental Health Act 1983, and Patients Subject to Supervised Community Treatment, Annual Figures, England, 2011/12*. London: Health and Social Care Information Centre.

NIMHE (National Institute for Mental Health in England) (2005) *NIMHE Guiding Statement on Recovery*. London: Department of Health.

Office for Disability Issues (2008) *Independent Living: Cross Government Strategy about Independent Living for Disabled People*. London: HM Government.

O'Hagan, M. (2007) 'Parting Thoughts', *Mental Notes*, 18: 4–5.

O'Hagan, M. (2009) 'Living well', *Open Mind*, 118: 16–17.

Oliver, M. (2004) 'If I had a hammer: the social model in action', in J. Swain, S. French, C. Barnes and C. Thomas (eds), *Disabling Barriers – Enabling Environments*. London: Sage.

Perkins, R. (2010) 'Professionals: from centre stage to the wings', in Sainsbury Centre for Mental Health (eds) *Looking Ahead: The Next 25 Years in Mental Health*. London: Sainsbury Centre for Mental Health.

Perkins, R. (2012) 'UK mental health policy development – an alternative view', in P. Phillips, T. Sandford and C. Johnston (eds), *Working in Mental Health: Practice and Policy in a Changing Environment*. Abingdon: Routledge.

Pilgrim, D. (2008) ' "Recovery" and current mental health policy', *Chronic Illness*, 4 (4): 295–304.

Reeves, A. (1998) *Recovery: A Holistic Approach*. Runcorn: Handsell Publishing.

Repper, J. and Carter, T. (2011) 'A review of the literature on peer support in mental health services', *Journal of Mental Health*, 20 (4): 392–411.

Repper, J. and Perkins, R. (2003) *Recovery and Social Inclusion*. London: Ballière Tindall.

Repper, J. and Perkins, R. (2012) Recovery: a journey of discovery for individuals and services', in P. Phillips, T. Sandford and C. Johnston (eds), *Working in Mental Health: Practice and Policy in a Changing Environment*. Abingdon: Routledge.

Roberts, G., Davenport, S., Holloway, F. and Tattan, T. (2006) *Enabling Recovery*. London: Gaskell/Royal College of Psychiatrists.

Sayce, L. (2000) *From Psychiatric Patient to Citizen: Overcoming Discrimination and Social Exclusion*. London: Macmillan.

Spaniol, L. and Koehler, M. (eds) (1994) *The Experience of Recovery*. Boston: Center for Psychiatric Rehabilitation.

Spaniol, L., Gagne, C. and Koehler, M. (1997) 'Recovery from serious mental illness: what it is and how to assist people', *Continuum*, 4 (4): 3–15.

Szmukler, G. (2010) *How Mental Health Law Discriminates Unfairly Against People with Mental Illness*. Paper presented at Barnards Inn Hall, Gresham College, 15 November.

Warner, R. (2009) 'Recovery from schizophrenia and the recovery model', *Current Opinion in Psychiatry*, 22 (4): 374–80.

# 13

# Stress Vulnerability and Psychosis

## LORRAINE RAYNER

### Learning Objectives

- Understand vulnerability factors that may make people more susceptible to developing a psychosis.
- Consider environmental factors that may increase the risk of developing a psychosis.
- Explore how stress vulnerability theories can be applied in practice.
- Identify limitations with the illness model of psychosis.
- Consider the strengths and limitations of a multi-factorial framework approach to psychosis.

## Introduction

This chapter will focus on stress vulnerability theories and their role in our understanding of psychosis and the care and treatment of people who have these experiences. It is important for the reader to have some understanding of the nature of psychosis, so the chapter starts with a brief overview of what is meant by psychosis. It considers the limitations of the illness model of psychosis and then presents stress vulnerability theories and the supporting evidence base. Stress vulnerability theories provide a framework to analyse the situations that people with psychosis may find themselves in and the problems they face. This framework also provides a guide to the nature and process of interventions that mental health nurses can provide. A case study will illustrate this. The overall purpose of this chapter is to provide the reader with an evidence-based explanation of our contemporary understanding of the complex nature of psychosis.

# Psychosis

Psychosis is a term used when someone's reality is not shared by people around them. It has been used since the 1840s as an alternative to terms like madness or insanity. Psychosis most frequently occurs in schizophrenia, bipolar disorder (sometimes called manic depression) or as a result of drug or alcohol misuse. The person with psychosis may experience a range of different things.

## Hallucinations

Hearing voices is the most common hallucinatory experience but people can experience hallucinations through any of the five senses: visual – seeing things which others cannot see; tactile – invisible people touching them; olfactory – experiencing unusual smells that others do not detect; gustatory – experiencing unusual unpleasant tastes.

## Delusions

Delusions are unusual beliefs that a person firmly holds on inadequate evidence, that is not affected by rational argument or contrary evidence and is not a belief that a person might be expected to hold given their educational and cultural background. The nature of these unusual beliefs vary but the most common are persecutory or paranoid beliefs in which the person feels him or herself to be the victim of some kind of malevolent plot. Delusions have been described as attempts to make sense of the world (Maher, 1974).

## Thought disorder

This is where the amount and speed of thought is changed and is particularly seen in schizophrenia and sometimes mania. Individuals with thought disorder may be incoherent, they may experience their thoughts suddenly stopping or they may experience thoughts arising very quickly and passing through their mind very rapidly.

Experiences of thought disorder are difficulties with the stream of thinking, whereas delusions are difficulties with the form of thought.

Hallucinations, delusions and thought disorder are often called 'positive symptoms' of schizophrenia (though of course they do not feel positive to the person experiencing them).

From a medical or pathogenic viewpoint, hallucinations, delusions and thought disorder are symptoms of a mental disorder, for example schizophrenia. The psychiatrist will often seek to find out if a person is having any of these experiences in order to make an accurate diagnosis and provide the most appropriate treatment. Difficulties with this approach will be explored later in the chapter.

People with psychosis may also experience mania, anxiety and depression. They may have motivational difficulties, find it difficult to interact with other people and feel they have lost the ability to feel and express emotions (known as 'negative symptoms'). The experience of psychosis can be terrifying, confusing, highly distressing, or at times magical and uplifting for the person experiencing it. Experiencing psychosis can have a negative impact on all aspects of a person's life and suicide rates are high. Some social consequences of psychosis may include:

- In social and interpersonal relationships, the person may find it difficult to form and maintain relationships.
- The person may find it difficult to get and keep a job. This may be due to the difficulties that the person actually experiences, i.e. he or she finds it difficult to concentrate due to hearing voices or it may be due to discrimination.
- People may experience a loss of meaningful role. They may have difficulties with relationships and their occupation and these may lead the person to lose a sense of purpose; previous hopes, plans and ambitions for life may be lost or altered radically.
- People may experience stigma, discrimination and exclusion. Being given a diagnosis of a mental disorder or labelled as mentally ill, with its sense of victim-blaming and the discrimination and the exclusion that may follow, can lead to a loss of a sense of self-worth.

## Psychosis: a historical perspective

Written descriptions of what is now described as psychotic experiences have been available for many centuries. In the Middle Ages these experiences were often viewed as part of a religious experience. People hearing voices were viewed as visionaries and having especial closeness to God; consequently they may have been treated in a special way (this is still the case today in some cultures). Alternatively, these experiences were sometimes interpreted as the work of the Devil and as a consequence the person was subject to cruel, inhuman treatment. People were generally looked after by their own communities and later by religious communities and by the middle of the nineteenth century hospitals, with the medical profession taking the lead for their care and treatment. Emil Kraepelin (1856–1926), a German psychiatrist, is credited with developing the first diagnostic system for psychiatry. He studied his patients' symptoms, seeing which symptoms occurred together and how they changed over time. His observations on thousands of cases led to his conclusion that he was seeing two different diseases: one characterised by a progressive, deteriorating course, which he called dementia praecox (senility of early life) and the other he named manic depression, which had a more positive outcome. Dementia praecox was renamed schizophrenia by Swiss psychiatrist Emil Bleuler early in the twentieth century. Manic depression as described by Kraepelin included not only what is now called bipolar disorder but what we today consider as unipolar depression.

It is difficult to underestimate Kraepelin's influence on psychiatry and the treatment of mental illness. Acceptance of his theories began to lead to some clarity about diagnosis and the influence of Kraepelin can still be seen in the diagnostic manuals used in psychiatry today. These manuals provide the standard criteria for the classification of mental disorders. *The Diagnostic and Statistical Manual of Mental Disorders-V* (DSM-V) (APA, 2013) is the most commonly used and has been since 1952. Kraepelin's ideas that schizophrenia had a progressive and deteriorating course – prognosis was poor – have been influential in the treatment of people given this diagnosis. It has led to a pessimistic viewpoint that schizophrenia is largely incurable or untreatable, despite there being evidence for many years, particularly from studies in the developing countries, that people can improve and lead meaningful lives (Bhugra, 2006).

Though classification and the use of diagnostic manuals provides a means to describe and communicate what is happening to the person with psychosis, albeit in a simple, medicalised way, questions remain about the legitimacy of the classification system. The scientific validity and reliability of the diagnostic system has been challenged (for an example, see Bentall, 2004). The whole concept of mental illness as being fundamentally different from normal experiences has been questioned. Studies have shown that psychotic experiences like hearing voices are relatively common, belief in 'unscientific' phenomena like astrology and alien abduction are shared by many (Kingdon and Turkington, 1994). This understanding seems to suggest that these kinds of experiences are not qualitatively different but lie somewhere on a continuum between common and unusual experiences. From this we may conclude that we all have the capacity to have these kinds of experiences.

Just as the validity of the diagnosis has been challenged, and so too has reliability; for a diagnosis to be reliable we would expect that if two people assess the same person they would make the same diagnosis and we would also expect the same diagnosis to be made on different occasions. Studies have shown that this is not the case; for example Bromet et al. (2011) followed 470 patients from first diagnosis to 10 years later. They found 50% of patients had their diagnosis changed at some point in this period.

Diagnosis should also predict outcome, so we know what is likely to happen to the person and what the best treatment is: again psychiatric diagnosis fails (Bentall, 2003). Antipsychotic medication is not always effective and different medications are used to treat different disorders: lithium is used to treat both schizophrenia and bipolar disorder. Outcome is variable for both schizophrenia and bipolar disorder, with some people having only one episode in their lives and recovering fully; others have episodes throughout their lives, but have long periods of wellness, whereas others will continue to have problems throughout their lives. Diagnostic classification is viewed as flawed and not based on good science (Bentall, 2004, 2010).

In addition to the challenge of psychiatric diagnosis many aspects of the medical treatment of mental illness have been criticised and condemned as being dehumanising and exploitative, creating dependency for those diagnosed mentally ill (Laing, 1964; Szasz, 1960). So problems with the pathogenic view of psychosis make it necessary for us to consider alternative ideas. One that has received attention since the 1980s is that of focusing on particular, individual symptoms (Persons, 1986). Instead of energy being exerted into categorising symptoms, the focus is on looking at treating individual symptoms, like hearing voices or paranoid beliefs. Psychologists have led research into identifying the psychological processes that may underlie these experiences, and have then developed approaches to work with service users in clinical practice (Garety et al., 2001). Results from studies have been promising (Drury et al., 2000; Sensky et al., 2000). Critics of this approach highlight that most people with psychosis have more than one symptom and the psychological models formulated are general and do not include all the factors that may be involved in the development of psychosis, for example biological and social factors.

Until the development in the 1950s of the drug chlorpromazine, psychiatrists only had available to them medication that sedated those diagnosed with psychosis.

But with the advent of chlorpromazine and later other antipsychotic medication it seemed that there were treatments that could have a long-term effect on behaviour and could prevent relapse. By the 1970s these medications were the main treatment for psychosis and the pessimistic view for psychosis as being untreatable had been replaced to some degree by the belief that psychosis could be controlled, even though this meant taking powerful medications continually. But by the 1970s and 1980s it was apparent there were problems with medication: distressing side-effects were experienced by many (Barnes, 1992), this in turn had an effect on adherence: up to 60% did not take their medication as prescribed (Fenton et al., 1997) and often medication was not fully effective: Curson et al. (1985) found up to 23% of patients with psychosis experienced persistent symptoms resistant to medication. Even with the advent of the new second generation of antipsychotic medication, the initial promise of medications has not materialised (Allison et al., 1999; Leucht et al., 2009).

Alongside pharmacological developments in the 1950s and 1960s debate developed over the aetiological mechanisms causing psychosis. On the one hand there was evidence for a biological cause lying in genes, brain anatomy or the biochemical processes in the brain. On the other there was growing evidence for factors such as life events and the social environment. By the 1970s these debates had polarised into a nature versus nurture argument: did the cause of psychosis lie in the genes or in the environment, with both viewpoints providing only partial answers (Zubin and Spring, 1977). It was only with the development of the vulnerabilities model did these viewpoints unite and provide a multi-factorial framework of the processes that determine the risk and relapse of psychosis.

# The development of stress vulnerability theories

There are a number of vulnerability models but the best known is the one proposed by Zubin and Spring (1977). Developed at a time when there was a need for a fresh approach to the study of the causes of schizophrenia, Zubin and Spring drew on the common elements shared by the different theories. Also important in the development of the model was Zubin and Spring's focus on the episodic nature of schizophrenia. After reviewing the evidence they argued that the majority of those experiencing an episode of psychosis returned to normal functioning between episodes.

Zubin and Spring's vulnerability model (see Figure 13.1) proposes that we all have a degree of vulnerability that given certain circumstances may express itself in psychosis. Vulnerability in this model may be either inherited, through genes, or environmentally acquired. Environmental factors such as birth complications, early experiences and peer interactions are included by Zubin and Spring. According to the model psychotic episodes are triggered by 'challenging events' or environmental stress. This environmental stress might include social stress or stressful life events. If these stressors exceed a threshold, determined by the individual's vulnerability, then an episode may be triggered. The model also stressed the importance of the individual's capacity to adapt to future episodes and to learn from previous ones. The inclusion of a coping, assimilation and adaption model had important implications for future research and clinical practice (Clements and Turpin, 1992).

Nearly 40 years have passed since the development of this model, in which time it has become accepted as a way of understanding the causes of psychosis, providing a method of directing and assisting the development of research and practice. As it combines a number of theories the next section of the chapter will look at the supporting evidence for these.

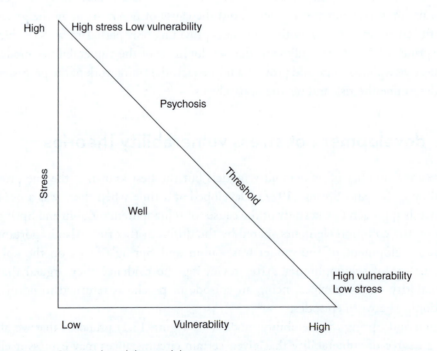

**FIGURE 13.1**   Stress vulnerability model

## Vulnerability: inherited

Zubin and Spring (1977) propose that vulnerability can be inherited or acquired. Genetic research indicates that the development of schizophrenia is influenced by heredity (Blows, 2011). This is based on the study of identical twins, adoption studies (where identical twins have been adopted soon after birth) and families where a number of members have developed schizophrenia. However, the initial optimism that a specific gene would be found for schizophrenia has been replaced by the current understanding that schizophrenia is polygenic – several genes are involved, interacting with the environment (Blows, 2011). Even so, critics have suggested that findings in the field of genetics and schizophrenia have exaggerated the size of associations between heredity and the risk of developing schizophrenia (Bentall, 2004).

## Vulnerabilities: acquired

Acquired vulnerabilities include a range of different theories: biological, concerning brain structure, neurodevelopment and biochemical changes; the impact of trauma and early experiences; the influence of the social environment; and personality traits.

### Biological explanations

Factors that influence the developing nervous system in utero may increase a person's vulnerability: birth traumas, such as prolonged periods of cerebral hypoxia during labour or problems like pre-eclampsia has been identified as significant (Mednick, 1970). The role of the influenza virus has also been the subject of much research and debate, with exposure to the virus in the early stages of pregnancy increasing the risk of developing schizophrenia later in life for the offspring (Brown, 2006). Low vitamin D levels have also been linked to schizophrenia (Furlow, 2001). There is a 10% increase in the number of infants destined to develop schizophrenia born in late winter and early spring, when there are low levels of ultraviolet light which may affect maternal levels of vitamin D (Blows, 2011).

The dopamine hypothesis of schizophrenia is one of the oldest biological explanations of the causes of the disorder. This hypothesis attempts to explain how biochemical changes lead to symptoms like hallucinations and paranoia. It was developed in the late 1950s when it was observed that taking drugs like cocaine and LSD caused acute psychotic symptoms and high levels of dopamine, a neurotransmitter, were implicated. Further research revealed that antipsychotic medication blocked dopamine receptors in the brain. Therefore it was hypothesised that excess dopamine was involved in the cause of hallucinations and delusions. Further research has revealed a more complex picture and currently it is considered a simple cause and effect is not the correct explanation (Howes and Kapur, 2009).

Some of the most compelling evidence to support a biological explanation of psychosis comes from CT (Computerised Axial Tomography) scanning. Imaging of the live brains of people with a diagnosis of schizophrenia and bipolar disorder showed that the ventricles – the cavities within the brain – are larger than those without a diagnosis of a mental illness (Weinberger et al., 1983). Critics have suggested that other factors like the effect of long-term use of antipsychotic medication on brain structures should also be considered and more recent research has shown brain structure is 'plastic' and can change as a result of experience (Kolb et al., 2011). Therefore the social environment must be considered in conjunction with biological theories. Research has continued to look at brain pathology, linking particular pathology with particular symptoms: for example, visual hallucinations (David and Busatto, 1999) and negative symptoms (Maier, 1999).

## Trauma

The evidence that early traumatic experiences can play a part in the causal role in psychosis is strong (Read et al., 2005). Childhood trauma, particularly sexual abuse, appears to increase the risk of developing psychosis in later life, and the experience of auditory hallucinations is especially associated with the early experience of sexual abuse (Hammersly et al., 2003; Morrison and Petersen, 2003). It is unclear how the experience of early trauma produces psychotic experiences in later life, but it is suggested that psychological trauma can contribute to oversensitivity to stress in individuals (Read et al., 2005). There is now acknowledgement that the environment influences brain structure and it has been argued that many of the biological abnormalities seen in people with psychosis are similar to those demonstrated in the victims of trauma (Read et al., 2001).

## Early experiences

Attachment theory developed by John Bowlby and Mary Ainsworth (Ainsworth and Bowlby, 1991) asserts that secure attachment – a close, continuous relationship with a care giver in early life – is necessary for healthy emotional development. Research has shown that emotional deprivation at an early age (poor attachment) can have a negative effect on developing relationships in later life and understanding the mental states of others (Meins et al., 1998). Research has shown that people with psychosis, especially those with paranoid thinking, have insecure attachments (Dozier and Lee, 1995).

## Social environment

Urban living is generally more stressful than living in a rural environment, with more social fragmentation, crime, vandalism and poverty (Paykel et al., 2000). The incidence of schizophrenia in deprived areas is significantly higher (Boydell et al., 2004). Pilgrim and Rogers (2008) maintain that the social and environmental features of extreme poverty are not only relapse factors but are causal factors in psychosis. Living in urban environments increases an individual's vulnerability to psychosis.

It has been known for more than 30 years that people of Afro-Caribbean descent are more likely to be diagnosed with schizophrenia (Fernando, 1988), but more recently it has been suggested that this is due to the experience of racism and discrimination. Other immigrant groups experiencing these kinds of social inequalities are more likely to experience mental health problems (Boydell et al., 2001).

## Personality traits

Research conducted first in the 1960s into the risk factors of developing schizophrenia identified a link between schizotypal personality types and psychosis (Meehl, 1962, 1989). This personality trait is characterised by eccentric beliefs, magical thinking, difficulties with forming and maintaining relationships and misinterpreting situations as strange or having special meaning.

Zubin and Spring's (1977) hypothesis proposes that psychosis emerges in vulnerable people when they are faced by challenging events. It is the interaction of vulnerability factors with these challenging events, usually referred to as stress, that brings about psychosis. In summary, inherited or acquired vulnerabilities make the person more sensitive to stress. Let us now look at the evidence to support the part that challenging events play in psychosis.

## Challenging events

Challenging events can be divided into life events and family relationships. Studies have shown that stressful life events that occur suddenly and unpredictably have preceded the onset of schizophrenia (Brown and Birley, 1968). It is accepted that the evidence indicates that stressful life events can trigger psychosis in a vulnerable person (Lukoff et al., 1984).

**TABLE 13.1** Summary of the model and theory

**Vulnerability**
Inherited
- Genetic

**Stress**
- Life events
- Family environment

**Vulnerability**
Acquired
- Biological
- Trauma
- Early experiences
- Social environment
- Personality traits

The impact of relationships within families where someone has psychosis has been studied for many years. One strand of research in this area has looked at the emotional environment and the effect on relapse rates. Initially looking at relapse rates for people leaving psychiatric hospitals in the late 1950s, sociologist George Brown looked at people who returned to live with their families and those who were discharged to hostel-style accommodation (Brown et al., 1958). Results rather surprisingly revealed those who returned to live with their families were more likely to become ill again than those who lived alone or in hostels. Brown and colleagues explored the reasons for this and came to the conclusion that it was the emotional environment prevalent in the family households. The term 'expressed emotion' was coined. 'High expressed emotion' is used to describe the responses of criticism and over-involvement displayed by some family members to their relative.

Research has shown that people experiencing psychosis who live with relatives and who display the characteristics of high expressed emotion are more likely to relapse (Brown and Rutter, 1966; Brown et al., 1972). Researchers in this area have always stressed that expressed emotion plays no part in causing the psychosis in the first place, however critics have suggested that as high expressed emotion is seen as a factor that maintains mental illness, families may still feel negatively labelled and alienated (Hatfield et al., 1987).

Zubin and Spring's model combines a number of theories derived from a number of disciplines – predominately medicine, genetics, neuroscience, sociology and psychology. As research has developed in the intervening years since Zubin and Spring's paper other theories have been added to the stress vulnerability framework, showing the strengths and longevity of the model. Table 13.1 summarises the theories and the model.

# Theory applied to practice

This section will look at two ways stress vulnerability theories can be applied to practice: first how the overall framework has been used with individual service users as part of a specific intervention, and second how working with families in a systematic, structured way can prevent relapse.

Stress vulnerability theories can be used with service users to develop an individual understanding of what is happening to them and possible reasons for this happening. Most people who have psychosis who are in contact with services will have been told that they have a mental health problem; they may have been given a specific diagnosis or told they have a psychotic illness. Some may find a diagnosis helpful but others may reject this explanation. Using the stress vulnerability model as a framework to discuss the person's background and significant life events provides an alternative to a medical diagnosis.

A number of authors writing about the use of cognitive behavioural techniques with voices and unusual beliefs advocate using the stress vulnerability model to engage the person (Brabban and Turkington, 2002; Fowler et al., 1995; Kingdon and Turkington, 2005). Fowler et al. (1995) suggest gaining information about the person's vulnerability factors, for example, family history, birth trauma or adverse early experiences and events and stresses associated with the onset of psychosis (see Table 13.2). This is done in an atmosphere of a trusting, collaborative working relationship and often developed over a number of sessions. This information is written down for the person to keep and added to as therapeutic work continues. The authors suggest that this can be a powerful tool for the person to re-evaluate their past experiences and consider their current difficulties; it can destigmatise the mental illness label. They do add that the process does not necessarily lead to a change in unusual beliefs or the frequency or distress of voices, but can act as a beginning for further work.

This individual summary, developed in collaboration with the person, could be described as a 'formulation'. A formulation is defined as a 'hypothesis about a person's difficulties, which draws from psychological theory' (Johnstone and Dallos, 2006). A formulation is an essential component of psychological work for voices and unusual beliefs. Though not strictly drawing on psychological theory, the stress vulnerability model does provide an alternative to a purely medical model. Indeed,

**TABLE 13.2**  Vulnerability, stress and coping

| Vulnerabilities: | Personal protectors: |
|---|---|
| • Inherited | • Coping strategies |
| • Acquired | • Social skills |
|   – Biological factors | |
|   – Adverse early experiences | • Problem-solving strategies |

| Environmental stressors: | Environmental protectors: |
|---|---|
| • Relevant experiences that immediately preceded the emergence of psychosis – life events, critical incidents | • Social supports – family, friends |
| • Ongoing sources of stress | • Mental health service interventions |

Kingdon and Turkington (2005) suggest that the model offers both service user and professional a different way of explaining what has happened. So instead of providing an illness explanation, 'you have an illness called schizophrenia', it is suggested that the person is offered an alternative account of being particularly vulnerable to stress. Kingdon and Turkington (2005: 69) recommend obtaining a balanced formulation, which includes vulnerability factors 'those issues that may make the person more sensitive to stress'; precipitating factors: the life events immediately prior to becoming unwell; perpetuating factors: those issues that make recovery more difficult; and protective factors: the strengths and resources that will aid the person.

Brabban and Turkington (2002) use the analogy of a bucket to demonstrate stress and vulnerability. The bucket represents vulnerability; fluid filling the bucket denotes stress and when the bucket overflows this signifies the emergence or exacerbation of psychosis. Again an individual explanation can be arrived at, working collaboratively to identify the individual history, life experiences and stress that make up the bucket and the amount of water required to overfill the bucket.

Using stress vulnerability in this way not only develops a collaborative understanding for the service user and the professional, and therefore aids the assessment process, but also assists with the identification of potentially useful interventions. Often this will take the form of managing stress more effectively either by problem-solving or by developing coping strategies. Let us now turn our attention to see how the stress vulnerability theories can benefit individuals, their families and have an impact on relapse.

The findings on expressed emotion in the 1950s and 1960s provided an impetus to investigate if specific interventions focused on the family could bring about a change in expressed emotion and in turn have an effect on relapse rates. The simplified hypothesis was whether there was something that could be done to change high expressed emotion relatives and would this have an effect on the likelihood of the service user relapsing. Subsequently, family intervention was developed and a number of studies showed that this kind of structured, intensive approach was effective in reducing relapse rates (Falloon et al., 1982, 1985; Leff et al., 1982, 1985; Tarrier et al., 1988, 1989). Though a number of models of family work have been developed over the years, one of the key elements is that the stress vulnerability model is used with the service user and family to explain how in a vulnerable person stress can bring on psychosis. It is used to provide the psych-oeducation element of the intervention. Problem-solving and stress management strategies are then used by the family, including the service user, to counteract the strains and tensions that can occur when someone is experiencing psychosis. Zubin and Spring's original paper emphasised the importance of a vulnerable individual's capacity to adapt and learn from previous episodes, and family inter-vention encourages this to occur.

Though not without its critics (Johnstone, 1993) and later studies have had less spectacular results in relapse prevention (Szmukler et al., 1996; Telles et al., 1995), family intervention has been influential in policy formation and the National Insti-tute for Clinical Excellence (NICE) guidance advocates its use with relatives who are living or who have close contact with a person with a diagnosis of schizophrenia (NICE, 2009).

This section has looked at two ways that stress vulnerability theories can be applied in practice, first with individuals as a way of gaining understanding of their situation and second with families to help manage the pressure and worry that often accom-panies the experience of psychosis. The final section of the chapter will present a case example of how stress vulnerability theories can be used to engage a person in thera-peutic work, form part of the assessment and help identify possible interventions.

John is 42 and lives alone in a housing association flat. He has been in contact with mental health services for over 20 years, and currently receives support from a community team. John describes daily occurrences of hearing voices that are having conversations about him. He also experiences daily distressing events, which can be traced back to people he knew in the past. Examples include a neighbour ignoring him, an overheard comment in the supermarket and a passenger moving seats on a bus. Apart from causing acute distress for John, these experiences impact on his capacity to do ordinary things, like shopping, enjoying friendships and leisure activities.

CASE EXAMPLE

*(Continued)*

*(Continued)*

John traces these experiences back to when he joined the army at 17 and believes that most of the local community know he was in the army and hold it against him, though he does not come from the area. He accepts that other people (staff from the community health team and the housing association) do not share his views.

Over the years John has been admitted to hospital a number of times; the last time, three years ago, he had threatened his neighbours with a knife, believing that they were spreading malicious rumours about him. John does feel he has a mental health problem, and he takes antipsychotic medication generally as prescribed. He describes feeling depressed and anxious most of the time.

The community team provide support in helping John manage daily life: shopping, managing the flat and his finances and helping to structure his time, but it was felt that a more focused approach on his voices and unusual beliefs may have an effect on the distress of these experiences. This was proposed to John and he agreed to see one of the mental health nurses on a weekly basis.

Following an initial discussion of why he thought he had developed these problems in the first place, the stress vulnerability model was introduced to John. Over a number of sessions John's individual stresses and vulnerabilities were identified and written down in the different boxes (see Table 13.3). This was started by talking about John's childhood. A number of vulnerabilities were identified: he had a difficult relationship with his father, describing him as overbearing and a bully to both him and his mother. He felt he lacked confidence. His father died just before he left school and he went into the army. He was deeply unhappy and describes the only reason for his decision to join was to please his mother, who was very keen for him to enlist. He also identified that he had an aunt who spent a number of years in a psychiatric hospital, though he did not know for what reason, and this was tentatively added with a question mark.

The events leading up to the time when he first experienced voices and paranoid thoughts were then added. He was 20, and his mother had suddenly died, he felt increasingly isolated and unhappy with army life. During these sessions the nurse gave information about how adverse early experiences can make a person more vulnerable and how life events can trigger this vulnerability in later life. As a picture was built up of past events and experiences the sessions began to look at stresses that were present currently: managing everyday life, feeling overwhelmed when there were a lot of things to do, always feeling the need to be hyper-vigilant. As well as identifying difficulties, John and the nurse looked at the strengths and resources that he had available.

John found the process of looking back over his life as helpful and he found having it summarised on one page an 'eye opener'. Once the boxes were complete the nurse explained that what might be needed to help improve John's situation was to increase the personal and environmental protectors in order to decrease the stress. John already used some coping strategies for his voices and paranoid thinking, so it was agreed that the focus would be on the enhancement of these, but looking at their use in particular situations like travelling on the bus and going to the supermarket.

Developing this 'formulation' took four sessions, and though John had discussed many of the events and experiences before with mental health professionals, this

**TABLE 13.3** Case example: John's stress vulnerability formulation

| Vulnerabilities: | Personal protectors: |
| --- | --- |
| • Inherited | • Uses different coping strategies to deal with voices and intrusive thoughts: uses MP3 player, avoids eye contact |
| ? family history | • Takes medication regularly (but not completely effective) |
| • Acquired<br>  – Difficult tense relationship with father<br>  – Lack of confidence with making friendships<br>  – Father's death | |

| Environmental stressors: | Environmental protectors: |
| --- | --- |
| • Stressful events leading up to the time when John first became unwell<br>  – Mother's sudden death<br>  – Unhappiness with army life<br>  – Feeling alone<br>• Current sources of stress<br>  – Managing everyday life<br>  – Feeling on edge all the time | • Has support from staff from mental health services<br>• Mental health service interventions |

had often been in the context of a formal mental state assessment. This time the focus was to try to help John make sense of things, with a view to identifying ways of making changes. Stress vulnerability theories made the evidence base explicit and complex theories were used in a simple but effective way to practice.

# Summary

The chapter has presented the historical development of stress vulnerability theories, and examined the contested nature of and arguments about mental illness and psychosis. Zubin and Spring developed this influential model at a time when separate biological and environmental hypotheses did not provide all the answers to the causes of psychosis. The strengths of stress vulnerability theories have been highlighted. The

*(Continued)*

*(Continued)*

model incorporates a range of theories developed by different disciplines. It integrates theories that are complex into a simple, assessable framework for service users, carers and professionals. Drawing on research developed over many years it unites research and treatment, providing a formulation that can help care planning and specific interventions. Providing an alternative to medical diagnosis it can be used to challenge a catastrophic view of psychosis.

However there are limitations: Bentall (2004) maintains that it still assumes that psychosis is caused by a biological process, though with the growing evidence for the influence of adverse life events on brain structure and chemistry this is perhaps a minor criticism. More significant is that it ignores a whole range of research that has looked at the psychological processes that are likely to be implicated in psychosis, particularly voices and unusual beliefs. So research like that into hallucinations being a consequence of faulty source monitoring – the person who hears voices is mistaking inner speech as being external – is ignored (Bentall, 2000). Therefore stress vulnerability theories do not provide any indication how voices or unusual beliefs might be treated psychologically with the exception of enhancing coping strategies (Bentall, 2004).

Finally the chapter has shown that the mental health nurse informed by stress vulnerability theories can work sensitively with individuals to make links between their current experiences and past events, identify vulnerabilities and recognise possible triggers and risk factors.

# References

Ainsworth, M.D.S. and Bowlby, J. (1991) 'An ethological approach to personality development', *American Psychologist*, 46: 331–41.

Allison, D.B., Mentore, J.L., Moonseong, H., Chandler, L.P., Cappeleri, J.C., Ming, C., Infante, M.S. and Weiden, P.J. (1999) 'Antipsychotic-induced weight gain: a comprehensive research synthesis', *American Journal of Psychiatry*, 156 (11): 1686–96.

APA (American Psychiatric Association) (2013) *Diagnostic and Statistical Manual of Mental Disorders–V* (5th edition). Washington, DC: American Psychiatric Association.

Barnes, T.R.E. (1992) 'Clinical assessment of the extrapyramidal side effects of antipsychotic medication', *Journal of Psychopharmacology*, 6: 214–21.

Bentall, R.P. (2000) 'Hallucinatory experiences', in E. Cardena, S.L. Lynn and S. Krippner (eds), *Varieties of Anomalous Experience: Examining the Scientific Evidence*. Washington, DC: American Psychological Association.

Bentall, R.P. (2003) *Madness Explained: Psychosis and Human Nature*. London: Penguin Books.

Bentall, R.P. (2004) 'An overview of psychosis', in A.P. Morrison, J.C. Renton, H. Dunn, S. Williams and R.P. Bentall (eds), *Cognitive Therapy for Psychosis*. Hove: Brunner-Routledge.

Bentall, R.P. (2010) *Doctoring the Mind: Why Psychiatric Treatments Fail*. London: Penguin Books.

Bhugra, D. (2006) 'Severe mental illness across cultures', *Acta Psychiatrica Scandinavica*, 113 (suppl. 429): 17–23.

Blows, W.T. (2011) *The Biological Basis of Mental Health Nursing* (2nd edn). London: Routledge.

Boydell, J., Van Os, J., McKenzie, K., Allardyce, J., Goel, R., McCreadie, R.D. and Murray, R.M. (2001) 'Incidence of schizophrenia in ethnic minorities in London: ecological study into interactions with environment', *British Medical Journal*, 323: 1–4.

Boydell, J., Van Os, J., McKenzie, K. and Murray, R.M. (2004) 'The association of inequality with the incidence of schizophrenia: an ecological study', *Social Psychiatry and Psychiatric Epidemiology*, 39 (8): 597–9.

Brabban, A. and Turkington, D. (2002) 'The search for meaning: detecting congruence between life events, underlying schema and psychotic symptoms', in A. Morrison (ed.), *A Casebook of Cognitive Therapy for Psychosis*. Hove: Routledge.

Bromet, E.J., Kotov, R., Fochtmann, M.D., Carlson, G.A., Tanenberg, M., Ruggero, C. and Chang, S. (2011) 'Diagnostic shifts during the decade following first admission for psychosis', *American Journal of Psychiatry*, 168: 1186–94.

Brown, A.S. (2006) 'Prenatal infection as a risk factor for schizophrenia', *Schizophrenia Bulletin*, 32 (2): 200–2.

Brown, G.W. and Birley, J.L.T. (1968) 'Crisis and life changes and the onset of schizophrenia', *Journal of Health and Social Behaviour*, 9: 203–14.

Brown, G.W. and Rutter, M. (1966) 'The measurement of family activities and relationships: a methodological study', *Human Relations*, 19: 241–63.

Brown, G.W., Carstairs, M. and Topping, G. (1958) 'Post hospital adjustment of chronic mental patients', *The Lancet*, 2: 685–9.

Brown, G.W., Birley, J.L.T. and Wing, J.K. (1972) 'Influence of the family on the course of schizophrenic disorders: a replication', *British Journal of Psychiatry*, 121: 241–58.

Clements, K. and Turpin, G. (1992) 'Vulnerability models and schizophrenia: the assessment and prediction of relapse', in M. Birchwood and N. Tarrier (eds), *Innovations in the Psychological Management of Schizophrenia*. Chichester: John Wiley.

Curson, D.A., Barnes, T.R.E., Bamber, R.W., Platt, S.D., Hirsch, S.R. and Duffy, J.D. (1985) 'Long-term depot maintenance of chronic schizophrenic outpatients', *British Journal of Psychiatry*, 146: 454–80.

David, A.S. and Busatto, G. (1999) 'The hallucination: a disorder of brain and mind', in M.A. Ron and A.S. David (eds), *Disorders of Brain and Mind*. Cambridge: Cambridge University Press.

Dozier, M. and Lee, S.W. (1995) 'Discrepancies between self- and other-report of psychiatric symptomatology: effects of dismissing attachment strategies', *Development and Psychopathology*, 7: 217–26.

Drury, V., Birchwood, M. and Cochrane, R. (2000) 'Cognitive therapy and recovery from acute psychosis: a controlled trial', *British Journal of Psychiatry*, 177: 8–14.

Falloon, I.R.H., Boyd, J.L., McGill, C.W., Razani, J., Moss, M.B. and Gilderman, A.M. (1982) 'Family management in the prevention of exacerbations of schizophrenia: a controlled study', *New England Journal of Medicine*, 306: 1437–40.

Falloon, I.R.H., Jeffery, L.B., McGill, C.W., Williamson, M., Razani, J., Moss, B.M., Gilderman, A.M. and Simpson, G.M. (1985) 'Family management in the prevention of the morbidity of schizophrenia: clinical outcome of a two-year longitudinal study', *Archives of General Psychiatry*, 42: 887–96.

Fenton, W.S., Blyer, C.R. and Heinssen, R.K. (1997) 'Determinants of medication compliance in schizophrenia: empirical and clinical findings', *Schizophrenia Bulletin*, 23 (4): 637–51.

Fernando, S. (1988) *Race and Culture in Psychiatry*. London: Croom Helm.

Fowler, D., Garety, P. and Kuipers, E. (1995) *Cognitive Behaviour Therapy for Psychosis*. Chichester: John Wiley.

Furlow, B. (2001) 'The making of a mind', *New Scientist*, 171 (2300): 38–41.

Garety, P.A., Kuipers, E., Fowler, D. and Bebbington, P.E. (2001) 'A cognitive model of positive symptoms of psychosis', *Psychological Medicine*, 31: 189–95.

Hammersley, P., Dias, A., Todd, G., Bowen-Jones, K., Reilly, B. and Bentall, R. (2003) 'Childhood traumas and hallucinations in bipolar disorder', *British Journal of Psychiatry*, 182: 543–7.

Hatfield, A.B., Spariol, L. and Zipple, A.M.C. (1987) 'Expressed emotion: a family perspective', *Schizophrenia Bulletin*, 13: 221–6.

Howes, O.D. and Kapur, S. (2009) 'The dopamine hypothesis: version III – the final pathway', *Schizophrenia Bulletin*, 35 (3): 549–62.

Johnstone, L. (1993) 'Family management in schizophrenia: its assumptions and contradictions', *Journal of Mental Health*, 2: 255–69.

Johnstone, L. and Dallos, R. (2006) 'Introduction to formulation', in L. Johnstone and R. Dallos (eds), *Formulation in Psychology and Psychotherapy: Making Sense of People's Problems*. London: Routledge.

Kingdon, D. and Turkington, D. (2005) *Cognitive Therapy of Schizophrenia*. New York: Guilford Press.

Kingdon, D., Turkington, D. and John, C. (1994) 'Cognitive behaviour therapy of schizophrenia', *British Journal of Psychiatry*, 164: 581–7.

Kolb, B., Muhammad, A. and Gibb, R. (2011) 'Searching for factors underlying cerebral plasticity in the normal and injured brain', *Journal of Communication Disorders*, 44 (5): 503–14.

Laing, R.D. (1964) *Sanity, Madness and the Family*. London: Penguin.

Leff, J., Kuipers, L., Berkowitz, R., Eberlein-Freis, R. and Sturgeon, D. (1982) 'A controlled trial of social interventions in the families of schizophrenic patients', *British Journal of Psychiatry*, 141: 121–34.

Leff, J., Kuipers, L., Berkowitz, R. and Sturgeon, D. (1985) 'A controlled study of social intervention in the families of schizophrenic patients: two-year follow-up', *British Journal of Psychiatry*, 146: 594–600.

Leucht, S., Arbter, D., Engel, R.R., Kissling, W. and Davis, J.M. (2009) 'How effective are second-generation antipsychotic drugs? A meta-analysis of placebo-controlled trails', *Molecular Psychiatry*, 14: 429–47.

Lukoff, D., Snyder, K., Ventura, J. and Nuechterlein, K.H. (1984) 'Life events, familiar stress, and coping in the developmental course of schizophrenia', *Schizophrenia Bulletin*, 10: 258–92.

Maher, B.A. (1974) 'Delusional thinking and perceptual disorder', *Journal of Individual Psychology*, 30: 98–113.

Maier, M. (1999) 'Magnetic resonance spectroscopy', in M.A. Ron and A.S. David (eds), *Disorders of Brain and Mind*. Cambridge: Cambridge University Press.

Mednick, S.A. (1970) 'Breakdown in individuals at high risk of schizophrenia: possible predisposing perinatal factors', *Mental Hygiene*, 54: 50–63.

Meehl, P.E. (1962) 'Schizotaxia, schizotypy, schizophrenia', *American Psychologist*, 17: 827–38.

Meehl, P.E. (1989) 'Schizotaxia revisited', *Archives of General Psychiatry*, 46: 935–44.

Meins, E., Ferryhough, C., Russell, J.A. and Clark-Carter, D. (1998) 'Security of attachment as a predictor of symbolic and mentalizing abilities: a longitudinal study', *Social Development*, 15: 51–63.

Morrison, A. and Petersen, T. (2003) 'Trauma and metacognition as predicators of predisposition to hallucinations', *Behavioural and Cognitive Psychotherapy*, 31: 235–46.

NICE (National Institute for Health and Clinical Excellence) (2009) *Core Interventions in the Treatment and Management of Schizophrenia in Primary and Secondary Care (Update)*. London: National Collaborating Centre for Mental Health.

Paykel, E.S., Abbott, R., Jenkins, R., Brugha, T.S. and Meltzer, H. (2000) 'Urban-rural mental health differences in Great Britain: findings from the National Morbidity Survey', *Psychological Medicine*, 30 (2): 269–80.

Persons, J. (1986) 'The advantages of studying psychological phenomenon rather than psychiatric diagnosis', *American Psychologist*, 41: 1250–60.

Pilgrim, D. and Rogers, A. (2008) 'Socioeconomic disadvantage', in R. Tummey and T. Turner (eds), *Critical Issues in Mental Health*. Basingstoke: Palgrave Macmillan.

Read, J., Perry, B.D., Moskowitz, A. and Connolly, J. (2001) 'The contribution of early traumatic events to schizophrenia in some patients: a traumagenic neurode-velopmental model', *Psychiatry: Interpersonal and Biological Processes*, 64: 319–45.

Read, J., Van Os, J., Morrison, A.P. and Ross, C.A. (2005) 'Childhood trauma, psychosis and schizophrenia: a literature review with theoretical and clinical implications', *Acta Psychiatrica Scandinavica*, 112: 330–50.

Sensky, T., Turkington, D., Kingdon, D., Scott, J., Siddle, R., O'Carroll, M. and Barnes, T. (2000) 'A randomized controlled trial of cognitive-behavioral therapy for persistent symptoms in schizophrenia resistant to medication', *Archives of General Psychiatry*, 57: 165–72.

Szasz, T.S. (1960) 'The myth of mental illness', *American Psychologist*, 15: 113–18.

Szmukler, G.I., Herrma, H., Coulsa, S., Benson, A. and Bloch, S. (1996) 'A controlled trial of counselling interventions for caregivers of relatives with schizophrenia', *Social Psychiatric Epidemiology*, 31: 149–55.

Tarrier, N., Barrowclough, C., Vaughan, C., Barmrah, J.S., Porceddu, K., Watts, S. and Freeman, H. (1988) 'The community management of schizophrenia: a controlled trial of behavioral intervention with families to reduce relapse', *British Journal of Psychiatry*, 153: 532–42.

Tarrier, N., Barrowclough, C., Vaughan, C., Barmrah, J.S., Porceddu, K., Watts, S. and Freeman, H. (1989) 'Community management of schizophrenia: a two year follow-up study of a behavioral intervention with families', *British Journal of Psychiatry*, 154: 625–8.

Telles, C., Karno, M., Mintz, J., Paz, G., Arias, M., Tucker, D. and Lopez S. (1995) 'Immigrant families coping with schizophrenia: behavioural family intervention vs. case management with a low-income Spanish-speaking population', *British Journal of Psychiatry*, 167: 473–9.

Weinberger, D.R., Wagner, R.L. and Wyatt R.J. (1983) 'Neuropathological studies of schizophrenia: a selective review', *Schizophrenia Bulletin*, 9: 183–212.

Zubin, J. and Spring, B. (1977) 'Vulnerability: a new view of schizophrenia', *Journal of Abnormal Psychology*, 86 (2): 103–26.

# 14

# Counselling and Psychotherapy in Mental Health Nursing: Therapeutic Encounters

## GARY WINSHIP AND SALLY HARDY

### Learning Objectives

- Understand the historical influences of counselling and psychotherapy to mental health nursing practice.
- Consider the practical issues of engaging with counselling and psychotherapy with acute adult mental health patients.
- Awareness of the processes and outcomes of engaging with counselling and psychotherapy in mental health settings.

## Introduction

This chapter provides an overview of how counselling and psychotherapy have influenced mental health nursing practice. We aim to inspire a renewed curiosity about the influence of counselling and psychotherapy in contemporary mental health nursing practice. The idea of interpersonal mental health nursing, as at the heart of a therapeutic encounter, is considered in how words are spoken, received and constructed during the relationship that develops between a nurse and patient (Altschul, 1958; Cormack, 1976; Nolan, 1999; Peplau, 1952). We outline how a nurse seeks to develop therapeutic interaction through all aspects of his or her communication, whether verbal or non-verbal. Yet this can often feel like navigating through an 'unimaginable storm' (Jackson and Williams, 1994) as there is a challenge when aiming to meaningfully engage with patients to help them express their distress in words rather than actions. The nurse requires effective use of words when confusion, hurt and rage often reign paramount in the people he or she interacts with.

Talking therapy at its most potent is about expressing meaning, articulating thoughts and emotions through a considered therapeutic encounter. A mental health nurse might need to sit for hours with a suicidal patient, in a cold silence that can become deafening; or be in a high secure hospital unit, listening intently to ramblings of an index offender where truth is seemingly dead in the woods. At other times in outpatients with a detox-reluctant patient, where hope hangs as threadbare as his clothes. In such situations, it may be words that find the therapist and not the other way around. Where there is an urge to spit, scratch, smash, to embrace ideas of dying, feeling dead and buried, or to be so furious, murderous with rage; words found to utter, to clearly articulate such intensity of feeling, can bring relief in contrast to immense distress that evokes a silence of inadequate words. Words can become containers, filters and conduits that can 'hold' emotions (Rey, 1994), giving them an outlet, a release, as if the pressure valve of internalised angst silently screams for verbal expression: *'speak to me please'* (Selima Hill: b.1945)

## Counselling is something all nurses do?

Since the 1980s there has been a tradition of teaching Rogerian person-centred principles in counselling training that has generally underpinned a humanistic application of talking therapies across a range of mental health professions (Rogers, 1998). There are a number of broad interpersonal principles that all nurses are introduced to in their education and probably try to adhere to in their daily practice (Stein-Parbury, 1993). Even if the application of counselling and psychotherapy principles are not clearly defined, they are for mental health nurses unanimously applied. Burnard (1992) reports that all nurses counsel.

In the UK, the National Health Service is demanding as a workplace; physically, psychologically and intellectually for any practitioner. To prepare practitioners with information on a humane and well-meaning approach to the challenge of being alongside patients in mental health care practice, without adequate consideration of the powerful subversive influence of transference, counter-transference and resultant self-expression, is a recipe for disaster (Barnes, 1968; Bowers et al., 2010b).

Many nurses remain detached from their patients (Cohler and Shapiro, 1964; Henderson, 2001; Menzies-Lyth, 1960; Moyle, 2003; Remshardt, 2012; Winship, 1995), whether as a conscious or unconscious decision. Many have studied the psychological impact of being 'hit' by a patient (Wykes and Whittington, 1991), with the implications of workplace stress (Hardy et al., 1998) and need for effective supervision as an ethical dimension of mental health nursing practice (Hardy and Park, 1997; Milne and Reiser, 2012). Group therapy has become a key strategy used in the toolkit of a mental health nurse, yet sufficient training for nurses running therapy groups remains poor (Burlingame et al., 2004; Garland et al., 2010; Weisz et al., 2006). However, there is potential to reinvigorate interest and expectation around formal counselling and psychotherapy training, research evidence and practice wisdom that can enhance the therapeutic environment (Mahoney et al., 2012), patients' level of engagement in their treatment (Hobbs, 2009), therapeutic optimism/hope (Elsom and McCauley-Elsom, 2008) and well-being (Newnham et al., 2010).

## Historical developments

Active and exploratory psychotherapeutic approaches in mental health nursing have been derived from the field of psychoanalysis, running deep foundations in the formation of the modern profession of mental health nursing. Hildegard Peplau (USA) and Annie Altschul (UK) from the 1950s developed an adapted psychoanalytic procedure as a way of ensuring that mental health nurses could operate as independent practitioners, applying the idea of talking therapy with novel possibilities (Winship et al., 2009). There is much more that could be said about the combination of feminism and anti-psychiatry that was refracted through the work of Altschul and Peplau which not only pushed forward the establishment and authority of mental health nursing in the latter part of the twentieth century, but also the whole field of mental health. Derived in part from the radical libertarian ambitions of psychoanalysis, not only as a means to therapeutic cure, but as a vehicle for social reconstruction (Fromm, 1941, 1962; Marcuse, 1955), Altschul and Peplau learned their trade under the wings of psychoanalysis (Winship et al., 2009).

There are notable parallels between the influence of Eileen Skellern (in the UK) and Suzy Lego (in the USA), especially in shaping autonomous nursing practice, with mental health nurses carrying clinical caseloads. Skellern worked in therapeutic communities (the Cassell and the Henderson clinics) informed by a combination of psychoanalysis and social psychiatry. She had seen how politically alert therapeutic systems could enfranchise not only the patient, but also the staff. With a therapeutic philosophy which challenged the hierarchical regimes of traditional authority, Skellern and Lego were part of a wave of mental health nurses who were able to reframe the patriarchal traditions of the medical model (Winship, 2008; Winship et al., 2009). Skellern's influence on UK government strategy in the 1970s laid the foundations for annual nurse-led awards and increased nurse autonomy (www.skellern.info/index.html).

In the USA, Suzy Lego, having completed a further training as a psychoanalyst, published numerous papers outlining the role of 'one-to-one mental health nursing practice', defining a professional identity for the discipline of 'nurse psychotherapist' (Lego, 1974, 1987, 1993). As one of Peplau's brightest students and a close confidante, Suzy Lego carried forward Peplau's vision for mental health nursing into the 1980s and 1990s, advocating for a professional identity of a dually qualified advanced mental health nurses who could enjoy parity with psychologists and psychiatrists, whether in private practice or state institutions. Lego's idea of integrating the practice of psychotherapy and mental health nursing was embedded in the journal *Perspectives in Psychiatric Care*, which carried the subtitle: 'the Journal for Nurse Psychotherapists'. The development in the role of nurse psychotherapists was inspiring to a number of colleagues in the UK and though there were significant problems with access to psychotherapy training outside London (McMahon, 1994), still an increasing number of mental health nurses in the UK began to complete formal analytical training, and for a time this resulted in a momentum to define the role of nurse psychotherapists in the UK (Winship, 1996, 1998).

Lego's death in 1999 (only a few months after Peplau's) foreclosed what might have been further significant contributions to a discourse on the role of the nurse psychotherapist as an internationally regarded discipline. Mental health nursing arguably remains the challenge of case management, control and restraint, medication adherence and so forth, where there may be less emphasis on the art of counselling and psychotherapy. Even where there is general acceptance of the value of talking therapy, the alliance between nursing and psychoanalysis, albeit with some significant intellectual and institutional cornerstones, has been one that has rested uneasily (Winship, 1995).

Rather than the more active ingredient of psychodynamic agency in mental health nursing, the idea of psychotherapy has been generally applied in terms of models of pastoral listening, reflection and befriending (Strang, 1981). Models of recovery have also tended towards a frame of counselling as a friendly ear that can support, advise and instil hope in clients on their journey to recovery (Repper and

Perkins, 2003). The rise of cognitive behavioural therapy has been identified as an essential talking therapy in the discourse of mental health nursing with resultant positive patient outcomes (Layard, 2006). Bowers et al. (2010b) assert that knowing how to talk to patients is a necessary, everyday, core contingent in the process of mental health nursing. The publication of the Social Exclusion Unit report *Mental Health and Social Exclusion* (2004) reclaimed a socially orientated reconstruction of mental health, but also the centrality of talking therapy. The report argued that health services needed to be less medically driven and more socially focused in their orientation; 'more than 80% of GPs admitted over-prescribing anti-depressants such as Prozac and Seroxat to patients suffering from depression, anxiety or stress' (Social Exclusion Unit, 2004: 36). The report emphasised the importance of talking therapy as not only a viable alternative to pharmaceuticals, but as a first choice intervention.

The fact that the UK government put aside money for the development of a workforce of cognitive behavioural therapists demonstrated that the government (Labour at the time) was to some extent willing to put its money where its rhetoric was. However, the fit between CBT and social recovery might seem to be less viable than other more socially focused counselling and psychotherapy approaches, such as group therapy, interpersonal therapy or therapeutic community practice. CBT, with a narrow individualist focus on mind and behaviour, might not vitalise the relational dimensions of the therapeutic encounter that are the seeds of a recovery process. Peplau's (1952) first principle is that mental health nursing is essentially an interpersonal process, and that the main agent of therapy is not a device, or a biological rebalancing act, nor is it derived from a manual that prescribes a particular set of techniques that can correct the patient. Instead, Peplau asserts the main agent of therapy is the nurses themselves.

## Theory in practice

We learn to play with sound and forming words from the very start of life (Peddar, 2010; Winnicott, 1988). Although taken with the idea of psychotherapy as play, many encounters in acute psychiatry with people deeply disturbed (as outlined previously) show that play is a long way from what is happening in the encounter. The acutely disturbed or depressed patient may have lost capacity to play, or may not have learned how to play at all. Instead, the therapeutic encounter can feel much more like an altogether more backbreaking physical undertaking. The therapeutic alliance can be experienced as heavy duty. Counselling approaches for the mental health nurse, at the sharp end of practice, may seem too passive, a game even. Though the skills of listening are rightly credited, merely holding up a mirror and reflecting back to patients (see the case example below) is not always enough to bring about therapeutic gain.

A common mantra might be that words speak louder than actions for the ambition of all mental health practice. That is to say, helping patients find the words to express their wish to self-harm or an urge to hurt others, or their need to express what it feels like to be abused; these words might express feeling states that mean future destructive acts can be lessened, more controlled, prevented even. Yet, a common concern for many nurses centres on not speaking of, or asking provocative questions, or saying something that might provoke a violent reaction, encourage delusions, persecutory thoughts, suicide even. Experience of working on an inpatient unit has proven to me that continuous critical reflection, pertinent clinical supervision and a willingness to feel, engage with and consider discomfort are all important for the mental health nurse. The unit in question was influenced by the psychodynamic psychotherapy principles of forming close working alliances between nurse and patient (Jackson and Crawley, 1992). We achieved this through close supervision and a daily clinical evaluation system that incorporated all members of the clinical team to come together to reflect and review their interpersonal encounters. Learning from each other's experiences enhanced the level of confidence to express oneself within difficult and demanding situations.

## CASE EXAMPLE

### I've lost my songbook

| | |
|---|---|
| Patient: | *I had a two hundred year songbook* |
| Nurse: | *Tell me about your songbook* |
| Patient: | *I don't know where it is now – I lost it* |
| Nurse: | *That's sad to hear* |
| Patient: | *My feet are bad today* |
| Nurse: | *What's happening with your feet?* |
| Patient: | *My feet burn up, it's when I did the test and walked on fire coals, I suffer now and cannot get out of bed. I burnt my feet* |
| Nurse: | *Can you remember a time when your feet didn't burn?* |
| Patient: | *I'm preparing to do an Arab-spring at school, I'm standing in front of a room full of people, getting ready. I feel nervous, but do it, I get really excited, there's a tingle down my spine* |
| Nurse: | *What are you feeling now?* |

| | |
|---|---|
| Patient: | *My Dad used to hit me when I was smaller, I never let out a scream, I just kept quiet. Even at school I never showed things, even in prison I learnt to bottle it all up inside.* |
| Nurse: | *Now the pain is coming out in your feet?* |
| Patient: | *I got the same excited feeling when robbing someone* |
| Nurse: | *Do you feel robbed of your past, having lost your songbook?* |

Can practitioners ever find the right words to soothe raw wounds like an ointment or at other times, risk words that might cut deeply, like a surgeon's scalpel? Sometimes words need to be blunt, they can feel like using a mallet, resonating pain without a physical touch. A patient spoke of wanting to throw himself in front of a train, the nurse replied: 'what about the driver, what about his family living with him afterwards, could you do that to someone else's children?' The patient accused the nurse of being insensitive. But he seemed literally stopped in his tracks, at least for a moment. The words hit him, rather than the train. Words can also be sweet, soothing or have to be swallowed, like a bitter pill. We all need to find the capacity to speak out, find a voice, as clearly as we can. Of course there is a lineage here that goes back to Freud's development of the talking cure, from the moment that Anna O discovered the idea that talking therapy is akin to chimney sweeping (Breuer and Freud, 1895), where sense can be gleaned from experiences which otherwise seem mad and incomprehensible.

Masson (1989) argued that a therapeutic encounter is only possible in a relationship where there is no concern with power and hierarchy; yet for most, engaging in a therapeutic relationship occurs between a patient and practitioner that will initially offer a level of dependency on the therapist as carer/enabler. Breggin (1991) recognised value in such a dependence, but qualified this by identifying the need for consistency between the practitioner's philosophy of care, and that of the patient. Yet, there remain sizeable gaps in our knowledge about the finer tunings of talking therapy. Bowers et al. (2010a, 2010b) completed a detailed analysis of the way in which mental health nurses talk to acutely disturbed patients, showing that respect and compassion are primary in the applied repertoire of the language of the nurses. There is perhaps something unique in the everyday procedure of mental health nursing in terms of the application of counselling and psychotherapy. Although some nurses may indeed carry individual caseloads, and see clients for a traditional sit-down face-to-face 50-minute therapy session, in mental health nursing practice there are otherwise manifold opportunities to apply counselling skills. Peplau referred to this as the 'other 23 hours'.

As part of mental health nurse training at the Maudsley, during the 1980s to 1990s, a session was allocated where students could explore patients' words, statements, phrases that the student had found difficult to respond to, understand or accept. For example, when patients said, 'I don't see the point of living', or 'my feet are on fire', finding the right words to respond in a therapeutic, engaged way – rather than a more natural reaction of wanting to ignore, dismiss, laugh at or recoil from – was considered central to a mental health nursing training experience. This struggle to respond, reply, engage with the intensity of emotional distress is an important part of the process required to understand and work alongside others; understanding the chaos and uncertainty within which people exist. In further developing educational approaches where practitioners can become versed in therapeutic encounters, the use of experiential learning strategies whereby students are exposed to therapeutic milieus (including free association in language and articulation) is encouraged. For example, sessions where students develop narrative group collages, where they might produce a collective sonnet/poem. In these sessions students develop their own lines of thought around a particular topic before cutting and pasting them together to form a longer collaboratively devised poem. Students are encouraged to interrogate their own words, interactions, interconnections, reflecting on the nuances of their exchanges with patients, closely scrutinising the co-construction of meaning in verbal exchanges as part of the therapeutic encounter between nurse and patient.

## Conclusion

We advocate in this chapter for a revived interest in the importance of counselling and psychotherapy, as central theoretical principles in mental health nurses' personal and professional advancement. We call for not just language acquisition as a rational measure of competency in clinical practice, but the learning of fluency of thought and accurate emotional reciprocity. This remains the challenge, where the intensity of contact with a patient offers immeasurable opportunities to demonstrate, through words, how nurses can reach the person, not just in the one-to-one or group therapy sessions, but in all aspects of the 'other 23 hours'. It is often said 'a picture can paint a thousand words', but this overprivileges visual dexterity. Rather, one word can paint a million pictures; some words like 'love' and 'hate' are infinite in their complexity and meaning, experienced as different for each of us. When we glance and gather words in our encounters with patients, the intricacies of meaning suggest endless possibilities for therapeutic exploration.

## Summary

This chapter has provided an overview of how counselling and psychotherapy has influenced mental health nursing practice. We have aimed to inspire curiosity and interest in the position and influence of counselling and psychotherapy in contemporary mental health nursing practice. Nursing models have drawn from principles of counselling and psychotherapy in notions of interpersonal skills, therapeutic nurse–patient relationships, and these remain at the heart of a therapeutic encounter. We have outlined how a nurse seeks to develop therapeutic interaction through all aspects of their communication. Yet there is a challenge when aiming to meaningfully engage with patients to help them express their distress in words rather than actions. The nurse interested in the effective use of words can gain much from further study, training and ongoing critical evaluation/supervision of the personal and professional aspects of a therapeutic encounter. We would encourage continuous curiosity into the infinite riches of counselling and psychotherapy for contemporary mental health practice.

# References

Altschul, A. (1957) *Psychiatric Nursing*. London: Ballière Tindall.

Barnes, E. (1968) *Psychosocial Nursing: Studies from the Cassell Hospital*. Fakenham, Norfolk: Cox and Wyman Ltd. London: Tavistock.

Bowers, L., Brennan, G., Winship, G. and Theodoridou, C. (2010a) *Talking with Acutely Psychotic People: Communication Skills for Nurses and Others Spending Time with People Who Are Very Mentally Ill*. Monograph. London: City University.

Bowers, L., Brennan, G., Winship, G. and Theodoridou, C. (2010b) 'How expert nurses communicate with acutely psychotic patients', *Mental Health Practice*, 13 (7): 24–6.

Breggin, P. (1991) *Toxic Psychiatry: Why Therapy, Empathy and Love Must Replace the Drugs, Electroshock and Biochemical Theories of the 'New Psychiatry'*. Glasgow: HarperCollins.

Breuer, J. and Freud, S. (1895) 'Fraulein Anna O.', *Studies on Hysteria*, 21–47.

Burlingame, G.M., Fuhriman, A., Johnson, J. (2004) 'Process and outcome in group counseling and group psychotherapy', in J.L. DeLucia-Waack, D.A. Gerrity, C.R.Kalodner and M.T.Riva (eds), *Handbook of Group Counseling and Psychotherapy*. Thousand Oaks, CA: Sage, pp. 49–61.

Burnard, P. (1992) *Counselling: A Guide to Practice in Nursing*. Oxford: Butterworth-Heinemann.

Cohler, J. and Shapiro, L. (1964) 'Avoidance patterns in staff–patient interaction on a chronic schizophrenic treatment ward', *Psychiatry*, 27: 377–89.

Cormack, D. (1976) *Psychiatric Nursing Observed*. London: RCN Publications.

Elsom, S.J. and McCauley-Elsom, K.M. (2008) 'Measuring therapeutic optimism', *Australian and New Zealand Journal of Psychiatry*, 42 (3): A51.

Fromm, E. (1941) *Escape From Freedom*. New York: Avon Books, 1965.

Fromm, E. (1962) *Beyond the Chains of Illusion: My Encounter with Freud and Marx*. New York: Simon and Schuster.

Garland E.L., Fredrickson, B., King, A.M., Johnson, D.P., Meyer, P.S. and Penn D.L. (2010) 'Upward spirals of positive emotions counter downward spiral of negativity: insights from the broaden and build theory and affective neuroscience on the treatment of emotional dysfunctions and deficits in psychotherapy', *Clinical Psychology Review*, 30: 849–64.

Hardy, S. and Park, A. (1997) 'Supervision and professional practice', in B. Thomas, S. Hardy and P. Cutting (eds), *Stuart and Sundeen's Mental Health Nursing, Principles and Practice*. London: Mosby International.

Hardy, S., Carson, J. and Thomas, B. (1998) *Occupational Stress: Personal and Professional Approaches*. London: Stanley Thornes.

Henderson, A. (2001) 'Emotional labour and nursing: an under-appreciated aspect of caring work', *Nursing Inquiry*, 8 (2): 130–8.

Hill, S. (1993) *A Little Book of Meat*. Newcastle: Bloodaxe Books.

Hobbs, J.L. (2009) 'A dimensional analysis of patient-centred care', *Nursing Research*, 58 (1): 52–62.

Jackson, M. and Cawley, R. (1992) 'Psychodynamics and psychotherapy on an acute psychiatric ward. The story of an experimental unit', *The British Journal of Psychiatry*, 160 (1): 41–50.

Jackson, M. and Williams, P. (1994) *Unimaginable Storms: A Search for Meaning in Psychosis*. London: Karnac.

Layard, R. (2006) 'The case for psychological treatment centres', *British Medical Journal*, 332 (7548): 1030–2.

Lego, S. (1974) 'Nurse psychotherapists: how are we different?', *Perspectives in Psychiatric Care*, 11 (4): 144–7.

Lego, S. (1987) 'The borderline patient: systemic versus psychoanalytic approach', *Archives of Psychiatric Nursing*, 1 (3): 172–82.

Lego, S. (1993) 'Gratification and failure to separate', *Perspectives in Psychiatric Care*, 29 (4): 25–30.

McMahon, B. (1994) 'Professionalism and the development of psychotherapy', *Mental Health Nursing*, 14 (6): 14–17.

Mahoney, J.S., Paylo, G., Napier, G. and Giordano, J. (2012) 'The therapeutic milieu reconceptualized for the 21st century', *Archives of Psychiatric Nursing*, 23 (6): 423–35.

Marcuse, H. (1955) *Eros and Civilization*. Boston: Beacon Press.

Masson, J. (1989) *Against Therapy*. London: William Collins and Sons.

Menzies-Lyth, I. (1960) 'Social systems as a defence against anxiety', *Human Relations*, 13: 95–121.

Milne, D. and Reiser, R.P. (2012) 'A rationale for evidence-based clinical supervision', *Journal of Contemporary Psychotherapy*, 42 (3): 139–49.

Moyle, W. (2003) 'Nurse–patient relationship: a dichotomy of expectation', *International Journal of Mental Health Nursing*, 12 (2): 103–9.

Newnham, E.A., and Page, E.C. (2010) 'Bridging the gap between best evidence and best practice in mental health', *Clinical Psychology Review*, 30 (1): 127–42.

Nolan, P. (1999) 'Annie Altschul's legacy to 20th century British mental health nursing', *Journal of Psychiatric and Mental Health Nursing*, 6 (4): 267–72.

Peddar, J. (2010) *Attachment and New Beginnings: Reflections on Psychoanalytic Therapy*. London: Karnac Books.

Peplau, H. (1952) *Interpersonal Relations in Nursing*. New York: G.P. Putman and Sons.

Remshardht, M.A. (2012) 'Do you know your professional boundaries?', *Nursing Made Incredibly Easy*, 10 (1): 5–6.

Repper, J. and Perkins, R. (2003) *Social Inclusion and Recovery*. London: Ballière Tindall.

Rey, H. (1994) *Universals of Psychoanalysis*. London: Free Association Books.

Rogers, C.R. (1998) *Client-Centred Therapy*. London: Constable and Robinson.

Social Exclusion Unit (2004) *Mental Health and Social Exclusion*. London: Office of the Deputy Prime Minister, HMSO.

Strang, J. (1981) 'Psychotherapy by nurses', *Advanced Journal of Nursing*, 7 (2): 167–71.

Stein-Parbury, J. (1993) *Patient and Person: Developing Interpersonal Skills in Nursing*. Edinburgh: Churchill Livingstone.

Weisz, J.R., McCarty, C.A., and Valeri, S.M. (2006) Effects of psychotherapy for depression in children and adolescents: a meta-analysis', *Psychological Bulletin*, 132 (1): 132–49.

Winnicott, D.W. (1988) *Babies and their Mothers*. London: Free Association Books.

Winship, G. (1995) 'Nursing and psychoanalysis – uneasy alliances?', *Psychoanalytic Psychotherapy*, 9 (3): 289–99.

Winship, G. (1996) 'Developing the role of the nurse psychotherapist in the United Kingdom', *Perspectives in Psychiatric Care*, 33 (1): 25–31.

Winship, G. (1998) 'The nurse/therapist split', *Psychoanalytic Psychotherapy*, 11 (3): 271–4.

Winship, G. (2008) 'Therapeutic communities', in P. Barker (ed.), *The Art and Craft of Caring*. London: Hodder Arnold, Health Sciences.

Winship, G., Repper, J., Bray, J. and Hinshelwood, R.D. (2009) 'Collective biography and the legacy of Hildegard Peplau, Annie Altschul and Eileen Skellern; the origins of mental health nursing and its relevance to the current crisis in psychiatry', *Journal of Research in Nursing*, 14 (6): 505–17.

Wykes, T. and Whittington, R. (1991) 'Coping strategies used by staff following assault by a patient: an exploratory study', *Work and Stress*, 5 (1): 123–6.

# 15

# Values in Practice

## GEMMA STACEY AND BOB DIAMOND

### Learning Objectives

- Consider the concept of values in relation to mental health nursing practice.
- Reflect upon personal values and how these might influence your approach to practice.
- Critically consider the role of externally prescribed values and how these may be interpreted and applied in practice.
- Apply the theoretical discussion to a case example and reflect on personal learning.

## Introduction

The term 'values' is defined in the Oxford Dictionary in two ways. First, it is conceptualised as a set of principles or standards of behaviour (Oxford Dictionary, 2012). This definition is reflected in the ethical ideals of society or of a specific organisation like the NHS. These values are often externally prescribed by law, professional codes of conduct or organisational philosophies. The second definition is stated as 'one's judgement of what is important in life' (Oxford Dictionary, 2012). This description reflects the internal concept of values and relates to individuals' own beliefs and morals which influence their attitudes and behaviour.

This chapter will aim to discuss how these conceptualisations of values combine to influence mental health nursing practice. It will enable you to identify the organisational values and recognise how they support or challenge the expression of personal values when applied to practice scenarios. The ways in which personal and organisational values can conflict will be critically explored and you will be prompted through reflective learning activities to consider strategies to manage this.

## Historical development

As early as 1796 the more pioneering care provision for people commonly referred to as mad included many values such as compassion and understanding. Moral treatment, as it became known under the guidance of the Quaker William Tuke at York (Porter, 1991), emphasised the significance of values in care with the inclusion and provision of benevolence, self-respect and esteem. This was in addition to a pleasant, comfortable physical environment for those suffering. However, throughout the nineteenth century, as the pursuit of scientific principles increased, the care for people suffering with mental health difficulties became dominated by physicians. Minimal respect was afforded to the exploration of diverse values. For instance dignity in individual meaning of experiences was somewhat overlooked and dismissed in pursuit of the professional opinion proffered. The relationship between doctor and patient varied greatly. The Victorian asylums incarcerated many people for what today would be considered injustices; a narrow perspective of values focusing on control and restraint dominated care. Although it is always possible to read occasional accounts where the personal significance and meaning for the person experiencing significant mental health difficulties were upheld. The earliest days of psychoanalysis and psychotherapy at the turn of the nineteenth century placed the person's experiences central but still relied on values that encouraged the professional as expert with the client as passive recipient. During the 1960s with the development of person-centred psychology and the more pervasive sociocultural values of liberty, a milieu of freedom of expression and equality ensued. The anti-psychiatry movement (Double, 2006) appeared to have gained a foothold within mental health care, arising within the general sociopolitical context of the 1960s and early 1970s. Certainly, the anti-psychiatry movement placed the person as central in the context of mental health care and endorsed the values of dignity, freedom and respect by encouraging people experiencing significant mental health difficulties to create space to accept and explore for themselves their distressing experiences. Perhaps as a reaction to the tensions created between the anti-psychiatry and the conventional mental health care of the day, the importance of values lost some of its significance over the following 30 years, arguably with the user movement the major influence in reminding us of the importance of values in our practice (Campbell, 2006).

The influence of values in health care has gained increasing attention over the past 10 years, which has been reflected in government policy and guidance. A set of competences, the Essential Shared Capabilities (ESCs), were developed by the government in consultation with mental health service users, carers, practitioners and service providers. These provide a framework for the whole of the mental health workforce across the NHS, social care and the statutory and non-statutory sectors (DH, 2004). The need for values-based practice is explicitly identified within this framework. Values-based practice is a relatively new way of conceptualising practice, recognising that decisions taken in mental health care are based on values as well as facts (Woodbridge and Fulford, 2004).

The emphasis upon values in mental health care is further reinforced by the *Chief Nursing Officer's Review of Mental Health Nursing* written in response to the recognition of the need for change amongst the mental health nursing workforce (DH, 2006). The review emphasises the importance of strengthening and developing mental health nursing in order to improve the outcomes and experiences of service users. It suggests this will be achieved through a process of putting values into action, and identifies that mental health nursing should incorporate the broad principles of a recovery approach into every aspect of practice (see Chapter 12). The recovery approach is based around a number of principles that emphasise the importance of working in partnership with service users and carers to identify realistic life goals and enabling them to achieve them. It stresses the value of social inclusion and the need for professionals to be optimistic about the possibility of positive individual change (DH, 2006).

## The theory of values in practice

The influence of values on the way we practise as nurses has recently gained recognition in mental health care (see Cooper, 2009; Woodbridge and Fulford, 2003). This school of thought identifies that the decisions that we make and the way that we work are not only influenced by research evidence and local and national policy but also by our values. This recognition prompts us to be aware of what influences our response to a particular person, their behaviour and how this might impact the direction of their care.

## Reflective Learning Activity

The concept of values is difficult to define.

To help you start to understand this concept, use the thought bubble below to identify any words, phrases or terms you link with the term values. We have started you off with some suggestions.

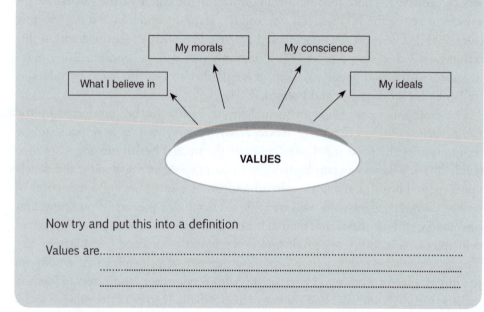

Now try and put this into a definition

Values are....................................................................................................................

........................................................................................................................................

........................................................................................................................................

Cooper (2009: 22) offers a definition of values:

> The worth, desirability, importance, or emotional investment (either for or against) we attach to something.

- How similar or different is this to your definition?
- What does this tell you about values?

You may have found that your definition of values is different to Cooper's. This does not mean that it is wrong but it does tell us that values are complex. Woodbridge and Fulford (2004) suggest this is for the following reasons:

- Values come in many varieties.

You may have found that your definition is more about ethics, human rights or virtues. Values often encompass all of these things and also go beyond them to take into consideration your own wishes, desires and dreams.

- Some values vary with time and place and others are more fixed.

Some values relate to the core beliefs that we tend to think of as with us from childhood and guiding us throughout life. These could be religious beliefs, family values or understanding of what society accepts as right or wrong. However they can be expressed in different ways or be fluid and changeable depending on life experiences which challenge our values and cause us to question them.

- Values vary from person to person.

We may have some consensus in what the term 'values' means to us but the individual values we hold may be very different. Also the importance we place on certain values may differ from colleagues, service users or friends. For example, you might feel that the value of honesty is highly important to you. However, a colleague may believe that honesty is less important than protecting the person from harm. In this situation you may want to give a person all the information but your colleague may want to withhold it if it could potentially lead to the person becoming distressed.

It is important to explore the values that you bring to your work as a student nurse in order to recognise how they are influencing your practice and identify why you may feel in conflict at times with people you are working with. This can include people who use mental health services, their carers and also your mentor or other professionals. A good way to start this process is by completing the activity below. This activity will help you to clearly define the values you bring to your work. It can become part of your portfolio and you may wish to reflect on it throughout your programme to identify when your values are challenged or reinforced in your practice and how you respond to this.

## Reflective Learning Activity

### Developing your nursing philosophy statement

A nursing philosophy is a personal statement that describes your own views, beliefs and theories about how nurses should practise and care for people who use

*(Continued)*

*(Continued)*

health services. There is not necessarily a 'right' or 'wrong' way to write your NPS. However, there are certain issues that you should probably consider when making the connections between what you believe about nursing, how you nurse and how you evaluate your practice.

Most simply, you can start by asking yourself:

- What are mental health services for?
- What do you think people who use mental health services should expect from nursing care?
- What are your values, attitudes and beliefs about people who use mental health services?
- So, what nursing approaches do you use that reflects this position (perhaps with a couple of examples)?

Woodbridge and Fulford (2004: 16) have developed the framework of values-based practice which aims to raise awareness of how values influence the decisions made in mental health care. It is defined as:

> ... the theory and skills base for effective health care decision making where different (and hence potentially conflicting) values are in play.

This framework recognises that in order for mental health practitioners to work with values they should:

- Raise awareness of values. Often, we are not aware of our values until they come into conflict or we feel our values are being ignored. As a professional, our values are usually advocated as a result of the power that is given to us in our role. However, people who use mental health services often feel their values are dismissed or viewed as less valid. Therefore it is important to consciously explore values in order to consider how they influence practice. This involves exploring personal values and creating forums for the discussion of values within teams.
- Adopt strategies for reasoning about values which enables the exploration of values which are influencing a situation and justify the outcome of a decision.
- Gain knowledge about the values which are likely to be influencing a situation. For example, gathering the past experiences of people involved, considering how

the media may have portrayed a similar situation, or exploring research which has been published on the issues arising.

- Adopt communication skills which enable people to give their views and feel listened to. This may involve some negotiation skills or resolution skills where there are conflicting values. This is important in order to ensure that each person's values are given equal attention.
- Start the decision-making process from the perspective of the service user to ensure that practice and policy is applied to the individual.
- Attend to the values of all others involved, including the service user's family, friends, informal carers, support workers and all mental health practitioners. This is known as multi-disciplinary practice. This will enable potential sources of misunderstanding or conflict to be converted into opportunities for discussion and creative working.
- Consider the influence of both the values and the facts when making decisions. This challenges the assumption that decisions made based on science, such as diagnosis, are not influenced by the values of the person conducting the assessment. Values are relevant to these decisions and can account for some of the inconsistencies in how different diagnoses are applied to the same symptoms or behaviours.

Values-based practice has been criticised however for not acknowledging the power, hierarchies and externally prescribed social constraints which will influence the decision-making process and outcomes. Houghton and Diamond (2010) have questioned the lack of importance given to issues of power and interest within values-based practice. The framework for values-based practice proposed by Woodbridge and Fulford (2004) refers to establishing a democracy in which all views are respected and balanced equally. There are few details about the structures and processes of how such a democracy would be established, expected to function and be sustained. Values in practice often refer to qualities of compassion, caring, dignity, kindness, but the values of justice, equality and fairness appear to be overlooked.

The common barriers to implementing values are summarised in Table 15.1 with some suggestions of how to manage these obstacles.

The moral choices we make in adopting a values-based approach require us as mental health nurses to justify our actions in the context of wider questions such as: *How does the action taken agree or conflict with my other moral values? How has the action taken enhanced the choice and well-being of the person I am working with?* What are considered reasonable actions will vary from person to person or situation to situation. However, there are some common principles which should underlie the approach taken to decision-making, and these are supported by the Nursing and Midwifery Council (NMC) Code of Professional Conduct (NMC, 2008):

- One ought not to harm physically or psychologically (non-maleficence).
- One ought to give positive help to people wherever necessary (benevolence or beneficence, and compassion).
- One ought to treat people fairly or equally (justice).
- One ought to produce the greatest happiness for the majority (utility) (Downie and Calman, 1994: 50).

When adopting a values-based approach to practice the principles above tend to encourage you to base your actions on duty and obligation, rather than care and compassion for the person you are working with. Such obligations need to be understood,

**TABLE 15.1**   Barriers and facilitators to Values Based Practice

| Barriers to implementing values-based practice | Helpful strategies to facilitate values-based practice |
| --- | --- |
| Forums for the discussion of values are not routinely in place in practice. | Clinical supervision, care reviews or multi-disciplinary team meetings can be reformatted to enable this discussion. |
| Decisions are sometimes made in an emergency situation which limits the time given to collaboration or effort to involve all parties. Also when the person who is using mental health service is in crisis, he or she may be seen as unable to contribute to decisions made about his or her care. | Crisis planning can allow for people to express their values in anticipation of an emergency situation. Therefore you can be assured that action taken is in line with a pre-agreed plan. This is where a relapse prevention plan can become very useful. |
| Some people you are working with may not see the value of considering other people's views or be unwilling to listen to alternatives which limits opportunities for negotiation. | This will require you to step into their shoes and question why they may find this way of working challenging. The individual may have personal support or professional development needs. |
| The wider organisation of mental health services places the responsibility and accountability of a decision with the professional. This may mean that some professionals are reluctant to consider others' views due to their accountability. | A multi-disciplinary approach to the decision-making process helps to share this responsibility as it enables concerns to be discussed, explored and strategies to be put in place which the whole team agree upon. It also allows for service users to take some responsibility for their actions and feel an increased sense of control. |

*Source*: Stacey et al. (2012).

interpreted and applied by you. This means they are inseparable from your character and the moral qualities and values you possess. Considering nursing practice as a moral quality or value that you hold allows you to consider caring towards another as a complex situation in which the moral character, the role of emotion and the significance of the relationship between you and the person with whom you are working should be fully acknowledged.

Relationships are central to our decision-making processes. The external principles defined above fail to fully acknowledge the interpersonal relationships that exist between practitioners and service users. An alternative approach to relying on external principles for decision-making in practice is known as *the ethics of care* and has routes in the feminist writings of Carol Gilligan (Allmark, 1995). This approach stresses the importance of attending to particular contexts rather than general principles. Accordingly, each practice-based dilemma is said to call for a unique response that cannot be summed up by universal principles. The ethics of care approach calls for 'engaged involvement' with clients and their goals rather that a detached consideration of theoretical concepts. This implies that rather than focusing exclusively on the use of reason, a combination of both reason and emotion is essential for decision-making. Therefore the consideration of how a client feels will introduce perspectives into our reasoning which may have been ignored by external principles.

This view is supported by *the virtue approach* to ethics which takes into account a person's character within decision-making (Armstrong, 2006). Rather than emphasising what a person should do in a given scenario, virtue ethics emphasises what a person should be in order to make ethically appropriate decisions. Armstrong (2006) recognises that working in this way will require the mental health nurse to demonstrate personal attributes such as compassion, patience and kindness. These qualities are identified as character traits and examples of moral virtues. They dispose the person to act and feel in certain ways as they are an integral part of a person's identity.

Mental health nurses will be aware of the distressing nature of the dilemmas they face in their work with service users and the potentially damaging consequences that may arise. Furthermore, it is morally appropriate to feel emotions such as regret, anguish, guilt, hurt or loss (Hursthouse, 1999). The use of principles to guide decisions places a firm emphasis on solving the ethical dilemmas. This simplistic view can be problematic as it assumes that all ethical dilemmas can be satisfactorily resolved by overlooking how the worker and client may feel during and after the decision has been made. Alternatively, virtue ethics acknowledges that conflicts between values will arise and it holds that exercising judgement is fundamental to good standards.

The acknowledgement of the dilemmas presented will involve the mental health nurse engaging in self-reflection and in-depth discussion with the service user. It will require the nurse to exercise moral perception and be able to see the morally relevant features of a situation such as rights, motives and beliefs. It will also necessitate the ability to identify the client's needs in a collaborative manner, demonstrating moral sensitivity. Finally, it will involve the mental health nurse exercising moral imagination. This refers to the nurse's ability to place him/herself in another's shoes and feel what it may be like to be that person in this specific situation (Armstrong, 2006).

The mental health nurse should acknowledge that making the decision in mental health practice is a values-based process and that our decisions are not those about which we are certain; they are those with which we can live. This uncertainty prompts us to reflect critically upon the decision-making process and our practice. This may result in making a decision without attempting to anticipate the outcome but being able to live with the consequences. Engaging in such a process will require the mental health nurse to negotiate rather than eliminate ethical uncertainty (McCarthy, 2006).

## Reflective Learning Activity

Using your nursing philosophy statement, circle any words or terms which reflect your moral virtues. These could be character traits, personal attributes or beliefs you bring.

Based on the discussion you have just read, what other traits do you feel would be essential to develop in order to implement a values-based approach to your practice? Some examples might include:

- Patience
- Willingness to listen to other views
- Self-reflection
- Modesty.

## The theory applied to practice

It is evident that there are several obstacles within the mental health care system which may obstruct a values-based approach to practice. You may be faced frequently with dilemmas which involve striking a balance between promoting recovery and the necessity to protect individuals and communities from harm. Currently risk is perceived as something that can be calculated and prevented (Freshwater and Westwood, 2006). This approach demands that mental health nurses are able to predict and develop measures to manage the behaviour of individuals experiencing mental health problems. In this professional context, it is likely that a more controlling rather than caring practice will be more easily justified. These circumstances often draw upon externally defined values to guide decisions and may leave the practitioner feeling that his/her internal values have been compromised or challenged.

A number of studies show that service users feel that professionals' priorities focus upon medication management and symptom monitoring in an effort to manage risk. This is at the expense of providing space and time for individual work, in which clients can raise issues that are important to them and feel appropriately heard and cared for (Dunn, 1999; SCMH, 1998). It is suggested that this dissonance of priorities can be explained by the continued dominance of a medicalised understanding of mental distress within mental health services. The consequence of this is a conflict of values and understandings which ultimately prevents shared decision-making and promotion of autonomy which are essential to the recovery approach to mental health care (Colombo et al., 2003). A values-based approach however focuses on the significance of the person, relationships and the context of the scenario, and it is the consideration of these factors which could provide the justification for adopting a more values-based driven approach health care practice.

## The nurse

When considering the person we are referring to the nurse's integral values and how the nurse influences his/her practice as suggested by the virtues approach (McKie and Swinton, 2000). In order to explore the significance of these values, the ability to reflect on practice is central. Values-based practice will require a reflective practitioner who is able to recognise the impact of the self on a situation and its ethical consequences, thus exemplifying the importance of such character traits.

Nurses may experience some anxiety around their perceived professional accountability in enabling service users to have more influence over their care at potentially risky times. They may also have genuine concerns for service users' safety. The experience of these emotions should be recognised as a morally appropriate response (Hursthouse, 1999). To take a positive risk nurses must place the service user's needs before their own and appropriately manage the anxiety this may create. Nurses may foster these skills through reflection within a clinical supervision setting. Clinical supervision is promoted as a mechanism to enable nurses to gain support and deal with the pressures of working in a demanding environment. This is achieved through discussion of practice in a supportive and confidential space. The supervisee is encouraged to identify and share emotions. They are also prompted to explore and challenge their assumptions (Jones, 2001; Wilken et al., 1997). This facilitates the exploration of both reason and emotion within decision-making as advocated by an ethics of care approach (Allmark, 1995).

## The relationship

The therapeutic relationship between the nurse and service user is essential. The ethics of care approach calls for engaged involvement with service users and their goals (Allmark, 1995). This should provide a vehicle for service users to voice their wishes and work towards the goals that they have identified. The trusting relationship has been described as the essence of mental health care. Much is written about the potential for the therapeutic relationship as a vehicle to support people to deal with their problems (Rogers, 1967). The existence of trust and acceptance within a therapeutic relationship can enhance hope, enabling service users to identify goals that can spark the collaborative decision-making process. The conditions within this relationship can facilitate service users to have the self-belief to follow these choices (Repper and Perkins, 2003). Collaboration between the service user and the nurse is essential to gain an in-depth understanding of a person's history and context. This will enable the personal meaning to be considered and the ethical dimensions to be explored.

The influence of trust extends further into agreeing upon a level of independence that the person is comfortable with. Once this has been established, the nurse has the responsibility to advocate for a service user's right to take back control. This demonstrates moral perception which refers to the practitioner's capacity to see the morally relevant features of a situation (Armstrong et al., 2006). Additionally, the ability to empathise is central to developing the trusting relationship, allowing the nurse to gain greater understanding of the person's perspective and to help make an informed judgement through exercising moral imagination (Armstrong, 2006). This will enable the nurse to advocate for the service user from a stronger position.

## Context

The principles framework is widely criticised due its tendency to ignore context (Armstrong, 2006; McCarthy, 2006; Rachels, 1999). The nurse is in a privileged position to comprehend context as a result of the trusting relationship and the amount of time spent with service users. This places nurses in an ideal position to communicate the complexity of the ethical situation to the multi-disciplinary team who are pressurised into making decisions based on a detached view. However, it is recognised that nurses do not make decisions in isolation. The multi-disciplinary team provides a context for mental health nurses and thus contributes significantly to their community. In this respect it is essential to consider their influence in the decision-making process (Morgan, 2007).

An open, democratic, multi-disciplinary approach to decision-making is central to challenging defensive practice that can block people taking opportunities for growth and personal development. Working with risk and developing plans to enable service users to exercise their autonomy can be a stressful aspect of practice. This is enhanced if a culture of blame and unresolved conflicts exist within the multi-disciplinary team, particularly if the risk taken doesn't have the outcome that would have been desired. Promoting positive risk taking is supported by open communication in which the ethical dilemmas are acknowledged and explored by teams.

Although the individual virtues of the practitioner are important, within mental health services these are insufficient in isolation. They require the nurture and support of the multi-disciplinary team in which a culture of a values-based approach to decision-making can be developed. For example, the ethical components of a situation could be explored within a team meeting. Within this forum the nurse may acknowledge his/her anxiety surrounding a service user's safety and share the burden of responsibility. This also involves viewing service users in the context of their own networks and community, considering communication with relevant family and friends who they recognise as important in their life. Acknowledging the significance of these relationships could help reduce the likelihood of long-term dependence on the services. This is in line with a recovery approach which advocates enabling people to maintain or re-establish roles and relationships outside mental health services.

You have been working with Anita during your placement. She is 24 years old and has had contact with mental health services since she was 14 due to disruptive behaviour in school and continual angry outbursts towards people in authority who challenged her. Anita now has a diagnosis of personality disorder and has support from a community mental health nurse who visits her once a week at her home where she lives with her parents. Over the years Anita has been violent towards her parents and has been arrested on several occasions due to antisocial behaviour.

You have been supporting Anita to attend a self-help group which is aiming to improve how she copes with her distress. She has been attending regularly and seems to be taking on board the help she is receiving. However, you are aware that Anita now self-harms more regularly by cutting her arms and burning her legs. She tells you that she finds it helps her manage her anger without taking it out on others.

You are concerned that this way of expressing her anger is not helpful and whilst you can see how others perceive her behaviour as improving, you feel that she is directing her anger towards herself. Her family are pleased with her progress and her consultant psychiatrist regards her as less problematic. You seek supervision from your mentor and reflect on the way your feel towards the situation.

## Reflective Learning Activity

In relation to the scenario above, consider how the following influences might affect both your emotions and values:

- Personal feelings towards Anita (relationship)
- Personal beliefs about your role as a student mental health nurse and how other members of the multi-disciplinary team may respond to your perspective (person)
- Professional obligations to manage risk and protect Anita and others from harm (external principles)
- The reaction of family and other professionals to the situation (context).

Your reflections in supervision confirm that you feel a responsibility to advocate for Anita and, with her permission, you feedback to her family and other members of the team on how she is managing her distress. They were unaware that she continued to self-harm and agree to attend a meeting in which suggestions for how to move forward can be discussed with Anita. Anita feels worried about the prospect of attending this meeting and so you work together to decide how it should be facilitated so that she feels part of the decisions that are made.

## Summary

This chapter provides an overview of values in nursing practice, including both the historical and theoretical frameworks to values and the applied practice. Throughout the chapter there are several reflective learning activities that elaborate values in practice and encourage the reader to explore their personal meaning and understanding of the importance of values in their practice.

# References

Allmark, P. (1995) 'Can there be an ethics of care?', *Journal of Medical Ethics*, 21 (1): 19–24.

Armstrong, A.E. (2006) 'Towards a strong virtue ethics for nursing practice', *Nursing Philosophy*, 7 (3): 110–24.

Campbell, P. (2006) *Some Things You Should Know about User/Survivor Action: A Mind Resource Pack*. London: Mind Publications.

Colombo, A., Bendelo, G., Fulford, B. and William, S. (2003) 'Evaluating the influence of implicit models of mental disorder on the process of shared decision making within community-based multi-disciplinary teams', *Social Science and Medicine*, 56 (7): 1557–70.

Cooper, L. (2009) 'Values-based mental health nursing practice', in P. Callaghan, J. Playle and L. Cooper (eds), *Mental Health Nursing Skills*. Oxford: Oxford University Press.

Department of Health (2004) *The Ten Essential Shared Capabilities: A Framework for the Whole of the Mental Health Workforce*. London: Department of Health.

Department of Health (2006) *From Values to Action: The Chief Nursing Officer's Review of Mental Health Nursing*. London: Department of Health.

Double, D. (2006) *Critical Psychiatry: The Limits of Madness*. Basingstoke: Palgrave Macmillan.

Downie, R.S. and Calman, K.C. (1994) *Healthy Respect: Ethics in Health Care* (2nd edn). Oxford: Oxford University Press.

Dunn, S. (1999) *Creating Excepting Communities: Report of the Mind Enquiry into Social Exclusion and Mental Health Problems*. London: Mind.

Freshwater, D. and Westwood, T. (2006) 'Editorial. Risk detention and evidence: humanizing mental health reform', *Journal of Psychiatric and Mental Health Nursing*, 13 (3): 257–9.

Houghton, P. and Diamond, R. (2010) 'Values-based practice: a critique', *Clinical Psychology Forum*, 205: 24–7.

Hursthouse, R. (1999) *On Virtue Ethics*. Oxford: Oxford University Press.

Jones, A. (2006) 'Clinical supervision: what do we know and what do we need to know? A review and commentary', *Journal of Nursing Management*, 14 (8): 577–85.

McCarthy, J. (2006) 'A pluralist view of nursing ethics', *Nursing Philosophy*, 7 (3): 157–64.

McKie, A. and Swinton, J. (2000) 'Community, culture and character: the place of the virtues in psychiatric nursing practice', *Journal of Psychiatric and Mental Health Nursing Practice*, 7 (1): 35–42.

Morgan, J.F. (2007) *'Giving up the Culture of Blame': Risk Assessment and Risk Management in Psychiatric Practice*. Briefing document for the Royal College of Psychiatrists. London: RCP.

NMC (Nursing and Midwifery Council) (2008) *The Code: Standards of Conduct, Performance and Ethics for Nurses and Midwives*. London: Nursing and Midwifery Council.

Oxford Dictionary (2012) Available at: http://oxforddictionaries.com/ (accessed on: 14/8/2012).

Porter, R. (1991) *The Faber Book of Madness*. London: Faber and Faber.

Rachels, J. (1999) *The Elements of Moral Philosophy* (3rd edn). New York: McGraw-Hill.

Repper, J. and Perkins, R. (2003) *Social Inclusion and Recovery: A Model for Mental Health Practice*. Edinburgh: Baillère Tindall.

Rogers, C. (1967) *On Becoming a Person*. London: Constable.

SCMH (Sainsbury Centre for Mental Health) (1998) *Acute Problems: A Survey of the Quality of Care in Acute Psychiatric Wards*. London: Sainsbury Centre for Mental Health.

Stacey, G., Felton, A. and Bonham, B. (2012) *Placement Learning in Mental Health Nursing: A Guide for Students in Practice*. London: Elsevier.

Wilken, P. (1998) 'Clinical supervision and community psychiatric nursing', in T. Butterworth and J. Faugler (eds), *Clinical Supervision and Mentorship in Nursing*. 2nd edn. London: Chapman & Hall.

Woodbridge, K. and Fulford, K.W.M. (2003) 'Good practice? Values-based practice in mental health', *Mental Health Practice*, 7 (2): 30–4.

Woodbridge, K. and Fulford, K.W.M. (2004) *Whose Values? A Workbook for Values-based Practice in Mental Health Care*. London: Sainsbury Centre for Mental Health.

# 16

# Employment and Mental Health: Theoretical Approaches to Gaining and Maintaining Work

## LOUISE THOMSON

### Learning Objectives

- Describe the historical background and current policy and legislation concerning employment and mental health.
- Understand the basic tenets of some of the key psychological theories explaining how work can improve or worsen an individual's mental health and how individual factors affect work performance and job retention.
- Consider how these theories have informed interventions including workplace-based stress management initiatives, job retention practices and vocational rehabilitation interventions.

## Introduction

> Iron rusts from disuse; stagnant water loses its purity and in cold weather becomes frozen; even so does inaction sap the vigour of the mind. (Leonardo da Vinci, 1452–1519, *The Notebooks*)

It has long been acknowledged that purposeful activity is important for people's mental health, as illustrated in the quote above. Research has also consistently demonstrated the positive link between employment and mental health, showing that people who are in work generally have better mental health and also that when people become unemployed or are absent from work for long periods their mental health is likely to deteriorate (Waddell and Burton, 2006).

Although we know that work is good for mental health, the reality is that people with enduring mental health problems often find it difficult to find or stay in work. Employment statistics show that the rates of employment for people with different mental health problems are considerably lower than those for the population in general and for those with other forms of illness and disability. Figures from 2009 estimated that 13.5% of people with any mental illness and 3.4% of people receiving secondary mental health services were employed (NHS Information Centre, 2009). This compares with an employment rate of 72.5% for the working-age population as a whole, and 47.5% for people with any disability.

On the surface, the relationship between employment and mental health appears to be a straightforward one – people with moderate and severe mental health problems are less likely to be able to hold down a full-time job because the nature of their illness may affect their ability to work to a consistent and high standard. However, there are other possible explanations for the low employment rates seen. First, it is often unemployment that leads to deterioration in a person's mental health. Also, mental health problems that develop in childhood or adolescence can impact on the educational and training opportunities an individual has during childhood and youth, and which subsequently impair the preparation for work. In addition, the stigma and discrimination associated with mental health can also be a barrier to employment.

Many people with mental health problems are able to work and have successful careers, and surveys suggest that 70–90% of people with mental ill health consistently say they want to work (Grove, 1999; Secker et al., 2001). Increasing the employment rates for people with mental health conditions is not only important to help their recovery and prevent relapse, but it is also essential in changing the way in which people with a mental health condition are viewed in our society, challenging the myths and stereotypes of mental illness (Perkins et al., 2009).

## Historical development

When looking at the historical development of employment and mental health interventions and approaches, there are two distinct perspectives to consider: the health and social care perspective, and the employer and organisational perspective. Both of these perspectives have been influenced by government policy and legislation, and also by pioneering individuals and organisations who have developed innovative practices and new ways of thinking.

For health and social care organisations and their staff, work has long been considered part of therapy for mental health service users. Manual work was a core part of therapy in the pre-NHS asylums of the nineteenth century (Gould, 2008). The Retreat at York, founded by William Tuke in 1796, was at the forefront of developing 'moral treatment' of the mentally ill, and included a variety of occupations including farming, carpentry and gardening (Paterson, 2008). The early pioneers of the discipline of occupational therapy promoted the use of occupational activities as a therapeutic practice with the mentally ill in the early 1900s. And with the closure of asylums from the 1950s onwards, occupational therapists were increasingly sought to help the mentally ill to become productive and independent members of society. As community care developed, enterprises or workshops providing sheltered employment within a segregated work setting were used to prepare people for competitive employment (Gervey and Bedell, 1994). However, success rates were low at only 5–10% (Bond and Boyer, 1988; Connors et al., 1987), and more recently this pre-vocational sheltered employment approach has been superseded by supported employment approaches, such as Individual Placement and Support (IPS), which aims to place clients into competitive employment as quickly as possible with ongoing support (Sainsbury Centre for Mental Health, 2009). This approach will be discussed in more detail later in the chapter.

These type of practices are now referred to as vocational rehabilitation. The field of vocational rehabilitation (VR) has developed as a multi-disciplinary approach aiming to 'help someone with a health condition or disability to stay in, return to or move into work' (TUC, 2000). As well as occupational therapists, other professions such as psychologists, physiotherapists, case managers, employment advisers and support workers all address VR as part of their work. The key principles of VR that these groups work to are:

- The need to intervene early to prevent people from losing their jobs, as the longer someone is off work, the greater the obstacles to a successful return.
- The need for good quality case management.
- The importance of a 'biopsychosocial' approach, recognising the biological, psychological and social causes of illness and which considers all of these elements when helping someone obtain or retain work.

However, VR is still a developing area and under the current government's welfare to work policies many of these services are being contracted out to private and voluntary sector organisations. This has led to calls for better accreditation and training to develop a skilled workforce and the creation of standards for rehabilitation service providers (Sainsbury Centre for Mental Health, 2008).

Although there is now general agreement about best practice in VR and increasing amounts of evidence about the effectiveness of approaches, the extent to which these practices are widely implemented and used is less certain. A recent independent review of mental health and employment (Perkins et al., 2009) sets out a number of recommendations for government to better help more people with mental health conditions who are workless into sustained employment. These recommendations fall into three broad groups:

- Increasing capacity and dispelling myths within existing structures so they are better able to meet the needs of people with a mental health condition.
- 'Model of more support': implementing IPS in a UK context.
- Establishing effective systems for monitoring outcomes and driving change.

The employers' perspective is rather different as the issue of mental health in the workplace has only received widespread recognition relatively recently. Increasing numbers of cases of workplace stress in the 1980s and 1990s, and the litigation that was often associated with them, led to organisations setting in place policies and procedures to manage mental health in the workplace. Responsibility for mental health in the workplace is traditionally shared by human resources departments, who oversee all aspects of personnel management, and occupational health physicians and nurses, who tend to be employed by larger organisations. However, in recent years there has been increasing recognition that line managers play a vital role in identifying and managing mental health problems in the workplace (Yarker et al., 2007). For all of these parties, the priority from the organisational perspective is to maximise employees' performance whilst maintaining a healthy work environment and a healthy and diverse workforce.

A few groups have played a significant role in the development of the employers' perspective. Over the last 40 years, occupational psychologists have led the development of theories of work-related stress, anxiety and depression, and interventions to manage and reduce their impact. Their approach has focused largely on identifying and reducing the hazards in the work environment that increase the risks of poor mental health, but also understanding the cognitive processes involved in appraising these hazards (Fingret, 2000).

Charitable and campaigning groups, such as Mind and the Centre for Mental Health (formerly the Sainsbury Centre for Mental Health), have played an important role in promoting employment for people with mental health problems, and working with both health care organisations and employers. As well as campaigning for and promoting better awareness and practices (e.g. Mind, 2011), they have also reviewed the evidence on the effectiveness of workplace interventions (Seymour, 2010; Seymour and Grove, 2005), and supported employment interventions through training and accreditation programmes for both health care staff and employers.

The differences in the overall purpose of these two parties (health care providers and employers) and the historical developments in their fields go a long way to explain their different perspectives. Where these perspectives merge is when considering health and social care organisations as employers, how they manage the mental health of their staff, and whether they recruit people with existing mental health problems, thus leading by example (Seebohm and Grove, 2006).

## The legislation

Another factor that brings the two perspectives of health care and employers closer together is the shared legal context. Both health and safety legislation and anti-discrimination legislation apply to employment and mental health. Two pieces of health and safety legislation place legal requirements upon employers to protect the health of their employees: the Health and Safety at Work Act (1974) and the Management of Health and Safety at Work Regulations (1999). Under this legislation employers have a duty to assess the risks of ill health (including mental ill health) arising from work activities and to take measures to control that risk.

---

### Box 16.1   The HSE Management Standards for stress

- Demand – workload, work pattern and the work environment.
- Control – how much say persons have about the way they do their work.
- Support – the encouragement, sponsorship and resources provided by the employer, line management and colleagues.
- Relationships – promoting positive working to avoid conflict and dealing with unacceptable behaviour.
- Role – understanding one's role within the organisation and avoiding conflicting roles.
- Change – how organisational change (large or small) is managed and communicated in the organisation.

To help to encourage employers to meet their legal obligations, the UK Health and Safety Executive (HSE) have developed a set of Management Standards – six key areas that, if not properly managed, are associated with poor health and well-being, lower productivity and increased sickness absence (Box 16.1). The HSE (2007) has published a comprehensive risk assessment approach to identifying, exploring and tackling work-related stress to help employers using the Management Standards to manage the causes of such stress and other common mental health problems. These tools have given employers a firm basis to allow them to meet their legal obligations and duty of care to their employees.

The last 20 years have seen momentous changes in anti-discrimination laws in the UK that have had an impact on employment for people with long-term mental health problems. The Disability Discrimination Act (DDA) of 1995 was the first piece of legislation that dealt directly with the issue of discrimination due to disability. It defined a person with a disability as someone with a physical or mental impairment which has a substantial and long-term adverse effect on his/her ability to carry out normal day-to-day activities. The DDA enabled people with long-term mental health problems to take their employer to an employment tribunal if they felt they had been discriminated against because of their mental health problem. The employer would be deemed to have discriminated against the employee if:

- For a reason which relates to that person's disability, the employer treats that person less favourably than he/she treats or would treat others to whom that reason does not or would not apply; or
- The employer fails to comply with a duty to make reasonable adjustments imposed on him/her in relation to the disabled person; or
- The employer allows harassment of a disabled employee.

The DDA was amended a number of times during the 1990s and was in need of further updating. So in 2010 it was superseded by the Equality Act. This brought together disability discrimination with discrimination against other 'protected characteristics' including age, gender, race and religion. One of the main changes that the Equality Act brought was acknowledging an increased number of different ways in which discrimination can arise. For example, perception discrimination is included, which is direct discrimination against an individual because others *think* they have a mental health problem, regardless of whether they do or do not. Victimisation is also included. This occurs when an employee is treated badly because he or she has made or supported a complaint or raised a grievance under the Equality Act; or is suspected of doing so. The Equality Act also limits the circumstances when employers can use pre-employment health checks to ask health-related questions before offering an individual a job.

Developments in the legislation over the last 15–20 years have had a big impact on employers in particular. Not only has the threat of employment tribunals, HSE enforcements and legal cases brought by employees focused employers on their legal obligations, but the associated guidance has prompted and supported many employers (predominantly the larger organisations) to take progressive steps to deal more effectively with mental health problems in the workplace and the diversity of their workforce.

## Recent government initiatives

The UK government has recently increased its focus on supporting better employment for people with mental health problems. This is largely in light of the increasing costs of health care, unemployment and incapacity benefits and long-term sickness absence associated with mental health problems, which have been estimated as £26 billion per year (Sainsbury Centre for Mental Health, 2007). Employment and mental health has been the topic for recent cross-government reports and recommendations, which include: *Working our Way to Better Mental Health* (2009), the first national framework for mental health and employment; *New Horizons: A Shared Vision for Mental Health* (2009), a cross-government programme of action for mental health; and *Work, Recovery and Inclusion: Realising Ambitions* (2009), the government's response to the Perkins Review, *Realising Ambitions: Better Employment Support for People with a Mental Health Condition* (Perkins et al., 2009). Together, these three documents set out a vision of employment as a central part of recovery from mental health problems, and provide three areas of focus for action:

- Promoting healthy workplaces to prevent mental health problems from developing or being made worse by work.
- Enabling job retention for people who develop mental health problems in work.
- Providing vocational rehabilitation support for people with mental health problems who want to gain employment.

We will revisit these three areas of intervention later in the chapter when we discuss how theory is applied to practice.

# Theories of employment and mental health

In this section, some of the psychological theories explaining the relationship between employment and mental health and well-being will first be described. Following that, we will turn our attention to some of the more individual-focused theories that have informed job retention and vocational rehabilitation practices. However, it is worth noting at this point that many vocational rehabilitation practices in particular are more evidence-based and practical in nature rather than theoretically based (Elliott and Leung, 2005).

Theories on the role of work in maintaining mental health and well-being have largely focused on the environmental factors to do with the nature of work and employment more generally. One of the earliest theories was developed by Marie Jahoda, an Austrian psychologist. Jahoda (1979, 1982) studied the impact of large-scale unemployment on the small industrial community of Marienthal. She looked beyond the obvious economic consequences of job loss to explore the psychological meaning of employment and unemployment. Through her observations, she developed the theory of the latent benefits of work which identified five categories which she said were vital to feelings of well-being (see Box 16.2). These latent benefits that work provided were the structuring of time, social contact outside the family, a wider purpose or goals, social status or identity and regular activity. She maintained that the unemployed were deprived of all five, and that this accounted for much of the reported mental ill health among unemployed people.

---

## Box 16.2   Jahoda's five latent benefits of work

- Time structure
- Social contact
- Collective purpose
- Social identity
- Regular activity

---

Other theorists have argued that Jahoda's approach is too simplistic as not *all* employment has a positive psychological impact. More complex theories have since been proposed that look at the component characteristics of a job, rather than its mere presence or absence, and how these impact on mental health and well-being. Warr (1987) identified nine job characteristics which were features of 'psychologically good' employment (see Box 16.3). He recognised that many of these job characteristics could both promote and impair mental health, depending on their level and duration. Some of the job characteristics have constant effects, with increases in these leading to ever improving well-being and mental health (e.g. money, valued social position). But as other job characteristics increase, they do not lead to further improvements in well-being but start to have a detrimental effect (e.g. variety, skill use, job control). Warr calls these 'additional decrement' factors. Because of the similarity of these effects to the actions seen by vitamins on physical health (vitamins A and D being beneficial up to a certain point at which they start to become harmful, but vitamins C and E having a constant effect), Warr called his theory the Vitamin Model.

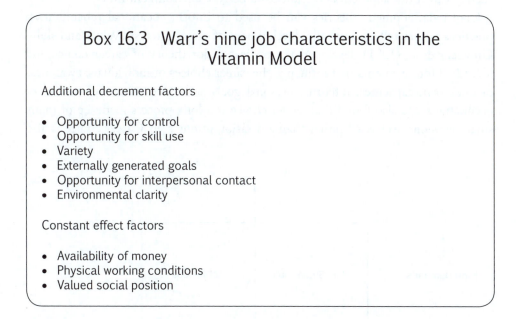

## Box 16.3   Warr's nine job characteristics in the Vitamin Model

Additional decrement factors

- Opportunity for control
- Opportunity for skill use
- Variety
- Externally generated goals
- Opportunity for interpersonal contact
- Environmental clarity

Constant effect factors

- Availability of money
- Physical working conditions
- Valued social position

One of the most widely studied and empirically supported theories of work and health is the Job Demands–Control Model (Karasek and Theorell, 1990). This model (Figure 16.1) focuses on the important role of two work characteristics in determining individuals' health and well-being – that of job demands and control over work. Job demands refer to the psychological demands and requirements at work, the difficulty of tasks and the pressure associated with them. Job control is the extent to which employees have the potential to control their tasks and conduct their working day. The central tenet of the theory is that having high levels of control over your work is good for health and mitigates the negative effects of having high levels of job demand. 'High strain' jobs are worst for health, i.e. a combination of high demands and low control. However, there is some debate as to which combination of demands and control is best for health – the low demands and high control of 'low strain' jobs or the high demands and high control of 'active' jobs.

The theories described above focus on the qualities and functions of the work environment and the impact they have on mental health. As we shall see in the next section, these theories have informed interventions for developing healthy workplaces and the management of common mental health problems in the workplace.

An additional set of theories inform job retention practices and vocational rehabilitation practices. These theories tend to focus more on aspects of the individual such as career development and choice and person–environment fit.

Career development theories can be used to inform vocational rehabilitation practices as they tell us about the development of career interests, values and skills. Ginzberg et al. (1951) developed the earliest major theory of career choice and identified four elements that influence the career choices of individuals: awareness of one's own capacities; interests; personal goals and values; time perspective of occupations. He also found that career choice is a long process made up of many small decisions over years rather than a decision in one step. Career choice is also

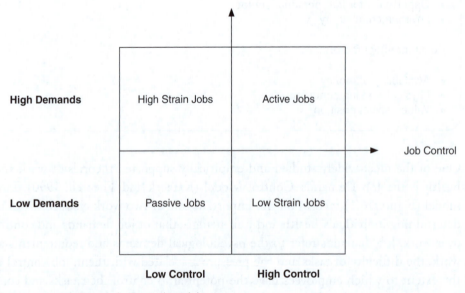

**FIGURE 16.1**   Job Demands-Control Model

determined by the opportunities available to an individual, and his or her knowledge about how to access them.

Person–environment fit theories go further to acknowledge the complex ways in which the characteristics of the person, their values, interests and skills, interact with the work environment. The Minnesota Theory of Work Adjustment (Dawis and Lofquist, 1984) is an example of this. According to this theory, work is conceptualised as an interaction between an individual and a work environment. The work environment requires that certain tasks be performed, and the individual has skills, values and personality traits that enable them to perform the tasks. In return, the individual requires compensation for work performance (i.e. a wage) and certain preferred conditions, such as a safe and comfortable place to work. The requirements of both the individual and the work environment need to be met, and the degree to which this happens is called 'correspondence'. Work adjustment is the process of achieving and maintaining correspondence. If there is a good match between the two, this will lead to increased levels of satisfaction in the individual and ongoing tenure with the organisation. If the individual becomes unable to meet the requirements of the work environment, either the work can be adjusted to meet the skills and abilities of the individual, or the individual can be trained or developed to be able to perform the tasks necessary in the work environment.

# Theory applied to practice

Here we will explore how the theories described above have influenced and informed the policies and practices concerning employment and mental health.

## Healthy workplace practices

Theories of work characteristics that promote and impair mental health have led directly to many of the key interventions to prevent work-related mental health problems. Aspects of Warr's Vitamin Model (1987) and Karasek and Theorell's Job Demands–Control Model (1990) have been tested empirically in numerous studies over the last 25 years and consistent relationships between these work characteristics and work-related health have been found. Based on this evidence, approaches to the prevention and management of work-related stress have used a variety of methods to assess the presence of these work characteristics in the organisation and make recommendations to control or reduce them. Some of these approaches have used standardised checklists (e.g. Occupational Stress Indicator; Cooper et al.,

1998) whilst others have used more context-specific measures to make risk assessments of the psychosocial hazards (Cox et al., 2000).

Following a review of the evidence on the effects of these work characteristics (Rick et al., 2002), the HSE developed and published its Management Standards for preventing and managing work-related stress (HSE, 2007). This national guidance on how to assess and manage work-related stress, and the associated measurement tools, are based on the theories of work characteristics and health described above.

## Job retention practices

Current practices to support job retention for people who develop mild to moderate mental health problems lean heavily on principles of person x environment fit theories. In particular, the Theory of Workplace Adjustment has informed a number of the key elements of job retention practices.

When someone has been absent from work due to mental health problems, their return to work needs to be carefully managed and coordinated in order for them to successfully retain their job. Best practice in this area has highlighted the importance of flexible return-to-work options and work adaptations and adjustments in achieving a successful return to work (Thomson et al., 2003). Flexible return-to-work options include a phased return which allows individuals to come back part-time initially and to gradually increase their hours as they feel able. It can also include amended duties, where individuals return to certain aspects of their job, and gradually increase the tasks or responsibilities that they have at an appropriate and agreed time. Workplace adaptation could include providing additional equipment or training, relocating work to a different premise or to the individual's home, providing a mentor or buddy, giving additional supervision or support for a task, allowing additional breaks. All of these job retention strategies acknowledge that, after a period of mental ill health, the person and environment may not achieve a good fit, or 'correspondence'. To enable the fit between the person and environment to be restored, temporary adjustments need to be made to the environment to accommodate the recovery needs of the person.

## Vocational rehabilitation practices

Vocational rehabilitation involves the provision of services to enhance the employability of an individual who has been limited by a disabling health condition (Elliott and Leung, 2005). Traditional approaches to vocational rehabilitation have been characterised by pre-employment training in sheltered settings. The aim of these 'train then place' approaches was to improve the skills and prepare people for competitive employment. However, there were a number of problems with this approach.

It was argued that, not only was it ineffective in developing the skills necessary for employment, but it also promoted dependency and deterred clients from finding competitive employment (Bilby, 1992; Bond et al., 1997).

In traditional approaches to VR the principles are drawn from a variety of sources, including general medical rehabilitation traditions, disability support service practices, assertive and strengths-based case management and other established principles in psychosocial rehabilitation (Waghorn et al., 2009). Traditional practices often take a step-by-step approach, gradually moving towards employment with little urgency. They also demonstrate segregation between the health care treatment and the vocational services.

A new approach to vocational rehabilitation emerged during the 1980s which focused on placing clients in paid work in normal work settings as quickly as possible and then providing them with training and support in those jobs (Becker and Drake, 1994). This 'place then train' approach became known as supported employment. The most carefully specified and well-established form of supported employment is Individual Placement and Support (IPS). The IPS approach has eight key principles, shown in Box 16.4, which should be closely followed in order for it to be effective.

---

## Box 16.4   Core principles of IPS supported employment

1 Every person with severe mental illness who wants to work is eligible for IPS supported employment.
2 Employment services are integrated with mental health treatment services.
3 Competitive employment is the goal.
4 Personalised benefits counselling is provided.
5 The job search starts soon after a person expresses interest in working.
6 Employment specialists systematically develop relationships with employers based upon their client's work preferences.
7 Job supports are continuous.
8 Client preferences are honoured.

---

A number of high quality studies (randomised controlled trials) have examined the effectiveness of IPS in comparison to other 'train then place' approaches to vocational rehabilitation. Bringing together the results of these studies, Bond et al. (2008) found that sites most closely following the principles of the IPS approach were most effective, with an average of 61% of participants gaining employment compared to a 23% employment rate in sites that followed other approaches. A more recent review of the effectiveness of IPS looked at the results of 18 high quality studies, and again found that supported employment approaches were significantly more effective than pre-vocational training in obtaining employment, but also that supported employment clients earned more and worked more hours per month than those in pre-vocational training (Crowther et al., 2010). For example, at 18 months 34% of people in supported employment were employed versus 12% in pre-vocational training.

Although IPS is promoted as an evidence-based approach (i.e. evidence shows that it works, so we should use it in practice) it does have some basis in theory. In particular, IPS is much more in line with career development theories than traditional VR approaches as it acknowledges the importance of a person's career interests, values and goals rather than just their abilities. A key feature of IPS is co-location of vocational services and the mental health team. A dedicated employment specialist has primary responsibility for implementing the intervention, but works closely with the community mental health team to address individual vocational needs and help to ensure that vocational goals are given a high priority within the mental health care plan (Rinaldi et al., 2008). Thus individual occupational goals and motivations are given high priority in this approach, rather than basing the intervention on a health professional's assessment of a client's ability to work.

## CASE EXAMPLE

John had been working in a warehouse since leaving school at the age of 16. In his early twenties he suffered a number of episodes of moderate depression which coincided with significant life events including the death of his father and the breaking up with his partner of three years. He did not tell anyone at work about the problems he was having, and his poor performance and attendance at work during this period were put down to 'laziness and bad attitude' by his managers. He ended up losing his job, and the increased financial hardship, lack of purpose and isolation he then experienced led to a more severe bout of depression. He was finally admitted to a psychiatric hospital after a failed suicide attempt. Once in the care of the community mental health team, John was asked if he wanted to talk to the employment specialist in the team about getting back into work. Initially John was sceptical as he felt that he would not be able to hold down a job as he had good days and bad days. But the employment specialist, working closely with John's care coordinator, helped to build his self-esteem and explore the kind of work he could envisage doing. He helped John with his CV and interview technique, and found some job vacancies that John was interested in applying for. After a few months, John got a part-time job at a local supermarket. His employment specialist continued to help him by teaching him coping strategies to use at work, talking to John's new employers about how they could give him the support he needed at work, and being there for John when he a needed some extra help and support. John and his line manager developed a good working relationship which allowed John to be open about the difficulties he may be experiencing and ask for help when he needed it. His line manager maintained enough flexibility to be able to let John work in the store rooms – where there was less pressure and no customer interaction required – if he was having a bad day. As John grew in confidence, he took on more duties and hours and also developed new friendships among his workmates. John's employment has provided him with more money, a structure and routine, relationships and a sense of personal fulfilment – all of which have made a contribution to his recovery.

## Summary

Employers and society in general have a responsibility to prevent mental ill health where possible, accommodate mental health problems in the workplace, acknowledge the capacity for work that people with mental health problems have and support their recovery through work where possible. There are three key areas to target in achieving this: the promotion of healthy workplaces providing well-designed and well-managed work which is good for mental health; early intervention for people who develop mental health problems whilst employed, to support their job retention and recovery; and help for people who want to work to find competitive jobs and to retain them with ongoing support. As we have seen, a number of theories have informed current practice in these areas. In addition to the theory, there are very practical elements that are needed to make these interventions work – many of which concern effective interactions between people with different roles. For example, an understanding line manager who can talk sensitively to his or her employees, a dedicated case manager who can juggle the needs of the employee returning to work with the demands of the human resources department or line manager, and an employment specialist working closely with the community mental health team to find work for his/her patients. To achieve better employment rates and more healthy workplaces for people with mental health problems it is not only vital that we have theoretically based interventions the effectiveness of which are empirically tested, but it is also crucial that all parties involved in delivering or receiving these interventions work together towards these aims.

# References

Becker, D.R. and Drake, R.E. (1994) 'Individual placement and support: a community mental health center approach to vocational rehabilitation', *Community Mental Health Journal*, 30 (2): 193–206.

Bilby, R. (1992) 'A response to the criticisms of transitional employment', *Psychosocial Rehabilitation Journal*, 16 (2): 69–82.

Bond, G.R. and Boyer, S.B. (1988) 'Rehabilitation programs and outcomes', in J.A. Ciardiello (ed.), *Vocational Rehabilitation of Persons with Prolonged Mental Illness*. Baltimore: Johns Hopkins University Press.

Bond, G.R., Drake, R.E., Mueser, K.T. and Becker, D.R. (1997) 'An update on supported employment for people with severe mental illness', *Psychiatric Services*, 48 (3): 335–46.

Bond, G.R., Drake, R.E. and Becker, D.R. (2008) 'An update on randomized controlled trials of evidence-based supported employment', *Psychiatric Rehabilitation Journal*, 31 (4): 280–9.

Connors, K.A., Graham, R.S. and Pulso, R. (1987) 'Playing the store: where is the vocational in psychiatric rehabilitation?', *Psychosocial Rehabilitation Journal*, 10 (3): 21–33.

Cooper, C.L., Sloan, S.J. and Williams, S. (1998) *Occupational Stress Indicator*. Windsor: Nelson.

Cox, T., Griffiths, A., Barlow, C., Randall, R., Thomson, L. and Rial-Gonzalez, E. (2000) *Organisational Interventions for Work Stress: A Risk Management Approach*. London: HSE Books.

Crowther, R., Marshall, M., Bond, G.R. and Huxley, P. (2010) *Vocational Rehabilitation for People with Severe Mental Illness (Review)*. Cochrane Library. Available at: http://onlinelibrary.wiley.com/doi/10.1002/14651858.CD003080/pdf (accessed on: 5/9/2012).

Dawis, R.V. and Lofquist, L.H. (1984) *A Psychological Theory of Work Adjustment*. Minneapolis: University of Minnesota Press.

Elliott, T.R. and Leung, P. (2005) 'Vocational rehabilitation: history and practice', in B.W. Walsh and M.L. Savickas (eds), *Handbook of Vocational Psychology* (3rd edn). Mahwah, NJ: Lawrence Erlbaum Associates.

Fingret, A. (2000) 'Occupational mental health: a brief history', *Occupational Medicine* 50 (5): 289–93.

Gervey, R. and Bedell, J.R. (1994) 'Psychological assessment and treatment of persons with severe mental disorders', in J.R. Bedell (ed.), *Supported Employment in Vocational Rehabilitation*. Washington, DC: Taylor and Francis.

Ginzberg, E., Ginsburg, S.W., Axelrad, S. and Herma, J.L. (1951) *Occupational Choice: An Approach to a General Theory*. New York: Columbia University Press.

Grove, B. (1999) 'Mental health and employment: Shaping a new agenda', *Journal of Mental Health*, 8 (2): 131–40.

Gould, M. (2008) 'Mental health history: taking over the asylum', *Health Service Journal*, May. Available at: www.hsj.co.uk/resource-centre/mental-health-history-taking-over-the-asylum/1136349.article (accessed 21/3/2013).

Health, Work and Well-being Programme (2009) *Working our Way to Better Mental Health: A Framework for Action*. Norwich: TSO.

HM Government (2009) *New Horizons: A Shared Vision for Mental Health*. London: COI.

HM Government (2009) *Work, Recovery and Inclusion: Realising Ambitions*. London: NMHDU.

HSE (Health and Safety Executive) (2007) *Managing the Causes of Work Related Stress: A Step-by Step Approach Using the Management Standards*. London: HSE Books.

Jahoda, M. (1979) 'The impact of unemployment in the 1930s and the 1970s', *Bulletin of the British Psychological Society*, 32 (2): 309–14.

Jahoda, M. (1982) *Employment and Unemployment: A Social-psychological Analysis*. Cambridge: Cambridge University Press.

Karasek, R.A. and Theorell, T. (1990) *Healthy Work: Stress, Productivity and the Reconstruction of Working Life*. New York: Basic Books.

Mind (2011) *Taking Care of Business: Employers' Guide to Mentally Healthy Workplaces*. London: Mind.

NHS Information Centre, Adult Social Care Statistics Team, Community and Mental Health Team (2009) *Social Care and Mental Health Indicators from the National Indicator Set – Further Analysis 2008–09*. Leeds: NHS Information Centre.

Paterson, C.F. (2008) 'A short history of occupational therapy in psychiatry', in J. Creek and L. Lougher (eds), *Occupational Therapy and Mental Health*. Philadelphia: Elsevier.

Perkins, R., Farmer, P. and Litchfield, P. (2009) *Realising Ambitions: Better Employment Support for People with a Mental Health Condition*. London: The Stationery Office.

Rick, J., Thomson, L., Briner, R., O'Regan, S. and Daniels, K. (2002) *Review of Existing Supporting Scientific Knowledge to Underpin Standards of Good Practice for Key Work – Related Stressors: Phase 1*. London: HSE Books.

Rinaldi, M., Perkins, R., Glynn, E., Montibeller, T., Clenaghan, M. and Rutherford, J. (2008) 'Individual placement and support: from research to practice', *Advances in Psychiatric Treatment*, 14 (1): 50–60.

Sainsbury Centre for Mental Health (2007) *Mental Health at Work: Developing the Business Case*. London: Sainsbury Centre for Mental Health.

Sainsbury Centre for Mental Health (2008) *Vocational Rehabilitation: What is it, Who can Deliver it, and Who Pays?* London: Sainsbury Centre for Mental Health.

Sainsbury Centre for Mental Health (2009) *Doing What Works: Individual Placement and Support into Employment*. London: Sainsbury Centre for Mental Health.

Secker, J., Grove, B. and Seebohm, P. (2001) 'Challenging barriers to employment, training and education for mental health service users: the service user's perspective', *Journal of Mental Health*, 10 (4): 395–404.

Seebohm, P. and Grove, B. (2006) *Leading by Example*. London: Sainsbury Centre for Mental Health.

Seymour, L. (2010) *Common Mental Health Problems at Work: What We Know about Successful Interventions. A Progress Review.* London: Sainsbury Centre for Mental Health.

Seymour, L. and Grove, B. (2005) *Workplace Interventions for People with Common Mental Health Problems.* London: British Occupational Health Research Foundation.

Thomson, L., Neathey, F. and Rick, J. (2003) *Best Practice in Rehabilitating Employees Following Absence due to Work-related Stress.* London: HSE Books.

TUC (Trades Union Congress) (2000) *Getting Better at Getting Back: Consultation Document on Rehabilitation.* London: TUC.

Waddell, G. and Burton, A.K. (2006) *Is Work Good for Your Health and Well-being?* Norwich: The Stationery Office.

Waghorn, G., Lloyd, C. and Clune, A. (2009) 'Reviewing the theory and practice of occupational therapy in mental health rehabilitation', *British Journal of Occupational Therapy*, 72 (7): 314–23.

Warr, P. (1987) *Work, Unemployment, and Mental Health.* Oxford: Clarendon Press.

Yarker, J., Donaldson-Feilder, E., Lewis, R. and Flaxman, P.E. (2007) *Management Competencies for Preventing and Reducing Stress at Work: Identifying and Developing the Management Behaviours Necessary to Implement the HSE Management Standards.* London: HSE Books.

# 17

# Solution Focused Nursing

## MARGARET McALLISTER

### Learning Objectives

- Observe the quality of your interactions with consumers or colleagues.
- Reflect on how you have been or could be more future-focused about ways these people are living and working.
- Cultivate and share strategies to assist people to live and work more productively.
- Understand and appreciate the thinkers that came before and influenced the development of solution focused nursing, as well as those who are practising solution focused work today.
- Expand your communication skills repertoire to include some of the solution focused strategies that are explained.

## Introduction

Solution focused nursing is a postmodern and middle range (as compared with a grand) theory for nursing. Theory development in nursing has been influenced by modernist and postmodernist schools of thought. Modernism as it relates to nursing has an emphasis on producing an overarching description of what nursing means, in order to differentiate itself from medicine and to promote the profession's development. Such theories have been useful in describing the nature, mission and goals of nursing. Because they offer a large, conceptual view of nursing they have been termed grand theories. Examples include Roy's Adaptation Model, Gordon's Functional Health Patterns and Leininger's Theory of Culture Care Diversity and Universality (Peterson and Bredow, 2013).

In mental health, modernist therapeutic approaches have been heavily influenced by biological determinism and stage theories of human development. Both tend to suggest that people experience things in similar ways. Whilst this might be true from a macro-perspective, at the individual level, people are different and will see their situation and handle their difficulties in unique ways.

Postmodernism does not believe in universal truths that exist and persist regardless of context, preferring instead the notion that theories can be meaningful for some groups, at some times, for some issues (Reed, 1995). Thus, middle range theories are those that are more focused on specific areas of nursing. They tend to be less abstract and more open to testing and verification. Middle range theories sit between grand theories that provide a conception of the whole of nursing, and hypothesis development that occurs during day-to-day research to find answers to problems.

Solution focused nursing provides a rationale and strategies for communicating with people in purposeful ways so that improvements are envisioned and specific goals are worked towards. Improvement approaches that take a 'solutions focus' have been applied in many fields – with children in schools, employees in workplaces, processes in business and with consumers in the therapeutic context. It is a practice that emerged around the 1970s, during a time when there was significant questioning about the superiority of problem-oriented thinking and on what helps people change. To understand solution focused nursing, it is therefore useful to consider historical developments in thinking that took place in the mid- to late twentieth century.

This chapter will summarise the body of work that preceded the emergence of solution focused nursing (SFN) (McAllister, 2007) as a separate concept unique to nursing, and show how learners can use it to empower their practice. Unlike some of the other chapters in this book, this one starts with a case example which explains why a theory such as SFN can enhance professional practice.

Whenever anyone begins to use a conceptual framework to guide their practice, practice becomes more strategic and less vulnerable to becoming directionless. It's sad that too many nurses fail to consciously use a theory to drive their practice – instead preferring to rely on their gut feelings, personal experiences, or acquired strategies absorbed in the process of watching how peers or predecessors have acted. Of course not all of these ways of acting are necessarily bad or ineffective, but they aren't easily able to be articulated, shared or open to revision. And the public, consumers, clients and professional colleagues deserve more than this from someone purporting to be a professional nurse.

In my experience, students of nursing are eager to learn the ideals for nursing, and want frameworks and structures to help them stay focused, encourage clear thinking and are helpful during complex health care situations. It's just that some of the theories, and, importantly, *how they are explained to students*, have failed in their objective of illuminating practice. Consider Paula's story.

Paula is a first year university nursing student who, like many students in Australia, works as an assistant in nursing (AIN) at a large nursing home as a way to provide income to support her full-time studies. She recalled a recent experience.

At the nursing home the other day, I had a guy (Mr Smith) who buzzed and called out that he wanted a shower because he had wet himself. I was carrying a mountain of linen and had already showered three people by this stage. I asked another AIN to lend a hand, but she refused. 'I'm not going near him!' She retorted, 'He's so rude! He just called me a bitch. So sorry, but I'm not helping you. You'll have to work that one out for yourself.'

Because of the things I had been learning at university, I knew that I couldn't ignore him. My attitude is that everyone deserves good quality care. But I still had no clue how to deal with him. I felt scared. I didn't want to get punched. But what could I say to him? He was bigger than me, he had dementia, and he hated being touched!

This situation is the perfect example of when a memorable and simple framework to guide nursing would be an immediate asset to Paula, and of course to the consumer who needs her care. She has no role models to guide her, no previous experience, not even gut feeling is telling her what to do. She went on:

Anyway, somehow I just had to pull it all together. Then and there I had to make a decision as to whether to shower or change him. I had to try and compose myself so that I wasn't upset and make the whole thing worse. I knew I needed to be calm, and be nice. I knew I needed to be a leader for the other nurses, but I just didn't know how!

The thing about coming to university is that I know now that it's not good to be judgemental, and that attitudes most people have towards people who have illnesses like dementia are not good, they cause stigma. And I also knew that the gentleman's mood would only get worse if I responded the same way, but no one teaches you how to be non-judgemental and how to not take people's anger or frustration to heart.

There are two key insights in Paula's commentary here. The first is that Paula has an awareness of her own impact on a person's psychosocial well-being and the second point is that she has identified her knowledge gap. She has reached a teachable moment.

If only Paula had a guide with her, so that she could act proactively with Mr Smith, since she has been able to identify the weakness in being reactive. If she had a solution focused framework she might see that:

1 The decision she felt was hers to make would actually be a shared decision, one that the consumer could participate in.
2 Going in with a conscious intent to be genuine, accepting and empathic (Rogers, 1975), as well having a respectful curiosity about this person's unique needs and desires (De Shazer, 1985), will help her to put the anger in its place.
3 Having a view towards the future (and not what's happened in the past, or even what's occurring in the present) may be a way that Paula can stay focused, helpful and optimistic.

These are the principles that underpin solution focused nursing – and show people like Paula how nurses can be goal-directed with any challenge that they are likely to encounter.

Knowing how to nurse is an ability that encompasses a balance between knowledge, caring attributes and psychomotor skills. It may come naturally to some people, but most nurses will need a framework to provide them with nursing know-how. Without it, there is a very real risk that students, graduates and experienced nurses will have their professional behaviour and thinking shaped, constrained and perhaps reduced to the more dominant, and pervasive medical model. This is where theory of nursing can come into its own. Nursing theory is valuable in both articulating and protecting that which is fundamentally nursing in nature. Solution focused nursing is one such theory that aims to articulate and extend nursing know-how.

And it's easy to remember.

1 What is happening here that could be changed?
2 How can we give *more* space to this imagined change, than the present problem?
3 What are the steps being made towards change that we need to notice and reinforce?

So, solution focused nursing emphasises the future, not so much the problem at hand. It appreciates that even the most problem-laden person or issue has positives. By harnessing those strengths, and building them up, the problem part will start to become less dominating or pervasive, and people can begin to see themselves as more capable. By thinking about strengths in a situation and not just risks and vulnerabilities, people start to develop a hopeful vision which is motivating.

# Historical development

Two important philosophical assumptions that underpin solution oriented work are: social constructionism and a strengths perspective.

## Social constructionism

Social constructionism is a view that reality is not universal and unchanging, but rather constructed, shaped and experienced (Berger and Luckmann, 1966). Let's take gender as an example. If we want to talk about the social construction of gender, it means that gender, as currently understood, is not an inevitable result of biology, but dependent on social and historical processes. The idea that girls like to wear pink is a social construction. Less than a hundred years ago it was actually the reverse and girls more commonly dressed in blue (Frassanito and Pettorini, 2008). Thus, a social construction is not a given fact, but a commonplace understanding of the world, and when it is harmful might be better modified or replaced.

Social constructionist therapies acknowledge that mental health problems are not facts, or given illnesses that are unchanging, they are experienced differently by people, depending on social and historical processes. So in the helping context, there is a view that enduring change is unlikely to be made by the expert clinician applying his/her own diagnosis and treatment for a problem. Instead, people are more likely to feel supported and heard if the helper takes an empathic stance, acknowledges that people are the experts of their own experience, and works with them to develop skills for recovery.

On the other hand, alternative models of change, such as psychoanalytic therapy, tend to assume that causes of problems are best understood by finding out what the root cause is. In psychology these approaches are known as depth psychology. Compare the two images of therapeutic interactions shown in Figures 17.1 and 17.2.

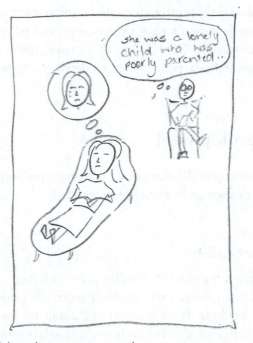

**FIGURE 17.1**  Traditional deep therapeutic approach

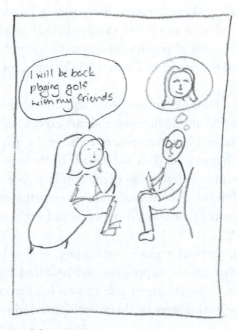

**FIGURE 17.2**  Solution focused therapy

In Figure 17.1, you might notice that it is the therapist who is doing the interpreting, the work is not really mutually distributed, it is the past that is being considered and the deficits about the person are the focus. In Figure 17.2, you will notice the client is engaged in the analytical work, the future is being imagined, and strengths not deficits are being explored.

Applied to the mental health nursing context, something like depression could be seen as socially constructed. Rather than consider that depression is a single illness that can only be diagnosed by expert therapists who must spend their time looking deeply into the patient's past, what matters is the person and the person's feelings of sadness, how that sadness is affecting the person's life, and what he or she wants to do about it. Solution focused therapy gives the past respectful recognition, but it doesn't dwell there. Instead, it builds on positive expectations for the future.

While all of this may make good sense, unfortunately most clinicians do not consciously view the world through a social constructionist lens. It remains quite a marginalised approach. The more dominant approach to health care and to helping people is to use a more deterministic approach – such as to favour biological theories over cultural theories. So in most clinical situations, depression is seen as an illness that can be diagnosed by an expert and treated with antidepressant medications. While this could be an effective way of looking at depression for some people, for the majority depression won't simply vanish by taking a pill. It requires individuals to agree that they are depressed, they need to work on ways to bring happiness into their life, and to keep doing what's working so that they will remain well.

Social constructionism applied to nursing means that nurses need to understand what the client thinks about his/her condition, identify what could be done to change or improve the situation, and then collaboratively work on specified goals. It also means that a therapist will not be successful unless able to see the problem from the client's point of view. If you insist on seeing the problem from the stance of the 'all-knowing' expert, then you are very unlikely to be effective and the problem will not be solved.

It may also be helpful to develop an understanding of how to take a social constructionist approach by thinking about when it is absent. Practices that involve nursing being done to people whether they like it or not, clients being left out of the decision-making process, or nurses applying standardised interventions in the belief that what worked for one person will work for the next, are all examples.

## A strengths perspective

The second important philosophical underpinning to solution focused nursing is the view that people have strengths and vulnerabilities operating in their lives at all times (Saleeby, 1997). Furthermore, most people, even though they may have experienced significant trauma, will survive. They are resilient. Such knowledge comes from a large body of research arising over the last 30–40 years (Rutter, 1989; Vaillant, 2002; Werner and Smith, 2001). Even when someone is at their very sickest, perhaps near death, they have assets and abilities. He or she might have good memories, a loving family, a safe place to be resting in, and so on. It is important that nurses work to identify those strengths so that the person can draw comfort from them.

The opposite perspective – to be observant mainly of people's deficits and deficiencies – is unfortunately still a widely held, although possibly subconscious attitude, driving the behaviours of nurses and clinicians. I argue, and so do those who advocate positive psychology, well-being, optimism, hope and resilience, that if we forget about what's going right, we will cement the *illness mindset*, triggering helplessness, despair and loss of hope (Bonanno, 2004; Saleeby, 1997; Seligman, 2011). Hospitals, health centres and nurses will become nothing more than illness-care workers. And in this model, health care is neglected.

Not only will nurses continue to limit their scope of practice to illness care, but consumers may be duped into thinking that once they have an illness there is nothing that can be done by them to facilitate recovery and well-being.

But consider this statement from WHO (2001: 1):

> Mental Health is more than the absence of disease. It is a state of wellbeing in which the individual realises his or her own abilities, can cope with the normal stresses of life, can work productively and fruitfully, and is able to make a contribution to his or her community.

To fully appreciate this concept, to become mental *health* workers, nurses need to be concerned about well-being, how people can be assisted to flourish in their lives: to enjoy what they do, to cope with difficulties, to believe in others, to feel they have a place in the world and to believe that they have something they can give to others. These are all the concerns of a strengths focused nurse.

The most famous of nurses, Florence Nightingale, said this over 150 years ago (cited in McDonald, 2004: 207):

> Health is not only to be well, but to use well every power that we have.

She beseeched her students to not take health for granted, to not assume that it is something that either exists or not. She knew then, as we do now, that health takes work, it involves setting goals, and making an effort and that nurses have an active role in helping people to develop the powers of self-care.

However, throughout the twentieth century, it would appear that many of us have failed to heed Nightingale's messages. Instead of seeing people as resilient, surviving and enduring, the illness-care approach has become more dominant. This has constrained our vision so that many nurses tend to see people as patients – and in weakened, debilitated, damaged or deficient states. And indeed, when the medications have been distributed, or the showers completed, some nurses think, 'My work here is done.' But of course, this is not the full picture. Only the illness-care work is complete. Failing to see other dimensions of a person means that we are likely to miss aspects about the person that are going well and which could be harnessed to further strengthen the person and allow his/her well-being to flourish. Caring has long been a central concept for nursing. Solution focused nursing attempts to reclaim it.

Let's return to Paula, who is anxiously stalling outside Mr Smith's door – not knowing how to act, just knowing that she must. In her pocket she has a notebook, reminding her of important tasks. On the left you can see what she actually had. On the right is what she also could have had (Figure 17.3).

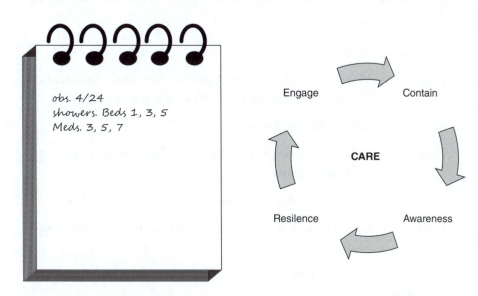

*obs. 4/24*
*showers. Beds 1, 3, 5*
*Meds. 3, 5, 7*

Engage

Contain

CARE

Resilence

Awareness

**FIGURE 17.3** The CARE Framework

Which of these do you think may have offered her a clearer direction for working with Mr Smith? Paula didn't tell me how her interaction with Mr Smith turned out, but I would imagine that it went something like this:

| | |
|---|---|
| Mr Smith: | Stop! |
| Paula: | What's the matter? (looking flustered) |
| Mr Smith: | I don't like the shower! |
| Paula: | Ok. I'll be fast |
| Mr Smith: | Noooooh!! (struggles and resists) |
| Paula: | I'm sorry. I'll be quick. (looking even more flustered) |
| Mr Smith: | You are a horrible nurse!!! Leave me alone! |

Using a solution focused approach to working with Mr Smith could have helped Paula to focus on *engaging* him in his own decision-making, getting his cooperation by talking about his interests, and aiming towards a more comfortable happy state (*resilience*), by thinking about what's ahead and not just the present battle over showers or baths.

With some training on solution focused nursing, the interaction could have gone more like this:

| | |
|---|---|
| Mr Smith: | Stop! |
| Paula: | What's the matter? (concern on her face, consciously slowed movements, aiming to **contain** the upset) |
| Mr Smith: | I don't like the shower. |
| Paula: | What would you rather have instead? (smiling, remaining calm, **raising awareness**) |
| Mr Smith: | I'd like to sit down and not have any water on my head. |
| Paula: | Ok. Let's do it that way. (smiling, letting him show the way, **engaging**). |

Paula turns on some Irish music (thinking about his strengths and **resilience**).

## The changing paradigm shifts to solution focused work

Solution focused work emerged from a paradigm shift that was occurring all across the world as the psychological, social work and counselling disciplines developed their knowledge and practice base and began to offer valid counterpoints to the prevailing medical model (Allan, 2003; Hofstetter, 2008; McKergow and Clarke, 2007; Mahlberg and Sjoblom, 2005).

Studies into vulnerable children and adolescents in the 1970s and 1980s revealed new insights into factors that facilitate resilience and verified the importance of compassionate care-giving (Aronowitz, 2005; Clark, 1984; Jacelon, 1997).

Family therapy began to emerge as an effective alternative to individual psychotherapy. Traditional psychotherapies, which aim to explore deep psychic structures, also tended to be locked into the problem orientation. Problem focused thinking came to be criticised for aiming for insight (i.e. individuals would acknowledge and accept their difficulties) but not necessarily change. Skilled mainly in problem-searching, clinicians who are problem-based tend to lack strategy in asking questions of a therapeutic nature that require the consumer to self-reflect, open up, consider other options and integrate changes (Polaschek and Polaschek, 2007).

The brief therapy movement grew out of this. Steve De Shazer and Insoo Kim Berg, as the main proponents, viewed therapeutic transformation as something that required the enactment of small changes, which would then have a ripple effect to create significant benefits (De Shazer, 1985).

Within psychology, the development of the positive psychology movement (Seligman, 2002) was examining characteristics of people who survive and overcome stressful situations to reveal knowledge about optimism, happiness and well-being. Most recently, Seligman's (2011) work on what makes people flourish happily in their lives, and not just endure, emphasises the importance of five measurable attributes: positive emotion, engagement, relationships, meaning and accomplishment (Figure 17.4).

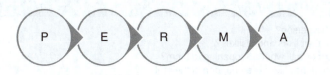

**FIGURE 17.4**   Seligman's theory of well-being

Together, these trans-disciplinary studies into resilience, brief therapy and well-being have converged into a view of helping that values taking a solution rather than a problem focus.

# The theory and practice of solution focused nursing

Similarly, solution focused nursing (SFN) has emerged from this paradigm shift about helping.

The studies on resilience and the importance of compassionate care validate nursing's identity and pursuit of the science of human caring. For quite some time in the twentieth century nursing tended to turn away from its location in the soft sciences, and for too long ignored the rising disillusionment with biotechnical care. SFN emphasises the role of nursing in providing compassionate, skilled care. Nurses work with vulnerable people and must understand that social justice is a realistic goal that can exist because of, not despite, the many differences that exist in this world. It understands that, as with life, not all health care experiences will be perfect or problem-free.

This is my definition of a solution focused nurse:

> Being skilled, helpful and supportive to people during significant and challenging life experiences so that they can make a successful transition from illness to adaptation, and therefore move on to happier, healthier and more connected lives.

---

**CONTAIN**

- What problems does the person want to change?
- What problems would be best contained?

**AWARENESS**

- How can self-knowledge of strengths and vulnerabilities be enhanced within the consumer, carer and clinicians?

**RESILIENCE**

- How can internal and external strengths such as coping mechanisms, resources and social connections be facilitated?

**ENGAGEMENT**

- Who is this person?
- What are their likes and dislikes?
- What do they call what's happening to them?
- What would they like to see happen in their future?

---

**FIGURE 17.5**   The concept of CARE

SFN values the importance of skilled illness work as well as strategic approaches to facilitate well-being. Problem-solving and solution-searching are part of a nurse's cognitive toolkit, so that problems can be identified and contained promptly, and solutions for restoring and maintaining health and well-being can be generated. SFN is interested in exploring and developing with clients their strengths and abilities rather than focusing solely on their weaknesses and disabilities.

The concept of CARE (McAllister and Walsh, 2003) provides a useful guiding framework for how a nurse can work in everyday interactions (Figure 17.5).

Table 17.1 shows that CARE fits snugly with the solutions focus.

**TABLE 17.1**   CARE and SFN

| The solutions focus | Fit with the CARE framework |
| --- | --- |
| 1  What is happening here that could be changed? | • With this focus we are moving beyond problem-identification, which is the illness containing aspect of our work, towards taking action.<br>• SFN emphasises an element to the problem-solving method that is often minimised or overlooked, and that is the solution generating phase (Johnson, 2005).<br>• In this sense, it has a broader and more creative set of strategies which are not limited to problems. |
| 2  How can we give *more* space to this imagined change, than the present problem? | • Problems are part of life, and because of the nature of the settings in which most nurses work, we are going to encounter people experiencing problems. Therefore, it's important not to dismiss or belittle clients when they wish to discuss the impact that such problems are having on their lives. (Be engaging, curious and respectful.)<br>• At the same time if nurses wish to act as a turning point for people, then it's important not to allow the conversation to stay stuck in the problem (raise awareness).<br>• Think of the problem as something that has played a part in the person's past, and the future will be a place where it plays less of a central part. |
| 3  What are the steps being made towards change that we need to notice and reinforce? | • Assessing a client and carers' strengths and resources will be key to moving on from the problem, towards coping, adaptation and better health (fostering resilience).<br>• Learning to use specific kinds of questions to achieve goals. |

## Specific questioning styles

The aim of a solution focused conversation with a client is to explore what the client wants to achieve, what he or she wants for the future. This might sound easy, but when you have spent a lot of your time and energy consumed with a problem, it is quite challenging to imagine a life without it. It takes creativity and persistence to find different ways to have conversations about this imagined future. It also requires a respectful curiosity and a hopeful stance. Five questioning or conversational styles are suggested below and the answers you receive during these conversations need to be put to use by individuals in creating that future for themselves. They become the subject for assignments to be worked on between sessions, or on discharge.

## Exception searching

This strategy reclaims previously existing strengths and abilities that may have become hidden by the problem. It replaces the distorted and false idea that the problem has always and will always exist. By having a conversation about these exceptions, more space can be made to imagine life without the problem playing a central and dominating role.

> Example: Before this anxiety came into your life, were there times that you can tell me about when you weren't feeling tense and were more carefree?

## Enduring question

This strategy helps individuals to see that they must have a lot of hidden strengths to have kept going the way that they have. It actually takes a lot of energy to bear a problem and this energy could be channelled and refocused, if it could be identified.

> Example: How have you managed to keep going in the face of this problem? You must have a lot of fortitude.

## The miracle question

This strategy invites clients to discuss what their life would be like if all their dreams could come true and everything was different. It's important to help them be specific in terms of feelings, behaviours, relationships, work, leisure,

Example: If I was to cast a magic wand, and take your problem away, describe to me what your world would look like, what you would be doing, how you would be spending your time.

## Externalising question

This strategy helps to the put the problem into an external space, where it can be noticed and analysed more impartially. It can help the person to see the problem as something separate and therefore not forever linked to him or her as a person.

Example: You called this anxiety the Big Worry. How has the Big Worry been playing itself out these last few days?

## Scaling question

This strategy helps to scale the problem down to size. By breaking the problem behaviour into manageable chunks, the person can be helped to see that change does not have to be enormous, or monumental. Little steps are signs of progress, more achievable, and can give you hope.

Example: Yesterday, you told me that the Big Worry was about a 5/10. If we were to bring that up to about a 6/10 where you were feeling a bit better, what would be different? And, what would a small step forward look like?

## The value of strategic communication

Nurses often complain that they do not want technical procedures to dominate their role, but yet technical procedures are by far the most common preoccupation among nursing students and are increasingly creeping into the undergraduate curriculum (Dijkstra, 2002). If consumers want more than a technically competent clinician, then students obviously need more than to learn nursing procedures.

Observational studies have also shown that nurses rarely interact verbally with consumers, and when they do they tend to be limited to prescriptive conversations, such as 'take this' or 'do that' (Leahy, 2004; Shattell, 2004). However, numerous studies have now been completed showing that solution focused communication strategies actually resolve these problems. They are brief strategies that do not take a lot of time, and they help the nurse feel more strategic and effective in helping the consumer move on from his or her problem.

Bowles et al. (2001), for example, found that simply learning the usual non-directive counselling techniques of empathy and active listening left students feeling directionless and lacking confidence with consumers. But after training in the solutions focus, students became more confident in their ability to listen and to redirect a client so that they could look beyond the problem.

In an intervention study, Boscart (2006) found that after students were given a lecture, role modelling and a reminder booklet on the strategies of the solutions focus, there were significant changes in three key areas. The quality of the introductory phase of their relationship significantly improved. That is, before the intervention, nurses introduced themselves rarely and only some of the time did they explain the purpose of their presence in the room. After the training these behaviours were significantly improved. Conversations about care also improved, with nurses giving consumers more choice, and less prescriptive advice.

In my own study (McAllister et al., 2008), where nurses were provided solution focused communication training in the emergency department, participants were more likely to engage with clients, to assess their strengths and vulnerabilities, and to be more future focused after the education than before. Prior to the training, nurses were not active health educators and nor did they consider the person's future support needs. Before, nurses tended to be concerned solely with the presenting problem. After learning solution focused nursing, participants were more able to demonstrate concern for a client's future.

## Summary

Solution focused nursing shifts the orientation towards the future, where the clinician is attempting to facilitate transition for consumers, transforming the present crisis into a turning point. From this standpoint, the clinician is not just interested in treating problems, but in preventing distress, and promoting health and well-being. Thinking about the future is one important change for nurses – to not become preoccupied with just what is happening in the present.

Solution focused clinicians do things slightly differently to others – they are interested in the person, apart from the problem, they are curious about the person's goals, and they are interested in finding out more about strengths and resources that will help the person get there.

The following mnemonic, adapted from Visser and Bodien (2003), summarises the power of the solution focus:

P      Problems are acknowledged but not indulged

O      Outcomes desired are specified

W     Where are you now on the scale?

E      Exceptions to the problem are keys to the solution

R      Relationships are enhanced and made productive

S      Small steps forward propel larger change

## Acknowledgement

I wish to acknowledge and thank Pauline May Lambert, the student who spoke with me and gave permission for me to fictionalise and relay her story of working in the nursing home, which gives more meaning to the struggle students of nursing face in responding to challenging situations in a confident, proactive and positive way. Pauline wants you to know of her passion for helping people within the community. She used to volunteer for St John Ambulance in Darwin and went to community events providing first aid. Now she volunteers for the Street Angels on the Sunshine Coast of Queensland, providing care to people who may be affected by alcohol or drugs. She still works in the nursing home and will complete her degree programme at the end of 2013.

Figures and tables are the author's own except where indicated.

## References

Allan, J. (2003) 'Practising critical social work', in J. Allan, B. Pease and L. Briskman (eds), *Critical Social Work: An Introduction to Theories and Practices.* Crows Nest, NSW: Allen and Unwin.

Aronowitz, T. (2005) 'The role of "envisioning the future" in the development of resilience among at-risk youth', *Public Health Nursing,* 22 (3): 200–8.

Berger, P. and Luckmann, T. (1966) *The Social Construction of Reality: A Treatise in the Sociology of Knowledge.* Garden City, NY: Anchor Books.

Bonanno, G. (2004) 'Loss, trauma, and human resilience: have we underestimated the human capacity to thrive after extremely adverse events?', *American Psychologist,* 59 (1): 20–8.

Boscart, V. (2006) 'A communication intervention for nursing staff in chronic care', *Journal of Advanced Nursing*, 65 (9): 1823–32.

Bowles, N., Mackintosh, C. and Torn, A. (2001) 'Nurses' communication skills: an evaluation of the impact of solution-focused communication training', *Journal of Advanced Nursing*, 36 (3): 347–54.

Clark, R. (1984) *Family Life and School Achievement: Why Poor Black Children Succeed or Fail.* Chicago: University of Chicago Press.

De Shazer, S. (1985) *Keys to Solution in Brief Therapy.* New York: W.W. Norton.

Dijkstra, K. (2002) 'My recaller is on vacation: discourse analysis of nursing-home residents with dementia', *Discourse Processes*, 33 (1): 53–76.

Frassanito, P. and Pettorini, B. (2008) 'Pink and blue: the colour of gender', *Child's Nervous System*, 24 (8): 881–2.

Hofstetter, D. (2008) *Solution Focused Selling.* Munich: Rainer Hampp Verlag.

Jacelon, C. (1997) 'The trait and process of resilience', *Journal of Advanced Nursing*, 25 (1): 123–9.

Johnson, B. (2005) 'Overcoming "doom and gloom": empowering students in courses on social problems, injustice and inequality', *Teaching Sociology*, 33 (1): 44–58.

Leahy, M. (2004) 'Therapy talk: analyzing therapeutic discourse', *Language, Speech, and Hearing Services in Schools*, 35 (1): 70–81.

McAllister, M. (2007) *Solution Focused Nursing: Rethinking Practice.* Basingstoke: Palgrave.

McAllister, M. and Walsh, K. (2003) 'C.A.R.E: A framework for mental health practice', *Journal of Psychiatric and Mental Health Nursing*, 10 (1): 39–48.

McAllister, M., Zimmer-Gembeck, M., Moyle, W. and Billett, S. (2008) 'Working effectively with clients who self-injure using a solution focused approach', *Journal of International Emergency Nursing*, 16 (4): 272–9.

McDonald, L. (2004) *Florence Nightingale on Public Health: The Collected Works of Florence Nightingale.* Waterloo, ON: Wilfrid Laurier University Press.

McKergow, M. and Clarke, J. (2007) *Solutions Focus Working: 80 Real Life Lessons for Successful Organisational Change.* London: Solutions Books.

Mahlberg, K. and Sjoblom, K. (2005) *Solution Focused Education.* London: Solutions Books.

Peterson, S. and Bredow, T. (2013) *Middle Range Theories: Application to Nursing Research* (3rd edn). Philadelphia: Lippincott, Williams and Wilkins.

Polaschek, L. and Polaschek, N. (2007) 'Solution-focused conversations: a new therapeutic strategy in well child health nursing telephone consultations', *Journal of Advanced Nursing*, 59 (2): 111–19.

Reed, P. (1995) 'A treatise on nursing knowledge development for the 21st century: beyond postmodernism', *Advances in Nursing Science*, 17 (3): 70–84.

Rogers, C. (1975) 'Empathic: an unappreciated way of being', *The Counseling Psychologist*, 5 (2): 2–10.

Rutter, M. (1989) 'Pathways from childhood to adult life', *Journal of Child Psychology and Psychiatry*, 30 (1): 23–54.

Saleeby, D. (1997) *The Strengths Perspective in Social Work Practice*. New York: Longman.

Seligman, M. (2002) 'Positive psychology, positive prevention and positive therapy', in C. Snyder and S. Lopez (eds), *Handbook of Positive Psychology*. Oxford: Oxford University Press.

Seligman, M. (2011) *Flourish: A Visionary New Understanding of Happiness and Wellbeing*. New York: Free Press.

Shattell, M. (2004) 'Nurse–patient interaction: a review of the literature', *Journal of Clinical Nursing*, 13 (6): 714–22.

Vaillant, G. (2002) *Aging Well: Surprising Guideposts to a Happier Life from the Landmark Harvard Study of Adult Development*. Boston: Little, Brown and Company.

Visser, C. and Bodien, G. (2003) *The POWERS of the Solution Focus: An Effective Approach to Individual and Organizational Development*. Available at: http://solutionfocusedchange.blogspot.com/ (accessed on: 28/5/2012).

Werner, E. and Smith, R. (2001) *Journeys from Childhood to the Midlife: Risk, Resilience, and Recovery*. New York: Cornell University Press.

WHO (World Health Organization) (2001) *The World Health Report 2001 – Mental Health: New Understanding, New Hope*. Geneva: World Health Organization.

# 18

# Risk

## ANNE FELTON

### Learning Objectives

- Recognise that the meaning of 'risk' has changed over time and understand the implications of this for people diagnosed with a mental health problem.
- Outline scientific, cultural and social theories of risk.
- Explain the relevance of theories of risk for mental health nursing practice.

## Introduction

'Risk' in many respects will be a concept that you are familiar with. Within contemporary western society we are surrounded by the presence of risk. This may be seen in the laws and informal codes that we live by that aim to promote safety and well-being, such as locking the door when we leave the house or wearing a bicycle helmet. Risk is also evident in those activities that we might be involved in that challenge these informal codes whether that is climbing a mountain, driving over the speed limit or jumping out of a plane.

Mental health services reflect this focus on risk within society. The assessment and management of risk associated with people with mental health problems has become a core part of mental health nursing practice (Godin, 2004). Yet the dominance of risk in mental health services is problematic. Professionals can feel that the quality of their work is judged on their ability to control risk and that this can get in the way of their therapeutic relationship with people who use mental health services (Godin, 2004; Repper and Perkins, 2003). For those experiencing mental health problems themselves, being subject to the measures put in place to control risk can be damaging and ultimately inhibit their recovery. In order to move beyond this position in which avoidance of risk can become the aim of mental health care it is important that there is a critical examination of where our understanding of risk comes from. In addition, we need to question how risk became such a dominant part of working with people with mental health problems.

This chapter uses a series of theories to explore these questions. It will examine those theories that suggest risk is something that we can calculate and predict. The discussion will also consider theories that offer an alternative view, that suggest risk is a product of our society alongside writers who claim that the function of risk is a system of blame and that people with mental health problems are used as scapegoats to be blamed for society's difficulties. This critical examination will be followed by a consideration of how these theories can be applied to mental health nursing practice. In order to make sense of these critical theories the chapter will start with a historical exploration of 'risk' and the role of risk in mental health services.

## Historical development

Take a moment to ask yourself – what does the term risk mean? When answering this question it's likely that some of the words that you came up with included harm, danger, injury or loss. The potential for harm is how we have come to understand risk in contemporary society, yet this has not always been the case.

### Evolution of risk

Lupton's (1999) historical examination of risk starts with early pre-industrial society which for many was a place fraught with danger, natural disasters, disease epidemics and war. However, the way in which these dangers were explained and managed for people inhabiting that society was through a system of superstitions, beliefs and customs. These belief systems are described as a means through which people felt some control over the dangers they faced. Lupton cites the first presence of the concept of risk appearing in the Middle Ages where it was associated with sea voyages, wherein dangers that could threaten a crossing were identified. One of the important elements of this early version of risk assessment was that the dangers that threatened a voyage were natural and as such were seen as a catastrophe, an act of fate over which humans had no control (Lupton, 1999; Muir-Cochrane, 2006).

The industrial revolution with the development of a capitalist economic system and scientific ideas contributed to a shift in the way that danger (and consequently risk) was viewed. The popularity of science meant that new ideas were emerging which suggested that society and to some degree nature followed set rules that could be calculated and consequently predicted. These ideas begin to form a new system of beliefs around danger, governed by calculations of the probability that an event might happen. Lupton (1999) highlights that as modern society continued to develop, risk also became associated with human behaviour. Like the system of superstitions and customs of early society, calculation, probability and prediction become the modern system through which people feel that they have some control over danger. But because this modern system is based on rules and calculations it also assumes that the action of human beings may be responsible for events rather than fate or an act of God as was previously believed.

The linking of risk with mathematics did provide the potential for risk to be considered in terms of hazards and loss but also in terms of gains. This was reinforced by the association with the insurance industry but also gambling theory (Kettles, 2004). The possibility that gains could be made by making a bet or taking a risk introduced a notion of 'good risk' (Douglas, 1992). However, as the question at the start of this section highlights, in the twenty-first century this potential for good associated with risk seems to have disappeared from our understanding. Instead, risk has become synonymous with the possibility of hazards and harm.

This section has provided a brief overview of the historical development of the concept of risk and how meanings of the term have changed over time. The next section summarises some important historical changes in mental health services and how these have influenced the focus on risk.

## Risk and the history of mental health services

The history of mental health care is to a degree dominated by the large public asylums that provided care and treatment for the mentally ill between the mid-nineteenth and late twentieth centuries. Yet it is in the creation of these asylums that the foundations for the association between people with mental health problems and 'risk' can be viewed.

Public asylums were created in response to concerns about mistreatment within privately run institutions (Porter, 2002). The newly built asylums were generally constructed away from cities where diseases were common and were amongst the first widespread social support systems for those who were too poor to pay for health and welfare support (Nolan, 1993). These institutions have, however, been seen to serve another purpose in the separation of those deemed to have a mental disorder away from the rest of society (Foucault, 2006). Morrall and Hazleton (2000) suggest that the function of asylums became one of 'custodial warehouses' for parts of the population who did not fit in with the dominant values in industrial society. Consequently, the mentally ill have been viewed as threatening the social and moral structures of this society due to a perception that they lack discipline and self-control. Integrated within the history of asylums is also the history of psychiatry as this new profession developed within the institutions to provide treatment for the mentally ill (Porter, 2002).

The consequence of this situation is to imply that people with mental health problems are a threat and therefore need to be separated from society. This is made explicit in more recent history as 'dangerousness' has been used as a criterion for involuntary detention in hospital (Steadman, 1983). This reinforces the view that there is something to fear from the mentally ill and that the psychiatric system has a role in controlling this threat. Theorists such as Andrew Scull (1979) and Michel Foucault consider this issue in terms of the networks that maintain certain power relationships in society. However, this position is clearly reflected on a more practical level when contemporary public attitudes towards people with mental health problems are considered. What was the view of your relatives and friends when you told them about your plans to become a mental health nurse? Fear and danger often dominate perceptions of people with mental health problems. It is the evolution of community care in the late twentieth century that cemented this perception within the public mind. During this time the link between mental illness and danger changed to one between mental illness and risk.

Between 1961 and the late 1990s there was a gradual period of de-institutionalisation in which the large psychiatric hospitals closed. The presence of people previously contained behind the walls of an asylum in the community setting was seen to create a number of challenges, taking into consideration the perceived function of these institutions. Stein (2002) claims that in closing the hospitals psychiatry lost its system of containing risk for people with mental health problems.

During the 1990s a succession of government policies introduced changes that increased monitoring of people with mental health problems in the community (DH, 1998; DH, 1999; NHS Management Executive, 1994) such as the care programme approach. It has been suggested that these changes were developed as a new system of containment in the community based on continued fears regarding the threat and danger that people with mental health problems posed (hence the need to assess and calculate the risk).

At this time there were also a number of tragic high profile suicides and in particular homicides committed by people with mental health problems that fuelled public fears about the danger they posed in the community (Kaliniecka and Shawe-Taylor, 2008), reinforcing views that there is a link between violence and mental illness (Paterson and Stark, 2001). The media's response to the homicides and their wider portrayal of people with mental health problems has been criticised for contributing to this climate of fear (Cutcliffe and Hannigan, 2001; Freshwater and Westwood, 2006).

Whilst each one of these homicides was a tragedy, in reality the number of murders committed by people with mental health problems in the 1990s during the advent of community care actually fell (Paterson and Stark, 2001; Taylor and Gunn, 1999). There is only a small percentage of murders committed by people with mental health problems (around 10%; James, 2006; Szmukler, 2000) making it more likely that a murder is committed by someone without mental illness.

This contributes to an unusual position in which there exists in mental health services a preoccupation with the risk of violence to others (Warner and Gabe, 2004). Ultimately there is a tendency for mental health care to focus on the assessment of risk in relation to violence, suicide and self-harm at the cost of recognising the risks that individuals are likely to be exposed to themselves (Kaliniecka and Shawe-Taylor, 2008; Muir-Cochrane, 2006). In this section it has been argued that the meaning and practice of 'risk' has changed as society has developed. The discussion has also established that throughout the history of mental health care people with mental health problems have been linked with danger and ultimately risk, recognising that a key role for mental health professionals in contemporary society is the assessment and management of risk. The following discussion goes on to examine some theories which may explain how this position has developed and why it is reinforced.

## Theories of risk

Each theory offers a different perspective on what risk means and how we can understand it. The theories do share one common element and that is the recognition that there is a relationship between scientists ('experts'), policy-makers and the public when it comes to defining, understanding and responding to risk.

## The scientific view of risk

The first theoretical position on risk originates from a scientific perspective. This perspective recognises the existence of risk as a fact. The Royal Society, an organisation of eminent scientists, in its report examining risks to health has defined risk as 'the probability that a particular adverse event occurs during a stated period of time or results from a particular challenge' (Royal Society, 1992: 2). This definition identifies some elements of risk including that it can be calculated giving rise to a probability, that it is associated with a negative, adverse outcome and that this can be confined to a set period of time. The Royal Society (1992) report on risk also defines two different types of risk, 'objective' and 'subjective'. Objective risk reflects the scientific stance that risks exist as fact and can therefore be measured; subjective risk is associated with the ways in which people respond to risk (Lupton, 1999).

From this position, risk therefore needs to be calculated scientifically by those who have the knowledge and expertise to do this. These calculations by experts are viewed as unbiased. The measurement of probability also has benefits for decision-makers as it gives the impression of reducing uncertainty (McDonald et al., 2005). Underlying scientists' distinction of risk is the assumption that giving people information will help them understand and respond accordingly to the real scope of the risk (Thompson and Rayner, 1998) and that this information needs to come from risk experts.

Non-experts or lay people are viewed as using unreliable mechanisms to make sense of risk, such as intuition. Researchers have suggested that lay people experience 'cognitive biases' in the way that they perceive probability that inhibit the accuracy of these perceptions of risk (Kahneman and Tversky, 1979; McDonald et al., 2005). Non-experts are more likely to base their judgements of risk on personal and historical experiences whilst the judgements of risk experts are based on probabilities and objective knowledge (Garvin, 2001). Lay people therefore require the knowledge of experts to help correct these biases as Thompson and Rayner (1998) highlight and inform them of the real nature of risk. Crucially, this approach assumes that by identifying and calculating a risk, steps can be taken to manage this risk with humans responding to such information about risk in a rational and logical way (Lupton, 1999).

Within mental health services this scientific perspective of risk is evident in a variety of ways. A number of psychiatric risk assessments are based on a type of risk calculation described as 'actuarial'. Actuarial approaches to risk assessment are based on statistical population information that is developed from research and incorporates analysis of a specific set of variables (Allen, 1997; McGuire, 2004), for example, that there is a higher risk of committing suicide if you are a young man or unemployed. This statistical information is used to make predictions in accordance with rules which are fixed (Buchanan, 1999; Doyle and Dolan, 2002). The origins of actuarial approaches lie in the insurance industry, though their use has been adapted for mental health risk assessments. Research from an actuarial perspective suggests the strength of these statistical approaches has been linked to their identification of variables that are associated with violence in the population and people diagnosed with mental health problems (Buchanan, 1999). However, further research has questioned the findings of this population information, in particular undermining a link between 'delusions' and violence (Appelbaum et al., 2000).

The influence of the scientific view is also seen in the creation of experts on risk in mental health practice. The role of mental health professionals as experts in risk is a conflictual one. However, the notion that assessment of risk is based on expert scientific knowledge effectively excludes service users from participating in judgements of risk as they are perceived as lacking in the required expert knowledge.

The existence of risk as an objective fact that can be measured by experts has been questioned. In this respect, the cultural perspective of risk offers an alternative interpretation.

## The cultural view of risk

The cultural approach emphasises the significance of the social and cultural contexts in which risk exists and is championed by anthropologist Mary Douglas. The cultural view suggests that what is and is not classed as a risk reflects shared values, beliefs and conventions within society. In this respect attempts to divorce judgements of risk from bias are impossible, so the cultural perspective of risk takes an opposing view to the scientific theories.

The cultural theory introduces the idea that culture helps inform shared, communal rather than individual notions of risk. Douglas's (1992) theories emphasise the selective nature of the risk process through the means in which certain risks are ignored whilst others create great anxiety. Selection is based on the values and ways of life that people live by and avoidance of certain risks serves as an attempt to try and protect the systems that underpin that way of life. This might be seen in the way in which western society accepts certain risk-taking behaviours, for example, bungee jumping, and not others such as being near train lines. For Douglas (1992) the relationship between policy-makers, scientists and the public is integral. Whilst scientists might claim to be objective and consequently aim to exclude bias and politics from their calculations of risk, this is impossible, not least because they are also part of a social and cultural system. In this respect risk cannot be separated from politics (Douglas, 1992). This becomes clear when you think about examples associated with possible risks that you may have seen on the news that have led to legal changes or financial investment by the government; an example acknowledged in the Royal Society risk report is that of wearing seat belts in the car, but there are also others that include use of nuclear power, genetically modified crops and dealing with toxic waste. All of which are where policy-makers draw on the work of scientists to examine risk.

The cultural theoretical perspective also suggests that the way in which risk is used results in the term essentially meaning danger. Douglas (1992) explains that this is partly as a result of the focus on risk by science but also extends this to suggest that in modern society it is part of a 'new set of ideas' in which there is a heightened awareness of the dangers around us. Douglas and Wildavsky (1982) highlight that there are differences between groups who are part of the same culture about what they accept as a risk. Increasingly, this is manifested through apportioning blame for a risk of danger that may threaten a particular social group. Risk therefore functions as part of a blaming system in which we look for lines of fault and responsibility, for someone to take accountability. This has replaced the systems that we used in early society where beliefs about the occurrence of unfortunate events were associated with morals or sin (Douglas, 1992; Lupton, 1999). Douglas (1992) identifies the manner in which blame for danger is apportioned to certain groups, suggesting that those groups perceived as deviant or risky are marginalised by more dominant social sets (Lupton, 1999). This process has significant implications for people with mental health problems, particularly when viewed in the light of the public fears explored in the historical development section of this chapter.

Douglas's (1992) cultural theory of risk also highlights that as the meaning of risk has changed over time the dominant view has developed that avoiding risks is 'normal' and therefore taking risk is seen as abnormal and pathological.

The cultural perspective of risk has highlighted that risk has to be viewed in a social and cultural context. It has also suggested that risk acts as a system of blame within modern society. Social perspectives offer further interpretations of how risk can be understood.

## The social perspective on risk

Risk is perceived as an important way of making sense of modern society (Beck, 1992; Giddens, 1990). Sociologists Ulrich Beck and Anthony Giddens have developed in-depth examinations of risk by adopting this position. From the social perspective within our modern technological age, the production of wealth is accompanied by the production of risk (Giddens, 1990). This occurs to the extent that we are described as living in a risk society in which there is a preoccupation with minimising the risks that are produced by the very structures and systems of that society (Beck, 1992). Similar to the cultural theory, Beck's (1992) work suggests that risk represents hazards and for him these are real and tangible, though differences in the way these risks may be perceived by, for example, the public are acknowledged.

These risks pose global threats. This is accompanied by a growing consciousness of risk within society in which the motivating force becomes achieving safety. Beck suggests this has led to a situation in which 'one is no longer concerned with attaining something good … rather preventing the worst' (Beck, 1992: 49). In a society with a greater awareness of risks, complicated and expert processes develop to quantify that risk. However, Beck (1992) maintains that while it may be possible to identify risks it is not possible to predict and control them through technological measures. The growth in consciousness about risk within society has led to a loss of trust in these technological and/or scientific systems and the experts that developed them (Giddens, 1990).

In the nineteenth and early twentieth centuries science was responsible for causing risk but also for defining it and offering possible solutions. In the risk society with heightened consciousness about risk this certainty in science is lost. Experts contradict each other and solutions to the large-scale and complex risks (much of Beck's analysis is concerned with environmental threats) have not been provided by scientists. Lupton (1999) highlights that this means that science has lost its authority. The consequences of this according to Beck (1992) result in the public making choices regarding the many possible interpretations offered by science. This leads to them becoming co-producers in defining this knowledge about risk. In this respect Beck (1992) criticises the way in which experts have defined 'lay people' as unreliable in their interpretation and response to risk – that their responses actually make sense in the face of the failure of science to offer any definitive solutions. Beck's (1992) work does recognise that there are social inequalities that impact on the access some social groups have to resources to respond to some risks and keep themselves safe, though he also acknowledges some risks are global and threaten us all in the same way.

Interestingly, Beck (1992) singles out the medical profession as escaping the challenges faced by science in modern society. He suggests it has succeeded in maintaining its power to define risk excluding the public and decision-makers.

It is important to recognise that these perspectives each has limitations in their theories explaining risk. Each theory has been challenged for a variety of reasons, including on issues such as whether risk is real or constructed, how useful the theory is in responding to the changes within society and how accurate their distinctions between pre- and modern society are. Nonetheless, these sometimes conflicting perspectives have a lot to offer in helping explain the ways that we understand risk and what this might mean in contemporary society. Their critical exploration of the relationship between politics, experts and the public is important, particularly as we move on to consider the implications of these theories for mental health practice.

## Theory applied to practice

The scientific, cultural and social theories of risk are valuable for mental health practice through the way in which they can expose the role played by the government, the public and mental health professionals in positioning people with mental health problems as the subjects of risk. They also provide a critique for the way in which risk assessment and management have come to dominate mental health nursing practice to help us find a way to move beyond this position.

As a registered mental health nurse, you will have responsibility for managing risk and 'where possible reducing it to an acceptable level' (NMC, 2006). In order to enable mental health professionals to work towards this goal there is a wealth of literature which examines the process of risk assessment. Much of this literature is geared towards evaluating the effectiveness of tools that are designed to measure risk. This is part of a drive to make risk assessment evidence-based and improve the quality of standardised risk assessment tools (Royal College of Psychiatrists, 2008). Actuarial risk assessment is also linked with this process as statistical information can be used with the aim of making this assessment more objective and therefore more accurate.

The scientific perspective on risk is clearly evident within this picture. Yet as this chapter has highlighted, the perception that risk is able to be calculated is only one way of viewing risk. Within mental health services the limitation of this perspective is apparent in the impact that it is having on the lives of people with mental health problems and to a lesser degree, mental health professionals. The inequitable focus on the risk of violence has already been highlighted; this is important as the response to these perceived risks by the state and consequently professionals has been to increase the level of surveillance of people with mental health problems and the legal powers available to mental health services to deal with these perceived risks.

Yet there are also problems with the scientific view of risk when this science is applied to reviewing the calculations of a perceived risk of violence itself. According to Szmukler (2000) the chances of someone with mental health problems killing a stranger are about the same as that of being killed by lightening. Goldacre (2006) also provides a mathematical analysis of the predictive value of the most sensitive risk assessment tool measuring risk of violence which suggests this tool would be inaccurate 86 times out of 100, this increases to being inaccurate 97 times out of 100 when attempting to predict serious violence (partly due to the problems of calculation when an event is so rare). These problems of using risk assessment tools to predict human behaviour are also emphasised by a large review of research in this area (spanning 13 countries and 24,847 participants) that concluded that there is a huge variation in the predictive ability of such tools (Fazel et al., 2012). A good level of accuracy is achieved in predicting those who are low risk, perhaps unsurprising given this is more likely but limited when predicting high risk. Indeed, the authors suggest that 'even after 30 years of development, the view that violence, sexual or criminal risk can be predicted in most cases is not evidence based' (Fazel et al., 2012: 5).

This critique has highlighted that the scientific view of risk is integral to mental health services and the expectations on professionals working in these services. Yet the limitations of this focus on predication have also been recognised. For some, the manner in which people with mental health problems are targeted as the perpetrators of risk (and therefore danger) including the way in which this risk is dealt with, essentially through containment, is a form of discrimination. Anti-psychiatrist Thomas Szasz (1963) points to the dangers posed by, for example, people who drink and drive, who are not subject to the same level of control, yet who may also be perceived as 'treatable' (Szmukler and Holloway, 2000). Rogers and Pilgrim (2010) suggest that this perception of dangerousness can influence how persons who have been diagnosed with a mental health problem see themselves. Additionally, they point to how the use of mental health legislation based on risk (potential rather than actual acts) means that people with mental health problems are exposed to restrictions to their liberty in ways other groups within society are not. It is within these arguments that we also discover the value of the cultural theory in understanding risk in relation to people with mental health problems.

What becomes apparent from recognising that the risks posed by people with mental health problems are overstated and like any risk related to human behaviour difficult to predict, is that the mentally ill are treated differently. Douglas's (1992) theory suggests that blame for danger is apportioned to certain groups and forms part of a blaming system. Here people with mental health problems are one of those marginalised groups seen at fault in a way other groups are not. Mechanisms such as official homicide inquiries which examine the conduct of mental health services following a homicide committed by someone in contact with mental health services become part of the blaming system in which accountability is sought. Szmukler (2000) highlights how this system also serves to exclude the role of others from this process of accountability, such as other agencies and the victims themselves.

Douglas (1992) also promotes risk as a politicised concept. This can be applied to mental health practice when reviewing the arguments promoted by the government for changes to both mental health policy and law which have led to increased monitoring of people with mental health problems and further legislative powers for mental health services. The arguments used to justify these increased powers and therefore potential threats to autonomy and liberty have focused on the risks posed by this group (Harper, 2004).

The cultural theory emphasises that the avoidance of risk is the accepted norm within society and therefore taking risks becomes abnormal, something to be avoided. Yet protecting someone with mental health problems from taking risks could be detrimental to their recovery (Stickley and Felton, 2006). Studies examining risk taking suggest that it can bring affirmation and positive social recognition, that it can have positive implications for self-improvement, emotional engagement and control (Lupton and Tulloch, 2002; Parker and Stanworth, 2005). Consequently, recognising the dominance of negative connotations of risk is important, in addition to understanding that risk can mean making a gain. This can help create the space for therapeutic (or positive) risk taking in which people with mental health problems have the opportunity to make choices, decide on and follow different options (Morgan, 2000). Examples of risk taking in this context might be to come off their medication, to move into different accommodation or to take a holiday. Positive risk taking is increasingly perceived as an important feature of risk assessment and management in mental health services, yet there are still a number of barriers to overcome before therapeutic risk taking becomes the norm.

Beck (1992) and Giddens's (1990) theories to a degree provide some insight into the existence of these barriers. Mental health services do not exist in a vacuum. They are part of and are influenced by wider society and in turn the government of that society. Remember how all the theories of risk rested on the existence of a relationship between the public, the government and scientists. This also has relevance when considering the development of policy related to community care as highlighted at the start of this chapter. We see a complex interaction between the public, the government and mental health services regarding the definition and response to risk in relation to people with mental health problems.

This case example is an extract from the reflective diary of a community mental health nurse. In this extract the nurse shares some of her thoughts and feelings about working with a woman named Iona. Iona's situation is one the nurse and the team have struggled with and that has prompted this reflection. In it the nurse explores the implications this situation has for risk.

Each week Iona invites me into her home where we converse about the weather, clothes and TV programmes or sometimes we don't converse at all. For many weeks I have attempted to take this conversation further, to offer Iona the opportunity to share the thoughts and experiences that are clearly causing her so much distress. I wonder whether the weekly invitation into Iona's home means that there is some level of a therapeutic relationship and that this is the first but important step towards supporting recovery. Given what Iona has lost from her life, perhaps the costs of engaging with me further and all that I represent as a mental health nurse are too high. Particularly as this might mean acknowledging her voices and distressing thoughts and all that this means.

However, this also leaves me with a feeling of discomfort; as we know so little about Iona's experiences, yet she appears so unhappy there is a concern that this means that she is a high risk. In many respects we don't really know her at all. This was emphasised during a conversation with the consultant in which we reflected upon this and our fears that Iona is someone who might end up as a headline in a local newspaper.

If things continue to deteriorate further I am not sure what will be the best thing to do. She has coped fairly independently with her distressing experiences up until now, yet what do we know about how much has really changed and what the implications of this are? I do know I need to update her risk assessment paperwork to reflect this change and all I have to go on is this feeling that myself and the team have that something isn't right. If Iona is admitted under the Mental Health Act, I suspect that this will significantly damage the already tenuous relationship with mental health services and I am not sure that she will engage with our team again. There is also a question about what an admission to hospital will really achieve other than increasing our monitoring of Iona. Could this enable a more detailed assessment of her mental health and the risks that there may be? Equally an admission offers a different therapeutic approach and might create a change in the situation which forces Iona to face up to the losses in her life, ultimately enabling her to move on. There is perhaps also a need to consider our own possible motivations for looking at a section, it may be that it helps manage our own anxieties about Iona's distress and the possible risks knowing that she is in a 'safe' environment where she can be monitored and the possibility of newspaper headlines can be avoided.

Within this example, the nurse outlines her responsibility for understanding and predicting the level of risk that Iona is seen to present. However, the nurse's struggle with providing an accurate assessment of risk are clearly with someone who doesn't appear to want to be part of mental health services. In these reflections on someone diagnosed with a mental health problem, the nurse is immediately aware of the potential for risk in relation to Iona whilst the nurse's consideration of public perceptions through the reference to newspaper headlines recognises the social context. In this brief explanation the contribution of the scientific, social and cultural theories of risk start to become evident.

## Summary

This chapter has provided an exploration of the way in which risk is understood in contemporary society. It has examined this in light of the changing nature of the term over time. In addition it has considered how the history of mental health services has contributed to the perception of people with mental health problems as 'risky'. It has outlined three different theoretical positions that have sought to examine risk and related these to mental health practice.

Within modern society we are focused on risk and a desire to avoid bad things happening. Within mental health services there has been a pressure to quantify and control the risks perceived to be posed by people with mental health problems. Yet in recent years there has been increasing debate within the literature about the utility of predictive risk assessment tools and calls for the individual experience of service users to be recognised in relation to this assessment process. The emphasis on recovery within mental health services has suggested a redefinition of risk to think about enabling people to keep themselves safe. Whilst others have suggested there should be increasing emphasis on mental health professionals' own intuitive judgement. We now have a vital opportunity to challenge the ways in which risk in relation to people with mental health problems has been defined, to move away from fear and danger towards enabling people to make choices about how they want to live their lives.

# References

Allen, J. (1997) 'Assessing and managing risk of violence in the mentally disordered', *Journal of Psychiatric and Mental Health Nursing*, 4 (5): 369–78.

Appelbaum, P., Robbins, P. and Monahan, J. (2000) 'Violence and delusions: data from the MacArthur Violence Risk Assessment Study', *American Journal Psychiatry*, 157 (4): 566–72.

Beck, U. (1992) *Risk Society: Towards a New Modernity.* London: Sage.

Buchanan, A. (1999) 'Risk and dangerousness', *Psychological Medicine*, 29 (2): 465–73.

Cutcliffe, J. and Hannighan, B. (2001) 'Mass media, monsters and mental health clients: the need for increased lobbying', *Journal of Psychiatric and Mental Health Nursing*, 8 (4): 315–21.

Department of Health (1998) *Modernising Mental Health Services: Safe, Sound and Supportive.* London: HMSO.

Department of Health (1999) *Effective Care Co-ordination in Mental Health Services: Modernising the Care Programme Approach.* London: HMSO.

Douglas, M. (1992) *Risk and Blame: Essays in Cultural Theory.* London: Routledge.

Douglas, M. and Wildavsky, A. (1982) *Risk and Culture.* Los Angeles: University of California Press.

Doyle, M. and Dolan, M. (2002) 'Violence risk assessment: combining actuarial and clinical information to structure clinical judgements for the formulation and management of risk', *Journal of Psychiatric and Mental Health Nursing*, 9 (6): 649–57.

Fazel, S., Singh, J., Doll, H. and Grann, M. (2012) 'Use of risk assessment instruments to predict violence and antisocial behaviour in 73 samples involving 24 827 people: systematic review and meta analysis', *British Medical Journal*, 345: 1–12 .

Foucault, M. (2006) *History of Madness.* London: Routledge.

Freshwater, D. and Westwood, T. (2006) 'Risk, detention and evidence: humanizing mental health reform, editorial', *Journal of Psychiatric and Mental Health Nursing*, 13 (3): 257–9.

Garvin, T. (2001) 'Analytical paradigms: the epistemological distances between scientists, policy makers and the public', *Risk Analysis*, 21 (3): 443–55.

Giddens, A. (1990) *The Consequences of Modernity.* Cambridge: Polity.

Godin, P. (2004) ' "You don't tick boxes on a form": a study of how community mental health nurses assess and manage risk', *Health, Risk and Society*, 6 (4): 347–60.

Goldacre, B. (2006) *It's not Easy to Predict Murder – Do the Maths.* Available at: www.guardian.co.uk/science/2006/dec/09/badscience.uknews (accessed 25/6/2013).

Harper, D. (2004) 'Storying policy: constructions of risk in proposals to reform UK mental health legislation', in B. Hurwitz, V. Skultans and T. Greenhalgh (eds), *Narrative Research in Health and Illness.* London: BMA Books.

James, A. (2006) 'Mind the gaps', *Mental Health Today*, (November): 8–9.

Kahneman, D. and Tversky, A. (1979) 'Prospect theory: an analysis of decision under risk', *Econometricia*, 47 (2): 263–91.

Kaliniecka, H. and Shawe-Taylor, M. (2008) 'Promoting positive risk management: evaluation of a risk management panel', *Journal of Psychiatric and Mental Health Nursing*, 15 (4): 654–61.

Kettles, A. (2004) 'A concept analysis of forensic risk', *Journal of Psychiatric and Mental Health Nursing*, 11 (4): 484–93.

Lupton, D. (1999) *Risk*. London: Routledge.

Lupton, D. and Tulloch, J. (2002) ' "Life would be pretty dull without risk": voluntary risk taking and its pleasures', *Health Risk and Society* 4 (2): 113–24.

McDonald, R., Waring, J. and Harrison, S. (2005) ' "Balancing risk that is my life": the politics of risk in a hospital operating theatre department', *Health, Risk and Society*, 7 (4): 397–411.

McGuire, J. (2004) 'Minimising harm in violence risk assessment: practical solutions to ethical problems?', *Health, Risk and Society*, 6 (4): 329–45.

Morgan, S. (2000) *Clinical Risk Management: A Clinical Tool and Practitioner Manual*. London: Sainsbury Centre for Mental Health.

Morrall, P. and Hazleton, M. (2000) 'Architecture signifying social control: the restoration of asylumdom in mental health care?', *International Journal of Mental Health Nursing*, 9 (2): 89–96.

Muir-Cochrane, E. (2006) 'Medical co-morbidity risk factors and barriers to care for people with schizophrenia', *Journal of Psychiatric and Mental Health Nursing*, 13: 447–52.

NHS Management Executive (1994) *Discharge of Mentally Disordered People and Their Continuing Care in the Community HSG (94) 5*. Leeds: NHS Management Executive.

NMC (Nursing and Midwifery Council) (2006) *Risk Management, Advice Sheet*. London: NMC.

Nolan, P. (1993) *A History of Mental Health Nursing*. London: Chapman and Hall.

Parker, J. and Stanworth, H. (2005) 'Go for it! Towards a critical realist approach to voluntary risk taking', *Health, Risk and Society*, 7 (4): 319–36.

Paterson, B. and Stark, C. (2001) 'Social policy and mental illness in England in the 1990s: violence, moral panic and critical discourse', *Journal of Psychiatric and Mental Health Nursing*, 8 (3): 257–67.

Porter, R. (2002) *Madness, a Brief History*. Oxford: Oxford University Press.

Repper, J. and Perkins, R. (2003) *Social Inclusion and Recovery*. Edinburgh: Ballière Tindall.

Rogers, A. and Pilgrim, D. (2010) *A Sociology of Mental Health and Illness* (4th edn). Maidenhead: McGraw-Hill/Open University Press.

Royal College of Psychiatrists (2008) *Rethinking Risk to Others in Mental Health Services: Final Report of Scoping Group*. London: Royal College of Psychiatrists.

Royal Society (1992) *Risk: Analysis, Perception and Management – Report of a Royal Society Study Group*. London: Royal Society.

Scull, A. (1979) *Museums of Madness: The Social Organisation of Insanity in Nineteenth Century England*. London: Allen Lane.

Steadman, H. (1983) 'Predicting dangerousness among the mentally ill; art, magic and science', *International Journal of Law and Psychiatry*, 6 (3–4): 381–90.

Stein, W.M. (2002) 'The use of discharge risk assessment tools in general psychiatric services in the UK', *Journal of Psychiatric and Mental Health Nursing*, 9 (6): 713–24.

Stickley, T. and Felton, A. (2006) 'Promoting recovery through therapeutic risk taking', *Mental Health Practice*, 9 (8): 26–30.

Szasz, T. (1963) *Law, Liberty and Psychiatry.* New York: Macmillan.

Szmukler, G. (2000) 'Homicide inquiries, what sense do they make?', *Psychiatric Bulletin*, 24 (1): 6–10.

Szmukler, G. and Holloway, F. (2000) 'Reform of the Mental Health Act: health or safety?', *British Journal of Psychiatry*, 177 (3): 196–200.

Taylor, P. and Gunn, J. (1999) 'Homicides by people with mental health illness: myth and reality', *British Journal of Psychiatry*, 174 (1): 9–14.

Thompson, M. and Rayner, S. (1998) 'Risk and governance Part I: the discourse of climate change', *Government and Opposition*, 33 (2): 139–66.

Warner, J. and Gabe, J. (2004) 'Risk and liminality in mental health social work', *Health, Risk and Society*, 6 (4) 387–99.

# 19

# Psychological Interventions in Primary Care

## MARIE CHELLINGSWORTH

### Learning Objectives

- Understand what psychological interventions in primary care are.
- Examine the historical development of psychological interventions in primary care settings.
- Consider the role of the nurse in the delivery of psychological interventions.
- Consider implications for practice.

## Introduction

The purpose of this chapter is to provide the reader with a contemporary understanding of psychological interventions within primary care. The chapter will give a definition of psychological interventions, provide an overview of the main interventions that are used and outline the role of the nurse in their delivery.

It is important that nurses have an understanding of the nature and evidence that supports psychological interventions in primary care and the commonly encountered problems that patients may present with. As many psychological interventions are provided as components of a holistic care package, with comprehensive care plans, including physical and social treatments, often the quality of the intervention is dependent on an organisation's ability to deliver these care packages in ways to ensure the components reinforce, rather than work against one another. Therefore, it is important that nurses are able to have a common and psychologically informed network around them drawing on their team's strengths and working towards each patient's needs, so an overall care plan can be formulated.

Many patients with mental health problems are cared for in primary care, with access to specialist services only if they are needed (Goldberg and Huxley, 1992). It is therefore important that all nurses have an understanding of primary care psychological interventions that they may need to refer to. Equally nurses may wish to undertake further training after qualification as the nurse has a long-standing role in the delivery of psychological therapies. The chapter considers the strengths and limitations of psychological interventions and the evidence base within primary care that supports them, and provides a theoretical overview of the development that underpins them as a framework. This framework also provides a guide to the nature and process of interventions that mental health nurses can provide and the history of nurses' involvement in psychological interventions in primary care. Psychological interventions require a supportive therapeutic relationship to be built and maintained between the practitioner and patient. The chapter will discuss how psychological interventions can be delivered in a patient-centred way, to ensure that patients understand their difficulties and the things that may be maintaining them. A case study of a patient and the nurse's role in providing psychological support will be used to illustrate this. Conclusions will be drawn about the role of the nurse in supporting psychological interventions and will synthesise the key points of the chapter.

## Psychological interventions

Psychological intervention is a broad umbrella term that is used to describe a range of heterogeneous interventions that are said to have a positive impact upon a person's well-being, delivered by a health care practitioner or therapist. There are many schools of psychological intervention and orientation. Many different types of interventions may be classified this way, from therapies with an underpinning model and structure to more simple interactions between a patient and health care practitioner that are supportive in the face of psychological distress. Table 19.1 summarises some of these interventions. However the term is most commonly applied to psychological interventions from a particular therapeutic model, of which behavioural and cognitive behavioural interventions are most commonly used in primary care and which are the focus of this chapter.

Most psychological interventions within primary care are those delivered for common mental health problems. The term common mental health problem refers to high prevalence and commonly occurring difficulties, namely depression and anxiety. The term common should not be misunderstood to mean that they are not as significant as other mental health problems as they can cause significant distress and be severely disabling to the person experiencing them.

**TABLE 19.1**  Examples of psychological therapies

| | |
|---|---|
| **Cognitive behavioural therapy (CBT)** | CBT is a time-limited, structured and problem-focused treatment. It looks at the person's difficulties in the 'here-and-now' and treatment involves active interventions to target maintaining factors in the person's behavioural, physical or thoughts. The patient undertakes active work between sessions, often known as 'homework'. CBT has been shown to be effective for a wide range of mental health conditions and is widely recommended in NICE guidelines for depression, anxiety disorders and other problem areas. |
| **Behavioural activation (BA)** | BA is a standalone treatment which targets negative reinforcement in depression and is highly effective when used as a treatment in its own right. BA is often wrongly thought of as a treatment under the CBT umbrella but it is not part of a treatment package, but is in fact a treatment in itself. When a depressed patient has symptoms (such as lethargy) he/she may avoid activities as a result. Initially this avoidance gives relief from the symptoms. Avoidance is therefore repeated to avoid anticipated further symptoms. This however leads to removal of the patient from positive reinforcement and can maintain low mood as a result. Treatment targets in a hierarchy routine, necessary and pleasurable activities to get back to routine regulation. It uses an outside-in approach, asking the patient to act according to an external goal rather than an internal feeling or thought. It can target rumination and increase problem-solving. |
| **Interpersonal therapy (IPT) for depression** | IPT is a psychological therapy which looks at the role of interpersonal relationships in treating the patient's difficulties. It has been shown to be effective for depression and anorexia. IPT is time-limited and structured. Its central idea is that psychological symptoms, such as depressed mood, can be understood as a response to current difficulties in relationships and affect the quality of those relationships. Typically, IPT focuses on conflict with another person, life changes that affect how individuals may feel about themselves or others, grief, loss, or difficulty in starting or keeping relationships going. A course of IPT treatment usually involves 8–16 sessions. |

*(Continued)*

**TABLE 19.1**    (Continued)

| | |
|---|---|
| Brief dynamic interpersonal therapy (DIT) for depression | DIT is a short (16 session) treatment for depression. DIT is a form of brief psychodynamic psychotherapy developed for treating depression. It can help people with emotional and relationship problems. It explores difficult things in the past that continue to affect the way people feel and behave in the present. It is also referred to as psychoanalytic psychotherapy. NICE guidelines for depression state that brief psychodynamic therapy is one option that can be considered for depressed patients either when the patient has not responded to CBT interventions, or where the patient actively opts for a psychodynamic approach. |
| Counselling for depression | Counselling in primary care is recommended within NICE guidelines for depression for patients who have not responded to or who do not want CBT or another treatment. Counselling can help people with emotional difficulties and problems in relating to people. Typically people with mild to moderate depression might receive between 6 and 10 sessions over 8–12 weeks. In cases of serious depression, up to 20 sessions of counselling is recommended. In most primary care services people are likely to be seen once a week for 50–60 minutes. |
| Behavioural couples counselling for depression | Behavioural couples counselling aims to help couples understand the ways in which difficulties in their relationship can contribute to depression or anxiety in one (or sometimes both) partners. Couple therapy can help people with their relationship and the emotional difficulties that sometimes flow from problems between partners. Behavioural couples counselling should be no more than 20 sessions over a period of 6 months. |

# Historical development of psychological therapies within primary care

In England in 2007 the last Adult Psychiatric Morbidity Survey (APMS) found that one in six adults were stated to be suffering from a high prevalence common mental health problem such as an anxiety disorder or depression. Medically unexplained symptoms are conditions where the patient complains of physical symptoms that cause excessive worry or discomfort or lead the patient to seek treatment but for which no adequate organ pathology or pathophysiological basis can be found (Fink et al., 2002). Many patients in primary care complain of physical symptoms not attributable to any known conventionally defined disease, i.e. medically unexplained symptoms (MUS). Individuals with such symptoms may have an underlying psychological problem, which, if correctly identified, may respond to one or more of a number of psychological interventions in primary care (Henningsen et al., 2007).

Individuals with long-term physical conditions such as diabetes and chronic obstructive pulmonary disease are also more likely to have depression or anxiety. In patients with diabetes, for example, depression is two to three times as common as in the general population, indicating increased use of health care services and increased contact with primary care services (Cohen, 2008).

A review conducted by the King's Fund in 2006 to estimate mental health expenditure, including depression, in England up to 2026 (McCrone et al., 2008) combined prevalence rates taken from the APMS, with population estimates for 2007 through to 2026. It was estimated then that there were 1.24 million people with depression alone in England, and this was projected to rise by 17% to 1.45 million by 2026. Based on these figures the total costs for depression, including prescribed drugs, inpatient care, other NHS services, supported accommodation, social services and workplace absenteeism were estimated to be £1.7 billion in England in 2007, while lost employment increased this total to £7.5 billion. By 2026, these figures are projected to be £3 billion and £12.2 billion, respectively.

Whilst mental ill health and common mental health problems are known to be high prevalence, costly and attributed to negative societal outcomes, positive mental health and well-being is seen as fundamental to quality of life. Positive mental health is defined as individuals thinking and feeling good about themselves and feeling able to cope with their problems (World Health Organization, 2005). It is argued to be an essential component of productivity, social cohesion, peace and stability in the living environment, contributing to social capital and economic development in society (World Health Organization, 2005). Tackling mental illness and increasing well-being in primary care is therefore an understandable government priority within the UK, with well-being in the general population becoming an important marker in appraising life quality (ONS, 2012).

For both anxiety and depression there are effective treatments available which are recommended within clinical guidelines developed by the National Institute for Health and Clinical Excellence (NICE). Whilst NICE guidelines and the evidence that is selected within them have come under some criticism (Mollon, 2009), increasing the availability of cognitive behavioural therapy (CBT) based psychological therapies in England has become a key government and health care priority as a result of the burden of illness anxiety and depression cause. Current policy on psychological therapy treatment services is unusual in that it is being influenced both by economic pressures and by psychological research on the factors of happiness, subjective well-being and life satisfaction (Cooper, 2009).

## The history of psychological interventions in primary care

Over 90 years ago, Sigmund Freud remarked that 'compared to the vast amount of neurotic misery there is in the world and perhaps need not be, the quantity we can do away with is almost negligible' (Freud, 1919: 166). This prophetic passage both recognised the limited number of people able to help those in distress at that time, something which would remain the case, but also foresaw a day when the state would come to accept its collective responsibility and psychological interventions would be available according to need. The high economic and social costs associated with common mental health problems and the need to scale up appropriate care services are now widely recognised (World Health Organization, 2008). It could be argued the prediction of Freud in 1919 may have been realised within the ambitious aims of the Improving Access to Psychological Therapies (IAPT) initiative. The IAPT programme was a Department of Health initiative to improve access to psychological therapies recommended within NICE guidelines. It was developed in 2005, after a White Paper commitment in *Our Health, Our Care, Our Say* (DH, 2006).

The IAPT agenda set out the government's plans to implement national guidelines for the regional delivery of psychological therapies for anxiety and depression. From the outset of the IAPT initiative it was recognised that there was a shortage of trained therapists who could deliver the treatments recommended within NICE guidelines and that this was the core deficiency preventing the routine delivery of them (DH, 2011a). Therefore the need for training more practitioners such as nurses to deliver treatment was established. A key role played in driving forward the initiative was played by NICE and Lord Richard Layard, Professor Emeritus of Economics at the London School of Economics. In 2006, the London School of Economics published their long awaited publication *The Depression Report: A New Deal for Depression and Anxiety Disorders*; in it they called for the increase in availability of NICE-approved therapies, particularly CBT, and, argued that mental illness has now replaced unemployment as Britain's biggest social problem with only one in four people with anxiety and depression receiving any kind of treatment. Layard and colleagues further asserted that the economic consequences of this phenomenon are grave and proposed that a national strategy was required to make psychological therapy more widely available (Cooper, 2009). They also argued that in doing so treatment could be implemented for just £750 per person. It was clearly highlighted within the report that the evidence-based treatments were not being delivered because of the shortage of trained therapists and they called for action in terms of training 10,000 therapists from backgrounds such as nursing to work in new teams of psychological therapists in a seven-year centrally funded plan (Layard, 2006).

Two IAPT demonstration sites were established in 2006 to ascertain if the creation of services in which trained therapists offered NICE-approved therapies in line with the clinical trials in which the evidence base was created would be efficacious. These were situated in geographically different areas of England, in Doncaster and Newham, to provide the CBT-based services to those in the community who required them. Findings relating to the two demonstration sites were published in 2009 by Clark et al., who within their initial evaluation of the two sites, suggested that during the 13 months in which both were studied, nearly 5500 people had been referred, and 3500 had concluded their treatment. Both demonstration sites were reported to have achieved good recovery rates (52%) for people who had depression and/or an anxiety disorder for more than six months. Cooper (2009) offers an alternative perspective, however, and states that of those referred to the demonstration sites, 40% were deemed unsuitable for treatment, declined therapy or dropped out after a single episode. Despite this, the results from the two demonstration sites do appear to suggest that CBT in the field can deliver rapid and effective results as proposed within the NICE guidelines. Moreover, the follow-up study reports that these gains are maintained 4–12 months later. Interestingly, at the end of treatment, 5% more of the treated population were also in employment than at the start of treatment. Subsequently as a result of the successfully viewed pilot sites, 11 so-called 'Pathfinder' sites were then established at locations across the country (IAPT, 2008). Nearly 12,000 patients were referred. Over 90% of them were referred from general medical practice with diagnoses of depression and/or anxiety. A majority of patients were judged to require step 2 interventions: most often guided CBT self-help supported by low intensity CBT practitioners (subsequently named psychological well-being practitioners [PWPs]). Only one-quarter (27.3%) were offered full CBT with high intensity trained therapists (IAPT, 2008).

In September 2007, the Department of Health published *The Competences Required to Deliver Effective Cognitive and Behavioural Therapy for People with Depression and with Anxiety Disorders* (Roth and Pilling, 2007). The publication was the result of a project commissioned specifically by the Department of Health, with additional funding from Skills for Health and the Centre for Outcomes, Research and Effectiveness (CORE), and appears to have stemmed from a recognition that the success of the initiative would rest on the success of competently trained practitioners who were able to offer effective CBT interventions at both low and high intensity level (Holland, 2009).

This was followed in October 2007 by the then UK Health Secretary Alan Johnson announcing a remarkable expansion of psychological therapies based on the pathfinders, after findings from numerous reports indicated the huge cumulative financial cost to the UK in terms of providing care and support to people with anxiety and depression (Druss et al., 2001; Kessler et al., 1999; Layard, 2006). The UK government as a result of the comprehensive spending review (CSR07) initiated a national roll-out of new psychological therapy services to every Strategic Health Authority area in an initial three-year centrally funded programme to run to March 2011. The government invested £173 million in the first three years, £33 million being paid in 2008/9; £70 million in 2009/10 and £70 million again in 2010/11. In return for this financial investment, however, the services were required to deliver:

1  900,000 more people treated for depression and anxiety disorders
2  450,000 anticipated to move to recovery
3  25,000 fewer people with mental health problems on benefits
4  3700 more newly trained therapists to provide evidence-based low and high intensity psychological interventions (Clark, 2011).

In addition to the clinical skills training of over 3700 therapists through the IAPT agenda in England, a further 2400 are expected to be trained by 2015 (DH, 2011a). A large number of nurses undertook the training to become accredited CBT or IPT (interpersonal therapy) therapists working at step 3 or psychological well-being practitioners delivering CBT self-help at step 2 of the stepped care model (Figure 19.1).

Nurses make up the largest group of trained professionals in the IAPT workforce. These trainees attend a university-based programme to undertake the national curriculum training in the psychological therapy skills required for their respective roles (DH, 2008, 2011b).

| | | |
|---|---|---|
| Step 3: High intensity service | Depression<br>mild, moderate and severe | CBT, IPT behavioural<br>activation |
| | Depression<br>mild–moderate | Counselling,<br>couples therapy |
| | Panic disorder | CBT |
| | Generalised anxiety disorder<br>(GAD) mild–moderate | CBT |
| | Social phobia | CBT |
| | Post traumatic<br>stress disorder (PTSD) | CBT, eye movement<br>desensitisation<br>and reprocessing (EMDR) |
| | Obsessive compulsive<br>disorder (OCD) | CBT |
| Step 2: Low intensity service | Depression<br>mild–moderate | cCBT, guided self-help,<br>behavioural activation,<br>exercise |
| | Panic disorder<br>mild–moderate | cCBT, guided self-help, pure<br>self help, |
| | Generalised anxiety disorder<br>(GAD) mild–moderate | cCBT, guided self-help, pure<br>self-help, psychoeducation<br>groups |
| | OCD mild–moderate | Guided self-help |
| Step 1: Primary care/IAPT<br>service | Recognition of problem | Assessment / Watchful waiting |

**FIGURE 19.1**   The stepped care model of psychological interventions in primary care (IAPT, 2011)

*Source*: IAPT (2011) Improving Access to Psychological Therapies, Annex 2. Available at: www.iapt.nhs.uk/silo/
files/guidance-for-commissioning-iapt-training-201112-201415.pdf (accessed 25/6/2013)

# The history of the nurse in delivering evidence-based psychological therapy in primary care

The concept of the mental health nurse might signal the emergence of a new vision for human services, but might also indicate the need for mental health nurses to negotiate a formal separation from the traditional 'psychiatric' family (Barker and Buchanan-Barker, 2011). Today, the nurse's primary functions remain much the same as a century ago: to keep people (and others) safe, to express medical treatment and in hospital settings, to manage the physical and social environment; the stereotype of the 'housekeeper'. Barker and Buchanan-Barker (2011) state that it is clear that nurses are almost indispensable and many nurses have also completed supplementary training, qualifying them to deliver different therapies.

Nurses delivering psychological interventions have proved, in many robust evaluations over the years, to play a key role in the effective delivery of psychological interventions (Gournay, 1989, 2000). Prior to the seminal work of Isaac Marks in developing training for nurses in psychological interventions, therapies such as CBT were delivered by psychiatrists and psychologists. The training of nurses in the delivery of behaviour therapy was at first highly controversial, but showed that nurses can provide effective psychological interventions. It also provided a springboard for many nurses trained in this way to enter research, teaching and management (Gournay et al., 2009).

The English Nursing Board Behavioural Psychotherapy course (ENB 650) was the first of such training initiatives in psychological interventions to be opened to nurses. It was initiated by the psychiatrist Professor Isaac Marks and colleagues at the Maudsley Hospital, London in 1972 in order to address the lack of therapists to deliver the then emerging behaviour therapies (Marks et al., 1977). The course was developed in the face of considerable opposition from across the mental health professions (including nursing itself) and aimed to prepare nurses to become autonomous in using behavioural techniques. The course trained nurses in the treatment of specific phobias, agoraphobia, social phobia, social skills problems, obsessive compulsive disorder, sexual problems and habit disorders. The training was rigorously evaluated and the data showed clearly that nurses were at least as effective as their colleagues from other disciplines in delivering behavioural therapy (Gournay, 2000).

Nurses have played a key role working within primary care for many years, both in delivering CBT-based interventions but also in providing support and medication management. Nurse practitioner roles in primary care were highly specialist positions for experienced nurses. Nurses have delivered a range of psychological interventions to support patients in this setting and now many continue to work in primary care.

## The development of psychological theories

There are a number of theories which underpin specific psychological interventions. Behavioural and cognitive behavioural interventions are rooted within classical learning theory (conditioning and operant learning) and in social learning (see Chapter 5). Contemporary research and practice recognise the strength of behavioural interventions as standalone treatments for depression with treatments such as behavioural activation as well as CBT-based treatments as packages of care. Indeed it is argued that cognitive approaches in their own right may have limited effect without the behavioural elements. For example, cognitive restructuring effects may be as a direct result of the impact on the patient's behaviour which in turn modifies his or her subjective state (Roth and Fonagy, 2005). Component analyses of CBT versus behavioural activation for depression have shown behavioural activation to be just as effective, briefer (Jacobsen, 1996) and is said to be more easy to train staff to deliver.

## Theory applied to practice

The nurse plays a vital role in the stepped care model, recognising high prevalence disorders, referring patients for psychological therapies and supporting patients with their difficulties. Nurses are able to refer patients within the stepped care model to either psychological well-being practitioners who are trained to deliver low intensity CBT interventions at step 2 or high intensity workers at step 3, but may also be delivering these treatments themselves. Nurses also form part of many patients' treatment programmes, through supporting physical health care in patients with long-term health conditions as well as anxiety and/or depression. Therefore, nurses are ideally placed within these fields to recognise and support patients with both their physical and psychological needs.

As nurses are front-line clinicians in both primary and secondary care it is imperative that they are psychologically minded and possess key skills and expertise in mental health, in order to help to raise the profile of psychological support within mental health through a holistic approach. As GP awareness continues to rise in psychological therapies, nurses are in a position to be able to support the primary care team to become better aware of them. This awareness is crucial for both ensuring that appropriate referrals to therapy services are made and that patients are adequately prepared to be able to engage with psychological treatments (Royal College of Psychiatry, 2008). It is therefore essential for nursing staff to raise their awareness of psychological interventions within the stepped care model.

Psychological mindedness is an additional requirement to the generic *Ten Essential Shared Capabilities of Mental Health Workers* (National Institute for Mental Health in England and Sainsbury Centre for Mental Health, 2004). Psychological mindedness can motivate nurses who have little previous training in psychological therapies to take an active interest in this area. Historically, attitudes have been major obstacles to the wider use of psychological therapies, as much as structure and resources. Changes in attitudes have been necessary to help improvement in service provision and focus on change.

In principle, the stepped care model ensures patients receive the least complex intervention from which they are likely to benefit. Due to the expansion of the voluntary sector, nurses and GPs have a responsibility to ensure patients are aware of these opportunities and make full use of them. Signposting is key and ensures patients receive a comprehensive care package to meet their needs accordingly.

The following case example illustrates the ways in which psychological interventions in primary care can be used in practice.

**CASE EXAMPLE**

John is a 61-year-old man who has been feeling increasingly tired and lethargic. He has been feeling this way for seven months since he retired. John struggles to get out of bed in the morning as he does not feel he has any routine or structure to his day anymore. He describes a lack of energy and can't be bothered to do the activities he used to enjoy or needs to do around his home. John was a keen gardener and took pride in his garden as well as being the captain of his local golf club. He had looked forward to becoming more involved with his hobbies once retiring; however he can't see the point of them anymore.

His wife died nine years ago and he never remarried. He lives alone, but has two children. His oldest daughter is a very successful solicitor living in London and his younger daughter emigrated to Australia to work as a nurse five years ago. He does not get to see his daughters much. John can see the garden is becoming more overgrown and feels he is letting his friends at the club down. He has also been avoiding speaking with his daughters on Skype and tends to ignore their phone calls. John tends to just sit in front of the television during the day but does not take in the content of the programmes as he struggles to concentrate. He finds himself lying awake at night thinking about how he is letting everyone down and how upset his wife would be if she could see him now. John was referred by his GP for an assessment with Jill, a nurse therapist in primary care, and although he discussed possible antidepressant medication with his GP, he has chosen to meet the nurse therapist first when his GP offered him this.

He met with Jill and her student nurse Sally for an assessment at his GP surgery. Jill and Sally conducted a brief 35-minute assessment of how his current problem was affecting him physically (autonomic), behaviourally and cognitively. John did not report any current or past suicide or self-harming thoughts, plans or actions and did not feel he posed a risk to anyone else. Although he was not having regular contact with his daughters at present, he still described them as strong preventative factors if he were to get thoughts of suicide. A summary of the model used for the assessment is provided in Figure 19.2.

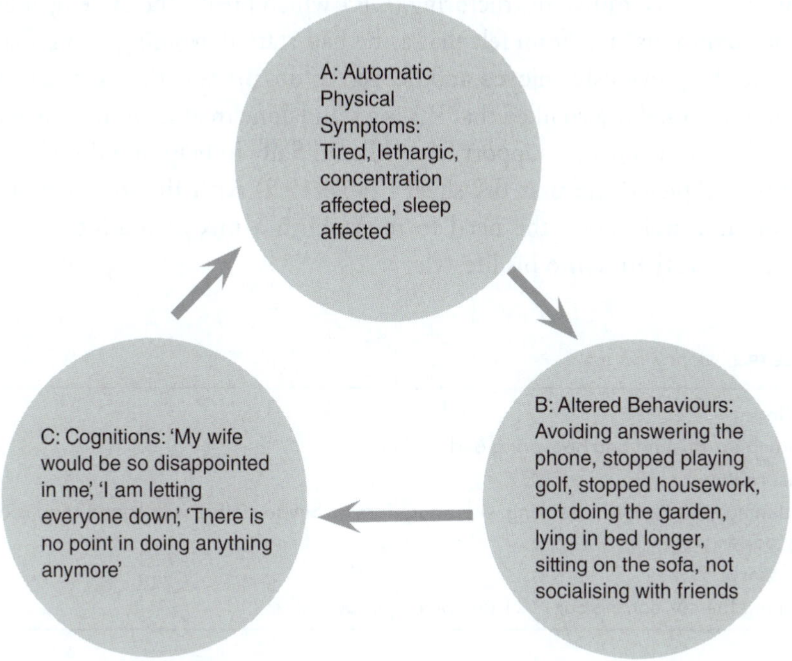

**FIGURE 19.2** John's ABC model

# John's treatment intervention

The information outlined in the ABC assessment model above is part of the information gathered during John's patient-centred assessment with Jill and Sally. Towards the end of the assessment, the student nurse and John devised a problem statement together using this information. The problem statement provided a shared understanding of John's current difficulties. The problem statement acted as a baseline for John, Jill and the student nurse to return to at each session to monitor progress. The symptoms described by John and summarised in his problem statement were indicative of depression. Jill and Sally gave John information about depression and talked through some low intensity evidence-based treatment options with him. In line with NICE guidelines (2009), the evidence-based treatment options discussed with John break into the areas identified in the diagram above.

The two primary treatment interventions discussed with John were behavioural activation (BA) which aims to break the cycle at the behaviours as a standalone treatment and cognitive restructuring (CR), which breaks the cycle by intervention in the cognitions area. John felt that as he had started avoiding doing many of the activities he previously enjoyed and needed to do, BA was the treatment he would like to focus on. He also liked that BA is a standalone treatment in its own right and he could have telephone support from Jill and Sally to help him do this.

John completed the first BA sheet (Table 19.2) with Jill and Sally in his next session and understood the need to re-establish a mix of routine, necessary and pleasurable activities into his lifestyle.

**TABLE 19.2**   John's BA list

| |
|---|
| **Routine:** |
| Washing up, dusting and hoovering and cooking |
| **Pleasurable:** |
| Gardening, playing golf, speaking with daughters on Skype, coffee with friends and reading the daily paper |
| **Necessary:** |
| Cleaning the car, sorting car MOT and paying paper bill. |

Jill and Sally then discussed with John putting a mix of the routine, necessary and pleasurable activities into a hierarchy according to the level of difficulty, i.e. easy, medium or difficult (Table 19.3). John initially took some time to do this as it felt to him as if all the tasks were difficult. However, with some encouragement he soon completed the second sheet.

**TABLE 19.3**   John's BA sheet 2·

| |
|---|
| **The most difficult:** |
| Cooking dinner, sorting car MOT, gardening, playing golf |
| **Medium difficulty:** |
| Cleaning the car, speaking with daughters on Skype, coffee with friends |
| **The easiest:** |
| Cleaning the car, paying paper bill, reading the daily paper. |

John liked the idea of then transferring these activities into a diary as it took him back to his working days of planning out tasks (Table 19.4). He also was able to grasp the principle of working according to his planned goals rather than how he was feeling and liked the phrase 'outside-in' rather than 'inside-out' as a reminder. John identified that he did not feel that he would gain pleasure from doing any of the activities straight away, so was reassured to hear that this was not the aim of BA and that initially BA aims to complete the activities just for the sake of doing them to help re-establish the routine he is aware he has lost. John reported that he felt better knowing in advance that his mood would lift in time as he said he would have been worried if he hadn't seen much change in himself otherwise.

John planned the activities into his diary for the following week and was clear to initially focus on the easier activities and to always ensure that there was a mix of routine, necessary and pleasure within the week.

**TABLE 19.4**  John's BA diary

| | | Mon | Tue | Wed | Thurs | Fri | Sat | Sun |
|---|---|---|---|---|---|---|---|---|
| Morning | What Where When Who | | | | | | Read daily paper, on own in summer house – 10 am | |
| Afternoon | What Where When Who | Pay paper bill – in village on own – 2 pm | | Clean car with Frank at home – 1 pm. | | | | |
| Evening | What Where When Who | | | | | | | |

Over the next three weeks, Sally the student nurse and Jill the primary care nurse met with John and reviewed his BA homework diary, which he completed and brought with him each week. John moved up the hierarchy and worked on some of the more difficult activities with the support and guidance of Jill and Sally. Over the next few weeks, John noticed an improvement in his mood and he reported a positive change and shift from the initial problem statement they devised together. It had become apparent that John had a much clearer routine to his day and he was beginning to enjoy some of the activities that he had been previously avoiding. John had begun seeing his friends at the golf club and speaking regularly with his daughters again on Skype. He felt more in control around the house and now felt like his 'old self again' and that through working on his behaviours he noticed that some of his negative thinking had changed as a result. Jill also asked John whether he had noticed any improvement in some of the initial physical symptoms he described and he reported sleeping much better and not feeling as tired and lethargic.

Jill and Sally spoke with John following their fifth session and it was agreed that he was ready to be discharged. John reported that he was pleased with how much progress he had made in a relatively short amount of time and felt he had a good 'toolkit' to take away from their sessions which he would continue to use and look over again as and when needed. Jill and John completed a recovery action plan for the future to help him to recognise early warning signs that his low mood may be returning and what he could do about it. John wrote on his recovery action plan that his main learning was 'you can't think your way out of depression, you act your way out of it and not to avoid things'.

## Summary

The chapter has presented the historical development of psychological interventions in primary care and the role of the nurse in their delivery. The strengths and limitations of psychological interventions have been examined and the historical development of psychological interventions in primary care explored. The role of the nurse within primary care has been discussed as important in understanding the stepped care model and the key part nurses can play in supporting and referring patients according to their presentations so they receive the most appropriate and least burdensome treatment first outlined. Finally, the case example of John has been used to illustrate how a nurse could easily deliver an evidence-based psychological intervention, in this case behavioural activation within a 35-minute assessment and five 25-minute treatment sessions, noting the key processes in assessing and treating a patient displaying symptoms of low mood and looking in more detail at how to support a patient through the step 2 evidence-based treatment option.

# Further learning

A web-based module is available for learning more about psychological interventions:

'Access to psychological therapies in primary care: an update'. BMJ Learning. http://learning.bmj.com/learning/search-result.html?moduleId=10014102

# References

Barker, P. and Buchanan-Barker, P. (2011) 'Myth of mental health nursing and the challenge of recovery', *International Journal of Mental Health Nursing*, 20 (5): 337–44.

Clark, D. (2011) 'Implementing NICE guidelines for the psychological treatment of depression and anxiety disorders: the IAPT experience', *International Review of Psychiatry*, 23: 375–84.

Clark, D., Layard, R., Smithies, R., Richards, D., Suckling, R. and Wright, B. (2009) 'Improving access to psychological therapies: initial evaluation of two UK demonstration sites', *Behaviour Research and Therapy*, 47 (8): 637–728.

Cohen, A. (2008) 'The primary care management of anxiety and depression: a GP's perspective', *Advances in Psychiatric Treatment*, 14 (2): 98–105.

Department of Health (2006) *Our Health, Our Care, Our Say*. London: DH.

Department of Health (2008) *Improving Access to Psychological Therapies: Implementation Plan: Curriculum for High Intensity Therapies Workers*. Available at: www.iapt.nhs.uk/silo/files/implementation-plan-curriculum-for-high8208intensity-therapies-workers.pdf.

Department of Health (2011a) *Talking Therapies: A Four-year Plan of Action*. London: DH.

Department of Health (2011b) *Curriculum and Commissioning Outline; IAPT Approved High Intensity Therapies (Additional to CBT)*. Available at: www.iapt.nhs.uk/silo/files/curriculum-and-commissioning-outline-march-2011-update-v0-6-final.pdf.

Druss, B. G., Rohrbaugh, R. M., Levinson, C. M., (2001) 'Integrated medical care for patients with a serious psychiatric illness', *Archives of General Psychiatry*, 58: 861–868.

Cooper, L. (2009) 'Values-based mental health nursing practice' in P. Callaghan, J. Playle and L. Cooper (eds), *Mental Health Nursing Skills*. Oxford: Oxford University Press.

Fink, P., Rosendal, M. and Toft, T. (2002) 'Assessment and treatment of functional disorders in general practice: the extended reattribution and management model – an advanced educational program for nonpsychiatric doctors', *Psychosomatics*, 43 (2): 93–131.

Freud, S. (1919) *The Uncanny*.

Goldberg, D. and Huxley, P. (1992) *Common Mental Disorders: A Biosocial Model*. London: Routledge.

Gournay, K. (1989) *Agoraphobia: Current Perspectives on Theory and Treatment.* London: Routledge.

Gournay, K. (2000) 'Nurses as therapists (1972–2000)', *Behavioural and Cognitive Psychotherapy*, 28 (4): 369–377.

Gournay, K., Denford, L., Parr, A.-M. and Newell, R. (2000) 'British nurses in behavioural psychotherapy: a 25-year follow up', *Journal of Advanced Nursing*, 32(2): 343–351.

Henningsen, P., Zipfel, Z. and Herzog, W. (2007) 'Management of functional somatic syndromes', *The Lancet*, 369 (9565): 946–55.

Holland, R. (2009) 'Assessing competences against the Cognitive Behavioural Therapy Framework', *CBT Today*, 39 (1): 12–13.

IAPT (2008) *The IAPT Pathfinders: Achievements and Challenges.* Available at: www.iapt.nhs.uk/silo/files/the-iapt-pathfinders-achievements-and-challenges.pdf.

IAPT (2011) *Improving Access to Psychological Therapies, Annex 2.* Available at: www.iapt.nhs.uk/silo/files/guidance-for-commissioning-iapt-training-201112-201415.pdf (accessed 25/6/13).

Jacobson, N.S., Dobson, K.S., Truax, P.A., Addis, M.E., Koerner, K., Gollan, J.K., Gortner, E. and Prince, S.E. (1996) 'A component analysis of cognitive-behavioral treatment for depression', *Journal of Consulting and Clinical Psychology*, 64(2): 295–304.

Kessler, R.C., Borges, G., and Walters, E.E. (1999) 'Prevalence of and risk factors for lifetime suicide attempts in the National Comorbidity Survey', *Archives of General Psychiatry*, 56(7): 617–626.

Layard, R. (2006) *The Depression Report.* London: London School of Economics.

McCrone, P., Dhanasiri, S., Patel, A., Knapp, M. and Lawton-Smith, S. (2008) *Paying the Price: The Cost of Mental Health Care in England to 2026.* London: King's Fund.

Marks, I., Hallam, R.S., Connolly, J. and Philpott, R. (1977) *Nursing in Behaviour Psychotherapy.* London: Royal College of Nursing.

Mollon, P. (2009) 'The NICE guidelines are misleading, unscientific and potentially impede good psychological care and help', *Psychodynamic Practice*, 15 (1): 9–24.

National Institute for Mental Health in England and Sainsbury Centre for Mental Health (2004) *The Ten Essential Shared Capabilities of Mental Health Workers.* London. Available at: www.mhhe.heacademy.ac.uk/silo/files/tenescpdf.pdf.

NICE (National Institute for Clinical Excellence) (2011) *Generalised Anxiety Disorder and Panic Disorder (with or without Agoraphobia) in Adults: Management in Primary, Secondary and Community Care.* London: National Institute for Clinical Excellence.

Richards, D. and Borglin, G. (2011) 'Implementation of psychological therapies for anxiety and depression in routine practice: two year prospective cohort study', *Journal of Affective Disorders*, 133: 51–60.

Roth, A. and Fonagy, P. (2005) *What Works for Whom? A Critical Review of Psychotherapy Research.* New York: Guilford Press.

Roth, A. and Pilling, S. (2007) *The Competences Required to Deliver Effective Cognitive and Behavioural Therapy for People with Depression and with Anxiety Disorders.* London: Department of Health.

Royal College of Psychiatry (2008) *Psychological Therapies in Psychiatry and Primary Care.* Available at www.rcpsych.ac.uk/files/pdfversion/cr151.pdf.

World Health Organization (2005) *Promoting Mental Health.* Available at www.who.int/mental_health/evidence/MH_Promotion_Book.pdf.

World Health Organization (2008) *mhGAP Mental Health Gap Action Programme.* Available at www.who.int/mental_health/evidence/mhGAP/en/index.html.

# 20

# Behaviour Change Theory

## PATRICK CALLAGHAN

### Learning Objectives

- Understand the development of behaviour change theories as they relate to health and well-being.
- Describe selected behaviour change theories.
- Evaluate behaviour change theories.
- Apply selected behaviour change theories in mental health nursing practice.

## Introduction

There is a strong evidence base showing that behaviour and lifestyle factors contribute to cancers, cardiovascular diseases and infectious diseases, the major causes of death in developed and developing countries today (WHO, 2010). People can enhance their health and well-being by adopting behaviours that improve their health such as taking regular exercise and avoiding behaviours harmful to health such as smoking. There are two main categories of factors that enhance or compromise people's health. Extrinsic factors include laws such as banning smoking in public places or penalising people who do not wear seat belts and impose restrictions that are designed to safeguard people's health and well-being and incentives such as public subsidies for sports and leisure services to encourage people to use such facilities. Taxing alcohol and tobacco products is designed to act as a deterrent against smoking and excess alcohol use. Intrinsic factors such as personality, behaviour, motivations, attitudes and beliefs are the focus of this chapter.

Understanding why people engage in behaviours helpful or harmful to their health can help us improve the health of individuals and societies and has long interested behavioural scientists and other researchers from whose studies behaviour changes theories have emerged.

Health behaviour change theories explain theoretically the links between behaviour and various health outcomes. These theories can be broadly categorised as stage theories or continuum theories; this chapter examines both categories. Stage theories, the most common of which is the Transtheoretical Model of Change, hypothesise that people move through discrete stages systematically towards a desired outcome and that different processes occur at each stage; these processes explain forward and backward movement between stages. It is assumed within stage theories that interventions to change people's behaviour must be matched to the stage of the person's behaviour. Continuum theories, the most widely researched of which is the Theory of Planned Behaviour, hypothesise that the likelihood of engaging in healthy behaviour depends on the individual's intention to do so on a continuum from weak to strong intentions. In continuum theories interventions to change people's behaviour do not need to be stage-matched.

Explanations inherent in health behaviour change theories allow us to develop behaviour change interventions that can reduce the prevalence of major diseases and deaths associated with these conditions and improve people's health and well-being. This chapter examines the historical development of health behaviour change theories, describes and evaluates theories of health behaviour change, and, using examples of work with people living with mental health issues, illustrates how mental health nurses can apply these theories to improve the health and well-being of people for whom they care.

# Historical development

The changing patterns of health and disease in the last hundred years show that the major causes of death in developed and developing countries have shifted from diseases related to microbial infections (e.g. tuberculosis) to diseases of the circulatory system and cancers (Ogden, 2007). In 1912 the major causes of death in the USA were pneumonia and influenza, tuberculosis and diarrhoea and other intestinal diseases. By 1940 these diseases were no longer the major killers that they were at the beginning of the twentieth century, having been supplanted by cancers and circulatory diseases (Levy and Moskowitz, 1982). Today, diseases of the circulatory system and cancers are the major causes of age-standardised deaths in most countries – with the exception of the African continent – from which there are recorded data. In Africa the major causes of death are infectious diseases, of which AIDS-related illnesses are the most prominent (WHO, 2010).

There are several explanations in the health literature for the changing patterns of health and disease in the last century. One explanation is that the changes arose from advances in medical care (e.g. more hospitals, dispensaries and midwifery services), improvements in medical education and doctors' understanding of anatomy and physiology, the development of health protective measures like vaccines, and the discovery of effective treatments like antibiotics (Griffith, cited in McKeown, 1976). These advances were thought to have significantly reduced diseases related to microbial infections and meant people lived longer and populations increased. However, McKeown (1976) argued that the changing patterns in health and disease in the early part of the century were largely the result of improved nutrition arising from better standards of living, and had little to do with medical advances. McKeown derived his evidence from epidemiological data showing that many of the diseases thought to be reduced by medical advances had been declining before these advances arrived. Szreter (1988) countered McKeown's criticisms by showing evidence that advances in medical and sanitary science and the rise of a public health agenda brought about significant changes in disease patterns. Evidence from the World Health Organization (WHO, 2010) suggests that the explanations reported by McKeown (1976) and Szreter (1988) have contributed to the changing patterns of health and disease in addition to environmental, political, personal, social and economic changes. The changes in health and illness in the twentieth century show a decline in diseases related to microbial and associated infections to conditions in which behaviour and lifestyle play an important part (Matarazzo and Leckliter, 1988).

## The role of behaviour and lifestyle on health

McKeown initially studied the late nineteenth to the early twentieth century, but in later work (McKeown, 1979) he also studied disease patterns in the latter part of the twentieth century. In his analysis of health and illness during the twentieth century McKeown argued that people's health depended upon their modification of behaviours like smoking, diet and exercise. In their review of evidence showing links between behaviour and health Matarazzo and Leckliter (1988) used the term behavioural pathogen to describe behaviours such as smoking, and behavioural immunogen, to describe behaviours such as regular exercise. Both of these behaviours are implicated in the major causes of death at the end of the twentieth century (WHO, 2000). Health psychology and behavioural medicine are predicated on the view that an individual's health is influenced by his/her behaviour. There is ample empirical evidence to support this view.

In 1954 statistics presented by the American Cancer Society (ACS) at the Sixth International Congress on Cancer in Sao Paulo, Brazil established the link between smoking and lung cancer. In a study of 187,000 male smokers aged between 50 and 70 years the ACS reported that 5000 participants died from cancer within two years. These figures were far in excess of any other cause of death among non-smokers (Gilbert, 1999). In 1981 Doll and Peto analysed the factors associated with deaths from cancer and showed that 70% of deaths could be attributed to behaviour such as tobacco use (30%), alcohol use (3%), diet (35%) and reproductive and sexual behaviour (7%). In his address to the British Association of Science Conference in 1998 Peto reported that HIV/AIDS and tobacco-related illnesses were the fastest growing causes of death in many parts of the world. Smokers are more likely than non-smokers to suffer coronary heart disease (CHD) and lung disorders and to die from these disorders (Matarazzo and Leckliter, 1988). Evidence also shows that cigarette smoking accounts for around 90% of deaths from lung cancer (Dougall, 2007). There are various modes of transmission of HIV, but the evidence shows that most people become infected with HIV through unsafe sexual practices and injecting drugs using equipment contaminated with HIV-infected blood (Mann and Tarantola, 1996).

The influence of emotion and attitude to disease processes such as CHD has been accepted for centuries (Matarazzo, 1984) but empirical evidence showing these links can be traced to the initial studies of Friedman and Rosenman (1959, cited in Matarazzo, 1984) into behaviour patterns associated with cardiovascular disease. Friedman and Rosenman identified a behavioural pattern that they called Type A. This typology describes a behaviour pattern that is highly competitive, unusually aggressive, highly work-oriented and with a persistent sense of time urgency. According to Friedman and Rosenman individuals showing consistent Type A behaviour had a higher risk of CHD; individuals showing consistently a so-called Type B behavioural pattern – relaxed, calm, unhurried and satisfied – had a lower risk of CHD. Two studies further tested Friedman and Rosenman's hypothesis of a link between behaviour pattern and CHD. In the Western Collaborative Group Study (Rosenman et al., 1975, cited in Matarazzo, 1984) 3524 males and in the Framingham Study (Haynes et al., 1980, cited in Matarazzo, 1984) 6000 males and females were assessed at baseline and followed up for two decades. Results from these studies show that even when controlling for classical risk factors (family history, age, hypertension), individuals showing consistent Type A behaviour pattern had double the risk of CHD and more than double the risk of death than individuals showing consistent Type B behaviour pattern.

Grossarth-Maticek et al. (1988) investigated the links between four behavioural patterns (i.e. psychosocial types) and cancer and circulatory disease in people living in Crvenka in (the former) Yugoslavia from 1965 to 1976 and Heidelberg in Germany from 1972 to 1982. In both countries the results show that people with Type 1 behaviour – emotional overdependence on an unattainable other – had a cancer mortality two to five times the national average, and below average rates of death from circulatory diseases. People showing Type 2 behaviour – a strong but unmet need to avoid a disturbing other – had a three- to fourfold increase in death from circulatory diseases. People showing Type 3 behaviour – ambivalence towards important others – had increased survival rates, but only in Heidelberg. People showing Type 4 behaviour – autonomous and independent – had increased survival rates in both countries. The Type 1 behaviour pattern emerged from this research as the so-called 'cancer prone personality'. However, more recent research (Amelang et al., 1996) failed to replicate this finding and the researchers rejected the notion of a cancer prone personality. Other personality factors and beliefs linked to health through empirical research include the hardiness (resilience) of the personality (Kobasa et al., 1985), locus of control (Wallston et al., 1993) and self-efficacy (Bandura, 1986; Schwarzer and Fuchs, 1996).

Arguably the strongest support for the links between behaviour, lifestyle and health derives from a study widely cited as a classic in health psychology literature (Steptoe and Wardle, 1994): the Alameda County Study (Belloc and Breslow, 1972). Alameda County is in Northern California and in 1965 researchers at the human population laboratory at the California Department of Public Health and the University of California studied the physical health of 6928 randomly selected adults aged from 16 to 85 and followed up after four-and-a-half and nine years. Data were collected by a questionnaire that measured health status (dependent variable) and physical health practices (independent variables). The researchers identified seven health practices – the so-called Alameda 7. These practices were seven to eight hours sleep per day, eating breakfast almost every day, never or rarely eating between meals, currently at or near one's prescribed height-adjusted weight, never smoked cigarettes, moderate or no use of alcohol and regular exercise. Researchers analysed the link between these health practices and health status. The results showed that people who reported following more of the health practices reported being in better health; people who reported following fewer of the health practices reported being in poorer health. The association between the health practices and health status held even when researchers controlled for age, sex, economic status and health status. Follow-up at four-and-a-half and nine years found that the practice of the seven health behaviours decreased the risk of death fourfold for males and more than twofold for females. The Alameda County Study had a seminal influence on future research investigating the links between behaviour, lifestyle and health and the findings from the study have been confirmed by subsequent, independent investigations (Wardle et al., 1997).

There is clear evidence of a link – and in many cases the link is strong – between behaviour, lifestyle and health. However, there is evidence that other factors also contribute to people's health status. These factors include exposure to stressful life events, like the death of a significant other, socioeconomic status (Bartley and Owen, 1996; Carroll et al., 1994), education level, macroeconomic conditions and legal restraints (Becker, 1993), human rights violations (Harlem-Brundtland, 1998), social support levels (Callaghan and Morrissey, 1993), age, work-related issues and poverty (Marmot, 2005). These social determinants of health were discussed in a WHO sponsored conference in Rio de Janeiro in 2011 (WHO, 2011) that led to the Rio declaration to take global action to address these determinants.

In the nine-year follow-up of Alameda County residents, Berkman and Syme (1979) reported epidemiological evidence showing that people who lacked social and community ties were more likely to die in the follow-up period than those with more extensive contacts. But the links between behaviour and health remain. Circulatory disease is the major cause of death in most countries and there is epidemiological evidence that exercise plays an important part in the aetiology of this disease (Paffenberger et al., 1986).

An important challenge for health psychologists and behavioural scientists is helping people adopt healthier behaviours so that they may lead healthier lives (Smedslund, 2000). A crucial part of this challenge is to understand factors thought to influence behaviour, explaining theoretically the links between behaviour and health and developing behaviour change interventions that might improve people's health and well-being. The next part of this chapter will examine theories of health behaviour change that seek to address this challenge.

# Theories of health behaviour change

Theories of health behaviour change seek to explain what motivates people to change, the role of learning in the change process and how people make decisions to change. In short they seek to explain the individual, psychosocial and environmental processes thought to initiate, maintain and modify health behaviour change (Carmody, 2007). Table 20.1 shows common behaviour change theories that are also widely researched.

**TABLE 20.1** Health behaviour change theories

| Theory | Category | Description |
|---|---|---|
| Theory of Planned Behaviour (TPB, Azjen, 1991) | Continuum | Individuals' behaviour is determined by their **intention** to engage in this behaviour. Intention is determined by individuals' *attitude* to the behaviour, *subjective norm* – their perceptions of whether significant others think they should perform the behaviour – and *perceived behavioural control* – their view of the level of difficulty of the desired behaviour. |
| Transtheoretical Model of Change (TTM, Prochaska and DiClemente, 1984) | Stage | There are five **stages of change**: movement between the stages is determined by people's level of *self-efficacy* (belief in their confidence), *decisional balance* – their assessment of the pros and cons of changing behaviour – and *processes of change* – conscious and unconscious activities that help people change behaviour. |
| Health Belief Model (HBM, Becker et al., 1972) | Continuum | Individuals' behaviour is determined by their **perceived vulnerability** to illness, their perceived *severity of the illness*, their *health motivation*, the *perceived benefits* of changing behaviour, *perceived barriers* to changing and *cues to action* – triggers that prompt behaviour change such as health promotion campaigns. |

| Theory | Category | Description |
| --- | --- | --- |
| **Protection Motivation Theory** (PMT, Rogers, 1975) | Continuum | Individuals' behaviour is determined by **protection motivation** (i.e. their intention to perform the behaviour). Protection motivation arises from people's *appraisal of the threat* to their health and their *appraisal of their coping* mechanisms to deal with threats. Threat and coping appraisals are in turn influenced by *severity of illness, perceived vulnerability* to the threat and *self-efficacy* (confidence). |
| **Health Action Process Approach** (HAPA, Schwarzer, 2004) | Stage[a] | There are two discrete phases: *motivation* (intention) and *volitional* phase (action). Intention is influenced by *self-efficacy, perception of risk and expected outcomes* of changing behaviour. Volition is influenced by making detailed action plans to turn intentions into action. |
| **Precaution Adoption Process Model** (PAPM, Weinstein, 1998) | Stage | There are seven stages to behaviour change: (1) being unaware of a health issue, (2) being unengaged with the issue, (3) thinking about acting or (4) not acting, (5) deciding to act, (6) acting and (7) sustaining the action (maintenance). Movement through the stages is influenced by media messages, messages from significant others, personal experience of risk, beliefs about the likelihood of being exposed to a health risk, fear and worry and time, effort and personal resources to act on risk. |

[a]Sutton's (2005) critical review of HAPA and other stage theories suggests that HAPA could be equally considered a continuum theory as most of the research testing the theory to date has treated it as such.

## Evaluation of behaviour change theories

If behaviour change theories are to have practical value, they need to inform the development of interventions that will ultimately lead to positive changes

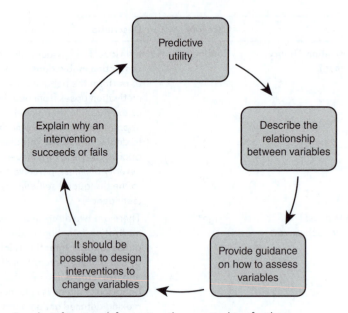

**FIGURE 20.1**    Brawley's framework for testing the practicality of a theory

in health behaviour (Norman and Conner, 2005). Brawley (1993) set five criteria against which to test the practicality of a theory. These are shown in Figure 20.1.

## Predictive utility

Predictive utility refers to whether the theories predict health behaviour as claimed and is one of the most common ways researchers test the theories, and the theories do relatively well on this criterion. However, there is variation in the predictive utility among the different theories. Also, the predictive utility of each theory will often depend on the target behaviour it is predicting. Systematic and meta-analytic reviews of literature are useful as they combine the data from many studies and this allows us to show the average predictive utility of each theory. In a widely cited meta-analysis, Armitage and Conner (2001) showed that the TPB had statistically significant moderate to strong predictive utility. The PMT performs similarly (Milne et al., 2000), the HBM performs moderately on predictive utility (Abraham and Sheeran, 2005) and the TTM appears to have moderate to good predictive utility (Sutton, 2005). At present there are too few studies testing the predictive utility of the PAPM and the HAPA, but the results from these studies are promising (Sutton, 2005).

## Theories should describe the relationship between their variables

This is strong in most of the theories; notable in the TPB and PMT and less developed in the HAPA, TTM and HBM (Norman and Conner, 2005).

## Theories should provide guidance for the assessment of key variables

The TPB and the TTM are excellent examples in relation to this criterion. Both have well-developed and widely available measures of their key variables which have strong psychometric properties. Other theories fair less well in this regard. It should be noted, however, that most of the theories have measures of their key variables that researchers have developed for individual studies; the reliability and validity of some of these measures are not consistently strong (Norman and Conner, 2005).

## It should be possible to design interventions to change the variables

Most behaviour change theories are weak in this regard; two exceptions are the self-efficacy construct of the TTM and the fear appeals process that is involved in the PMT. Several interventions have been shown empirically to improve self-efficacy including breaking a complex task into smaller discrete components and working through each of these parts systematically, observing a desired behaviour being performed successfully and including persuasive messages in self-help leaflets (Norman and Conner, 2005).

## Theories should explain why an intervention succeeds or fails

All behaviour change theories have this potential but it is a relatively untested area in the absence of well-designed intervention studies. For example, cognitive behavioural interventions succeed because they change cognitions that lead to changes in behaviours. The HBM has the potential to explain this relationship between these two variables.

The theories shown in Table 20.1 have been widely researched and there is a promising evidence base for each. The two theories focused on in this chapter provide clear guidance on how to research them, measure their constructs and show how these constructs can combine to develop interventions to produce meaningful change in health behaviours. However, there is a reliance on those constructs that comprise the theories at the exclusion of other variables that might effect behaviour change such as indulgent, impulsive actions. Also, the theories presuppose that individuals' behaviour change decisions are consciously driven by reasoned individuals; behaviours are just as readily driven by unconscious, irrational urges. The theories are also individually centric and overlook the role that economic, political, judicial and fiscal situations play in behaviour. In more recent research Abraham and Michie (2008), for example, have identified 26 behaviour change techniques, many of which are captured by the behaviour change theories presented here, and some of which are taken from other models, for example stress, time management and social comparison.

The TTM and the TPB are the most widely researched and cited health behaviour change theories. The next part of this chapter will focus on these two theories and illustrate how mental health nurses can apply them in clinical practice.

## The application of behaviour change theories to mental health nursing practice

### The Transtheoretical Model of Change

The TTM incorporates four related concepts considered central to behaviour change: stage of change, self-efficacy, decisional balance and processes of change. Stage of change reflects the temporal dimension in which attempts to change behaviours occur. It is proposed that individuals progress through five stages before they achieve a sustained change in behaviour: (1) precontemplation (i.e. not even thinking about changing); (2) contemplation (i.e. seriously considering changing); (3) preparation (i.e. making plans to change); (4) action (i.e. adopting the change); and (5) maintenance (i.e. maintaining the change for more than six months).

When applying the TTM in relation to the stages of change the mental health nurse has several tasks (Morrissey and Callaghan, 2010). Precontemplation: assessing the person's readiness to change; contemplation: assisting the person to identify reasons to change; preparation: working with the person to develop an action plan for change; action: helping the person make the change; and maintenance: helping the person to sustain the change.

In the TTM, progression through the stages of change is linked to differences in self-efficacy – the confidence individuals have in their ability to perform the target behaviour. Mental health nurses can assess the person's self-efficacy levels by asking them to complete a rating scale such as the one shown in Table 20.2 to assess self-efficacy for exercise.

**TABLE 20.2**  Self-efficacy for exercise questionnaire

| I am confident I can participate in regular exercise when: | | | | | | |
|---|---|---|---|---|---|---|
| | Not at all confident | | Moderately confident | | Extremely confident | |
| 1  I am tired. | 1 | 2 | 3 | 4 | 5 | |
| 2  I am in a bad mood. | 1 | 2 | 3 | 4 | 5 | |
| 3  I feel I don't have time. | 1 | 2 | 3 | 4 | 5 | |
| 4  I am on vacation/holiday. | 1 | 2 | 3 | 4 | 5 | |
| 5  The weather is bad. | 1 | 2 | 3 | 4 | 5 | |

Mental health nurses can use various techniques to improve people's self-efficacy levels in routine clinical practice by helping them break down complex tasks in smaller stages and working through each stage one by one.

The next construct of the TTM is decisional balance – assessing the pros and cons of changing behaviour. Using a problem-solving intervention (PSI) is a good example of applying the TTM in relation to decisional balance. In stage four of a PSI illustrated by Morrissey and Callaghan (2010) the person is asked to prioritise all potential solutions to a problem identified in a previous stage and select the most helpful. Weighing up the pros and cons of each potential solution will help the person to select the most suitable one for him or her.

The final construct of the TTM is processes of change – conscious and unconscious activities to try and change behaviour. Table 20.3 describes the processes of change and how a mental health nurse might use them in clinical practice to help someone stop smoking.

**TABLE 20.3**    Using the processes of change to help a person stop smoking

| Process | Description | Ask the person to identify |
|---|---|---|
| 1 Consciousness raising | Increasing knowledge about the benefits of giving up smoking | Some benefits of stopping smoking |
| 2 Dramatic relief | Reacting to warnings about the risks of smoking | Their typical reaction to warnings about the risks of smoking |
| 3 Environmental re-evaluation | Caring about consequences to others of smoking | How they feel their smoking affects how others see them |
| 4 Self re-evaluation | Comprehending benefits of stopping smoking | How they might *feel* if they stopped smoking |
| 5 Social liberation | Increasing opportunities to stop smoking | Smoking cessation clinics near where they live |
| 6 Self-liberation | Committing to stop smoking | Their readiness to stop smoking |
| 7 Helping relationships | Enlisting the support of significant others to stop smoking | Who they can turn to for help to quit, e.g. a friend who is an ex-smoker |
| 8 Counter-conditioning | Substituting alternatives | How they can take advantage of opportunities to quit smoking, e.g. attending the smoking cessation clinic |
| 9 Reinforcement management | Rewarding yourself | Systems of reward for stopping to smoke, e.g. saving money and buying themselves something with the savings |
| 10 Stimulus control | Controlling urges to smoke | Ways of controlling their urges, e.g. exercising, using nicotine replacement therapies |

## The Theory of Planned Behaviour

The key constructs of the TPB are intentions to adopt a desired behaviour, which are determined by *attitude* towards the behaviour; *subjective norm* – the perception of social norms and pressures to adopt the behaviour; and *perceived behavioral control* – the level of control people believe they have in adopting the behavior (Conner and Sparks, 2005). If a mental health nurse is working therapeutically with a person who is seeking help to understand and explain why they are struggling to moderate their alcohol use the TPB might prove useful. Two examples are apparent. In the first the nurse can use the TPB as an assessment tool using rating scales from the TPB manual that Francis et al. (2004) developed. These scales allow the nurse to assess the person's attitude by asking how likely, on a scale from 1, unlikely to 7, likely, that reducing alcohol use would benefit the person's health. To assess subjective norms the nurse can ask the person to respond from not all (1) to very much (7) to a series of statements such as: 'What my family think I should do matters to me'. To assess the person's perceived behaviour control the nurse presents a series of statements, an example of which is: 'I am confident that I could reduce my alcohol use if I wanted to' anchored from (1) strongly disagree to (7) strongly agree. Finally, to assess intention the nurse can pose a set of questions such as: 'I want to reduce my alcohol use' anchored from (1) strongly agree to (7) strongly disagree.

If mental health nurses wish to take a more qualitative approach to the assessment interview by applying the TPB they could use the TPB variable as an interview topic guide. Such use might involve open-ended questions such as:

1   Please take a few moments to tell me your thoughts about your alcohol use.
2   What do you believe are the advantages of reducing your alcohol use?
3   What other individuals or groups would disapprove of you reducing your alcohol intake?
4   What things would enable you to reduce your alcohol intake?
5   Are there any other things that come to mind when you think about your alcohol intake?

These examples show the many applications of the TTM and TPB to mental health nursing practice.

# Using motivational interviewing

Mental health nurses help people change from being overwhelmed by mental distress, to a position where they can lead meaningful and satisfying lives. People seeking mental health care are often looking to change aspects of their behaviour. However, people seeking change are often ambivalent, and may lack the will, ability or readiness to change (Hettema et al., 2005). Motivational interviewing (MI) is a person-centred, but directive, therapeutic intervention designed to help people improve their readiness to change (Miller and Rollnick, 2002). MI has its practical origins in humanistic approaches to therapy based upon the work of Carl Rogers (1961), but developed largely from the TTM. What follows is a case example of using MI approaches in a therapeutic encounter between a nurse and a service user in an acute mental health unit using the five basic principles of MI: expressing empathy, developing dissonance, avoiding arguments, rolling with resistance and supporting self-efficacy.

**CASE EXAMPLE**

David was a service user on an acute mental health ward and I had been assigned as his named nurse. David was diagnosed as having a borderline personality disorder. He struggled to engage with the mental health team, got angry and hostile as he felt it just did not understand how to help him. I invited David to spend some therapeutic time with me and decided to use the principles of MI to engage him.

## Expressing empathy

I made David aware that I understood the challenges he was facing on the ward. Statements such as 'It must be hard feeling that the team does not understand your difficulties' helped me demonstrate that I could relate to how he was feeling and that I cared enough to help.

On several occasions David's frustration at the team had caused him to cut his arms as a means to relieve the frustration he felt. As a result of this, he was restrained by staff and his access to time outside the ward was curtailed.

## Developing dissonance

I used the ABC – Antecedent, Behaviour, Consequence – approach as shown in Table 20.4.

**TABLE 20.4** The ABC approach

| Antecedent | Behaviour | Consequence |
| --- | --- | --- |
| David approached me to share that he was feeling frustrated. | David asked me for some therapeutic time to discuss how to deal with his frustration. | David got 60 minutes of therapeutic time with me. Both of us agreed he could have 60 minutes of therapeutic time with me away from the ward each day. As a result of this time, his frustration levels dropped and he stopped cutting his arm. His behaviour now had positive consequences. |

## Avoiding arguments

Initially David refused to meet with me for therapeutic time, arguing that it was a waste of his time as I did not understand his frustration. Statements such as 'you lot are all the same' was a common refrain. There was little point in engaging David in a war of attrition around dealing with those frustrations.

## Rolling with resistance

David was ambivalent about talking with me. This ambivalence led to resistance on his part. To start with I asked David to identify actions he thought might work and help him prioritise a list of what actions to take first.

## Supporting self-efficacy

To help David increase his belief in his ability to help himself I asked him to make a list of actions that had helped him successfully in the past. I encouraged him to try these actions again and when he succeeded praised him for this success.

## Summary

Changing patterns of health and disease in the last 100 years illustrate the role that behaviour and lifestyle factors contribute to the world's major diseases. Behaviour change theories explain the individual, psychosocial and environmental processes that initiate, maintain and modify health behaviour and researchers have used them

*(Continued)*

*(Continued)*

to develop interventions to enable positive behaviour change. The theories assume that behaviour change decisions are driven by conscious rational processes and overlook the role of unconscious and irrational urges. Mental health nurses often work with people seeking help to change aspects of their behaviour so that they may recover from incapacitating mental health difficulties. Behaviour changes theories offer techniques that mental health nurses can use to assess service users' needs and desire for change, explain how change might happen, and develop interventions to assist people change to a healthier lifestyle and reduce their risks of developing serious health problems.

# References

Abraham, C. and Michie, S. (2008) 'A taxonomy of behavior change techniques used in interventions', *Health Psychology*, 27 (3): 379–87.

Abraham, C. and Sheeran, P. (2005) 'The health belief model', in M. Conner and P. Norman (eds), *Predicting Health Behaviour* (2nd edn). Milton Keynes: Open University Press.

Amelang, M., Schmidt-Rathjens, C. and Matthews, G. (1996) 'Personality, cancer and coronary heart disease: further evidence on a controversial topic', *British Journal of Health Psychology*, 1: 191–205.

Ajzen, I. (1991) 'The theory of planned behaviour', *Organizational Behaviour and Human Decision Processes*, 50: 179–211.

Armitage, P. and Conner, M. (2001) 'Efficacy of the theory of planned behaviour: a meta-analytic review', *British Journal of Social Psychology*, 40: 471–99.

Bandura, A. (1986) *Social Foundations of Thought and Action: A Social Cognitive Theory*. Englewood Cliffs, NJ: Prentice Hall.

Bartley, M. and Owen, C. (1996) 'Relation between socioeconomic status, employment, and health during economic change, 1973–93', *British Medical Journal*, 313: 445–59.

Becker, M. H. (1993) 'A medical sociologist looks at health promotion', *Journal of Health and Social Behaviour*, 34 (March): 1–6.

Becker, M.H., Drachman, R.H. and Kirscht, P. (1972) 'Predicting mothers' compliance with pediatric medical regimens', *Journal of Pediatrics*, 81 (4): 843–854.

Belloc, N.B. and Breslow, L. (1972) 'Relationship of physical health status and health practices', *Preventive Medicine*, 1: 409–21.

Berkman, L.F. and Syme, S.L. (1979) 'Social networks, host resistance, and mortality: a nine-year follow-up study of Alameda County residents', *American Journal of Epidemiology*, 109: 186–204.

Brawley, L.R. (1993) 'The practicality of using social psychological theories for exercise and health research and intervention', *Journal of Applied Sport Psychology*, 5: 99–115.

Callaghan, P. and Morrissey, J. (1993) 'Social support and health: a review', *Journal of Advanced Nursing*, 18: 203–10.

Carmody, T. (2007) 'Health-related behaviours: common factors', in S. Ayers, A. Baum, C. McManus, S. Newman, K. Wallston, J. Weinman and R. West (eds), *Cambridge Handbook of Psychology, Health and Medicine* (2nd edn). Cambridge: Cambridge University Press.

Carroll, D., Davey-Smith, G. and Bennett, P. (1994) 'Health and socioeconomic status', *The Psychologist*, 7: 122–5.

Conner, M. and Sparks, P. (2005) 'Theory of planned behaviour and health behaviour', in M. Conner and P. Norman (eds), *Predicting Health Behaviour* (2nd edn). Milton Keynes: Open University Press.

Doll, R. and Peto, R. (1981) 'The causes of cancer: quantitative estimates of avoidable risks of cancer in the United States today', *Journal of National Cancer Institute*, 66 (6): 1191–1308.

Dougall, A.L. (2007) 'Cancer: lung', in S. Ayers, A. Baum, C. McManus, S. Newman, K. Wallston, J. Weinman and R. West (eds), *Cambridge Handbook of Psychology, Health and Medicine* (2nd edn). Cambridge: Cambridge University Press.

Francis, J.J., Eccles, M.P., Johnston, M., Walker, A., Grimshaw, J., Foy, R., Kaner, E.F.S., Smith, L. and Bonetti, D. (2004) *Constructing Questionnaires Based on the Theory of Planned Behaviour: A Manual for Health Services Researchers*. Newcastle Upon Tyne, UK: University of Newcastle, Centre for Health Services Research.

Gilbert, M. (1999) *Challenge to Civilization: A History of the 20th Century 1952–1999*. London: HarperCollins.

Grossarth-Maticek, R., Eysenck, H.J., Vetter, H. and Schmidt, P. (1988) 'Psychosocial types and chronic diseases: results of the Heidelberg Prospective Psychosomatic Intervention Study', in S. Maes, C.D. Spielberger, P.B. Defares and I.G. Sarason (eds), *Topics in Health Psychology*. New York: John Wiley.

Harlem-Brundtland, G. (1998) Press statement to the World Health Organization Accessed at: www.who.int/inf-pr-1998/en/pr98-93.html (accessed 1/5/2013).

Hettema, J., Steele, J. and Miller, W.R. (2005) 'Motivational interviewing', *Annual Review of Clinical Psychology*, 1: 91–111.

Kobasa, S.C.O., Maddi, S.R., Pucetti, M.C. and Zola, M.A. (1985) 'Effectiveness of hardiness, exercise and social support as resources against illness', *Journal of Psychosomatic Research*, 29: 525–33.

Levy, R.I. and Moskowitz, J. (1982) 'Cardiovascular research: decades of progress, a decade of promise', *Science*, 217: 121–8.

Mann, J. and Tarantola, D. (eds) (1996) *AIDS in the World II.* Oxford: Oxford University Press.

Marmot, M. (2005) 'Social determinants of health inequalities', *The Lancet,* 365: 1099–104.

Matarazzo, J.D. (1984) 'Behavioral health: a 1990 challenge for health sciences professions', in J.D. Matarazzo, S.M. Weiss, J.A. Herd, N.E. Miller and S.M. Weiss (eds) (1984) *Behavioral Health: A Handbook of Health Enhancement and Disease Prevention.* New York: Wiley, p. 1292.

Matarazzo, J.D. and Leckliter, I.N. (1988) 'Behavioural health: the role of good and bad habits in health and illness', in S. Maes, C.D. Spielberger, P.B. Defares and I.G. Sarason (eds), *Topics in Health Psychology.* New York: John Wiley.

McKeown, T. (1976) *The Modern Rise of Population.* London: Edward Arnold.

McKeown, T. (1979) *The Role of Medicine.* Oxford: Blackwell.

Miller, W.R. and Rollnick, S. (2002) *Motivational Interviewing: Preparing People for Change,* Vol. 2. New York: Guilford Press.

Milne, S., Sheeran, P. and Orbell, S. (2000) 'Prediction and intervention in health-related behavior: a meta-analytic review of protection motivation theory', *Journal of Applied Social Psychology,* 30: 106–43.

Morrissey, J. and Callaghan, P. (2010) *Communication Skills for Mental Health Nurses.* Milton Keynes: Open University Press.

Norman, P. and Conner, M. (2005) 'Predicting and changing health behaviours: future directions', in M. Conner and P. Norman (eds), *Predicting Health Behaviour* (2nd edn). Milton Keynes: Open University Press.

Ogden, J. (2007) *Health Psychology: A Textbook* (4th edn). Milton Keynes: Open University Press.

Paffenberger, R.S., Hyde, R.T., Wing, A.L. and Hsieh, C.C. (1986) 'Physical activity, all-cause mortality, and longevity of college alumni', *New England Journal of Medicine,* 314: 605–13.

Peto, R. (1998) Address to the British Association of Science Conference. Accessed at: http://news.bbc.co.uk/1/hi/health/166857.stm (accessed on: 1/5/2013).

Prochaska, J.O. and DiClemente, C. (1984) 'Toward a comprehensive model of change', in W.E. Miller and N. Heather (eds), *Treating Addictive Behaviours.* London: Plenum Press.

Rogers, C.R. (1961) *On Becoming a Person: A Therapist's View of Psychotherapy.* New York: Houghton-Mifflin.

Rogers, R.W. (1975) 'A protection motivation theory of fear appeals and attitude change', *Journal of Psychology,* 91: 93–114.

Rosenman, R.H., Brand, R.J., Jenkins, C.D., Friedman, M., Straus, R. and Wurm, M. (1975) 'Coronary heart disease in the western collaborative group study: final follow-up experience of 8.5 years', *Journal of the American Medical Association*, 25: 872–7.

Schwarzer, R. (2004) *Modeling Health Behaviour Change: The Health Action Process Approach*. Accessed at: http://userpage.fu.berlin.de/hapa.htm (accessed on: 12/1/2013).

Schwarzer, R. and Fuchs, R. (1996) 'Self-efficacy and health behaviours', in M. Conner and P. Norman (eds), *Predicting Health Behaviour*. Milton Keynes: Open University Press.

Smedslund, G. (2000) 'A pragmatic basis for judging models and theories in health psychology: the axiomatic method', *Journal of Health Psychology*, 5: 133–49.

Steptoe, A. and Wardle, J. (eds) (1994) *Psychosocial Processes and Health: A Reader*. London: Routledge.

Sutton, S. (2005) 'Stage theories of health behaviour', in M. Conner and P. Norman (eds), *Predicting Health Behaviour* (2nd edn). Milton Keynes: Open University Press.

Szreter, S. (1988) 'The importance of social intervention in Britain's mortality decline c. 1850–1914: a re-interpretation of the role of public health', *The Society for the Social History of Medicine*, 1–37.

Wardle, J., Steptoe, A., Bellisle, F., Davou, B., Reschke, K. and Lappalainen, R. (1997) 'Health dietary practices among European students', *Health Psychology*, 16 (5): 443–50.

Weinstein, N.D., Rothman, A.J. and Sutton, S.R. (1998) 'Stage theories of health behaviour: conceptual and methodological issues', *Health Psychology*, 17: 290–9.

WHO (World Health Organization) (2000) *The World Health Report 2000: Health Systems: Improving Performance*. Geneva: WHO.

WHO (World Health Organization) (2010) *The World Health Report 2010: Health Systems: Improving Performance*. Geneva: World Health Organization.

WHO (World Health Organization) (2011) *World Conference on the Social Determinants of Health*. Geneva, 19–21 October 2011. Available at: www.who.int/sdhconference/resources/Conference_Summary_Report.pdf (accessed on: 8/1/2013).

# 21

# Integrating Body and Mind

## ANN CHILDS

### Learning Objectives

- Consider the two-way influences between body and mind.
- Utilise evidence-based practice, clinical reasoning and an individualised, person-centred approach when considering any physical intervention.
- Consider how evidence and clinical practice can support your role from a body–mind perspective.
- Recognise and reflect on the meaning and changeability of your own embodied responses: be able to consider these in your responses to clients.
- Consider the relevance of touch, movement and body awareness to a person's whole sense of being.

## Introduction

The relationship between body and mind continues to be complex, contested and divisive, between philosophies, theories, health care professionals, academic departments, cultures and personal experience. This chapter does not critique theories, but looks at the many viewpoints from theorists, health care models and clinical practice to offer therapeutic significance. The two-way influence between body and mind is quoted in several formats including mind–body, bodymind and mindbody. There is no consensus of agreement. This chapter is primarily looking from a body perspective at the integration, thus body–mind.

We know without doubt we have a physical body including the brain which our senses tell us is real, and a mind which is thinking and feeling. In recent years the relationship and mutual influence between body and mind have become accepted within our society and health care culture, yet in personal lives we demarcate between headache and stress, and clearly we have totally separate mental and physical health care divisions, departments and trusts. This would imply duality, the two opposite poles of the body–mind. However, there is an inference that duality arises from the division of unity. Is this whole, non-dual state something to strive for? A state of integration or perfection? Is the body–mind just part of another system? Can they exist separately?

Western philosophy is comfortable with duality – cause/effect, objective/subjective, hypertension/hypotension – this is also reflected in the natural world of magnetic and electrical polarity. Within eastern philosophy, Tao is the expression of profound unity and Taoist philosophers consider everything has its complementary opposite, where everything can only be understood by comparing it to its opposite (Garbacz and Marshall, 2000). Yin and yang are expressions of opposites, yet cannot exist independently, only as a dynamic relationship where health is a balanced harmony (implying movement).

The intention of the chapter is to look at the body–mind, metaphorically with a wide lens, to illuminate a holograph from two-dimensional to three-dimensional, or perhaps as a fractal, infinitely repeating the self-similar pattern.

## Historical development

> The greatest mistake in the treatment of diseases is that there are physicians for the body and physicians for the soul, although the two cannot be separated. (Plato, Charmides, 380 BC)

Greek physicians over 2000 years ago understood how the mind was influenced by many processes, including the body (Gilbert, 2002). Yet, throughout western tradition, there has been no singular understanding of the body, other than ambivalence or love–hate relationships (Young, 2006). The current climate is becoming more receptive to a central focus of the body in health: 'body is now coming out of the closet' (Stam, 1998: 41–5). The history of the body–mind has been complex with divisions and cross-interconnections continuing to the present day. Historically physical activity for health benefits has been documented from the earliest records across cultures (Callaghan, 2004; Walach, 2007).

Most texts begin with René Descartes postulating the separation of the mind (thinking, feeling, conscious, aware, immortal) from the body (material, spatiotemporal, physical properties governed by mechanical law). This allowed science to continue medical exploration of the body, consigning the Christian church to claim the mind/soul, thereby minimising conflict. This 'Cartesian' mind/body split continues to be referred to as a divide in areas of health care, culture and society.

Current 'innovative' body work in mental health can be traced back through many historical roots. Dr Pierre Janet, who was influenced by Charcot, based his treatment approaches on the connection between emotional tensions and tissue changes, touch, visceral consciousness, channels of contact, the kinaesthetic sense, movement and intentionality and the importance of working with the body with traumatised patients (Boadella, 1997; Van der Kolk, 2006). Interestingly, these approaches are currently seen as 'innovative' and practised by body psychotherapists or experienced complementary therapists, usually working outside NHS services.

Freud's psychoanalysis grew partly out of body-oriented work, evolving into a verbal specialisation, a 'talking cure', thereby initiating a growing trend of disownment of the body in therapy, in parallel with the expansive growth of understanding about the mind. Janet's empathic and body-oriented concept of rapport was possibly the foundation of Freud's concept of transference (Young, 2006). Rather than just being ignored, the body was actively separated from psychotherapy. Interestingly, at a similar time, at the beginning of twentieth century, a counter health movement existed, widely embracing body-orientated philosophies, involving natural healing, dance and yoga (Young, 2006).

One of Freud's students, Wilhelm Reich (1897–1957), developed the concept of 'body' energy: the free flow of which is essential to good health, yet blocked by unresolved psychological and emotional traumas, physically manifested in specific, chronic muscular holding patterns. Directed body work and breathing techniques brought emotions back to consciousness for resolution. This formed a basis of Reichian body psychotherapy, the theory of which has continued to inform a plethora of therapeutic approaches addressing body and mind together. Currently, the physical techniques are more subtle and sensitive than the past deep tissue work (Levine, 2010).

In the 1980s, Stanley Keleman developed *emotional anatomy*, Boadella developed *psychotherapeutic biosynthesis* and Pat Ogden developed *sensorimotor psychotherapy* and Ron Kurtz developed a mindfulness-based *hakomi*, all working with the emotional constructs related to the physical patterns of the body tissues alongside the felt sense of the body and disconnection from trauma. This approach of working directly with the body to reveal and influence both mind and body was shaped by many, including Peter Levine, Ellert Nijenhuis, Stephen Porges, Dan Siegel, Bessel van der Kolk and Ken Wilber, and continues to evolve (Young, 2006). Further resources are available at www.body-psychotherapy.org.uk/resources/articles.html.

Phenomenology is the philosophical study of the subjective experience and consciousness, from the first-person point of view. It was founded in the early twentieth century by Edmund Husserl and expanded upon by many, including Martin Heidegger, Maurice Merleau-Ponty and Jean-Paul Sartre (Leder, 2005). Many treatment approaches focusing on the interrelationship of body and mind stem from the lived, personal meaning experience of the originator, therefore sit more comfortably within this phenomenological construct. Wilde (1999) explores how Merleau-Ponty's phenomenology is considered a philosophy of embodiment, with the focus on body–mind rather than just 'body', where embodiment is a form of experiencing and understanding the world through the body in lived experiences.

Throughout every culture, traditional, whole system health approaches such as Chinese medicine, yoga, shamanism and ayurveda, integrate the body, mind, spirit and total environment within their health care philosophies. They can be traced back over 4000 years to present-day use. Acupuncture, shiatsu, tai chi, qigong, yoga, breath training and mindfulness are some of the modalities from these ancient systems, utilised in current NHS mental health care. In China in the 1950s, under the People's Republic, 'old' classical medical systems were accepted, reorganised into a logical, consistent structure and renamed Traditional Chinese Medicine (TCM), which is now studied, practised and researched throughout the world (Garbacz and Marshall, 2000).

Within the UK NHS mental health services, physical body approaches have been provided by fitness and sports instructors, physiotherapists and occupational therapists. These have progressed from initially providing physically focused interventions to now including a person-centred, biopsychosocial, interprofessional working approach; supporting social inclusion, recovery and resilience, well-being and health promotion (CSP, 2008).

Scandinavian physiotherapists working in mental health have followed a different theoretical construct, completing several years of postgraduate training in body and movement awareness, to integrate body and mind. It is eclectically based on eastern philosophies of tai chi and western philosophies of movement, body work, modern dance, gymnastics, authentic movement, art, humanistic and existential psychotherapy, influenced by: Jaques Dropsy, Elsa Gindler, Mary Starks Whitehouse, Frederick Alexander, Moshe Feldenkrais and Alexander Lowen (Kolnes, 2012).

# Theories

The following theoretical approaches are highlighted: biopsychosocial, holism, well-being, complementary medicine (CM) and phenomenology informed by the embodiment of touch, movement and trauma.

## Biopsychosocial theory

The conception and acceptance of the biopsychosocial (BPS) model into health care were closely identified with the cardiologist George Engel. From the potentially dualistic biomedical model, BPS emerged as an inclusive, interdisciplinary, non-hierarchical model, where health and wellness emerge from a complex interaction of biological, psychological and sociocultural factors.

At a philosophical level, there are interactions between these domains in a wide sense (for example, how poverty affects rates of mental health disorders), yet also from molecular level to psychological (endorphins affect mood) and relational where clinicians utilise mindfulness in interactions (Borrell-Carrió, 2004; Gilbert, 2002).

Borrell-Carrió (2004) suggests that BPS can still have a dualistic view of human experience in which there is mutual influence of mind and body, suggesting the need to move beyond the linear thinking of mind–body duality by recognising that knowledge is multi-dimensional, multi-factorial and socially constructed, with a circular model of causality. Nevertheless, categories of 'mind' or 'body' need to be created to critically focus our thinking and action.

From a historically low profile, the therapeutic involvement of the body in mental health services has only recently emerged, driven by the statistics of poor physical health coexisting with mental illness, inequalities in health care, co-morbid pathologies, medication side-effects and high risk mortality. The government has responded by raising awareness and providing funding (NHS Confederation Briefing, 2006; Northey and Barnett, 2012; Russ et al., 2012). Further resources can be found at www.centreformentalhealth.org.uk/pdfs/not_all_in_the_mind.pdf.

The King's Fund and Centre for Mental Health (Naylor et al., 2012) report highlights co-morbidity of physical health and mental health in long-term conditions and relevance to current health care services, citing robust evidence. Physical and mental health care have traditionally been treated separately, with services designed around conditions rather than patients. Research evidence suggests that integrated approaches, with closer working between professionals responsible for patients' mental and physical health, can improve outcomes while also reducing costs. Failure to recognise and help a person's mental health problem is likely to delay his or her physical recovery (CSP, 2008). The BPS approach was proposed to provide a design for action in the real world of health care: in acute wards, liaison services (mental and physical health care working together) can improve care, outcomes and promote earlier discharge and reduce non-attendance (NHS Confederation Briefing, 2009). Screening for physical health is advised in all mental health settings (Bonfioli et al., 2012; Mailoo et al., 2011).

## Holism

In the early twentieth century Smuts describes the concept of a unified and coherent whole as: more than, and functions different from, the sum of the component parts. Natural systems and their properties will be inevitably interrelated and mutually dependent on each other, therefore a holistic approach to the human organism embraces and affirms complexity, inclusion, diversity, resisting reductionism, a separating into parts (Walach, 2007). There are similarities between holism and the BPS model, although it could be argued the BPS has many exclusions and pragmatically can be reduced to the separate health care departments.

## Complementary medicine

The therapeutic face of holism can be regarded as the use of complementary therapies (CM), representing a wide diversity of therapeutic philosophies and theories, shaped by culture, spirituality and meanings of health and illness. Users of CM report the importance of 'openness to the mind–body connection' (Long, 2009). Walach (2007) explores the philosophical debate around potential restrictions to holism relating to the transpersonal/spiritual and consciousness of the body–mind in terms of a mind–body–spirit or brain–consciousness–soul problem. This debate continues when considering therapeutic involvement of the recent explorations of biomagnetic fields around the body; subtle felt senses of tissues; communication through myo-fascial pathways (Oschman, 2003; Walach, 2007). 'Holism becomes an actual sensory perception rather than a philosophical concept' (Evans, 2007: 22).

## Quantum physics

Quantum mechanics questions the very nature of matter; at the subatomic level no particles exist except in relationship to others. These subatomic particles, from which all matter is made, are patterns of activity rather than things. The famous double split experiment can demonstrate how an electron can be either a particle or wave, but not both phenomena at the same moment. Based on extensive research, Oschman (2003, 2006) hypothesises how an understanding of cellular electronics within a connective tissue matrix forms a seamless dynamic web of interrelated parts and rhythmic process enabling extensive whole body communication, part explaining body–mind–conscious–unconscious interfaces. The theoretical construct of Chinese medicine has an absence of dichotomy between abstract/symbolic/concrete/material, or physical/mental, as all matter is not only interconnected but transmutes to different forms of Qi (energy) (Cassidy, 2004; Garbacz and Marshall, 2000).

The above discourse is complex and contested, however these metaphors capture some of its essence:

1  Compare thinking about body and mind together as in the *classic candlesticks and face* –to realise the challenge of experiencing both together, rather than separately (see Figure 21.1).
2  Many cultural concepts of bio-energy, for example Qi, are explained as a metaphor for changing states of water, steam and ice; the same but existing in different forms. Consider this as a metaphor for body and mind.

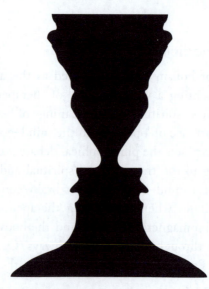

**FIGURE 21.1**  Classic candlestick and face puzzle

Acceptance of CM is not based on the intrinsic characteristics of the therapy, but its political marginality compared to medical orthodoxy. The orthodoxy of one period can therefore become the unorthodoxy of another, and vice versa. Forty years ago a discourse on Chinese medicine would not have happened, yet Niels Bohr (Nobel Prize 1922) looked at the teachings of Buddha and Lao Tsu to ground some of his understanding during his development of the *complementarity principle*: the effect of measurement on matter viewed as particles or waves of energy (Oschman, 2003). Therapists describe how 'Energy medicine works more with what is felt than measured' (Cassidy, 2004: 80). Patients are changing their language and personal meaning of their experience; 'restoring vital forces and self-healing energy' (Long, 2009: 8). Pike and Hald (2011) have considered these theoretical frameworks together with the intention, attention, attitude and the detached compassion of mindfulness, to suggest energy medicine may be a form of applied mindfulness.

## Well-being

Well-being is the positive outcome and optimum goal of the combination of good mental and physical health, a constructive body–mind approach. Well-being is not a static construct but rather a *dynamic process* considered by some to be an updated and more practical concept of holism. Government initiatives and an extensive review of evidence suggest for personal well-being: Connect, be Active, take Notice, keep Learning and Give (NHS, 2009).

## Embodiment

Reflecting on the philosophy of phenomenology, the personal lived experience and perception of life in this world, Wilde (1999) defines embodiment as how we live in and experience the world through our bodies, especially through perception, emotion, movement in space and action and response with the environment. Embodiment can be seen as a transformative way of moving on from body and mind dualism, where the person is situated within the world, being affected by social, cultural, political and historic forces (Wilde, 1999, quoting from Merleau-Ponty). Nicholls and Gibson (2010) suggest that rather than a theory, the notion of embodiment could be considered a viewpoint emphasising an orientation towards the whole person as part of the richness of life, providing a theoretically robust argument as guidance for 'embodied' manual and movement rehabilitation in current health care.

Skjaerven et al. (2010) suggest that embodied presence is a bodily felt sense, a form of personal knowing that evokes understanding and fosters meaning. Embodiment cannot be separated from awareness – defined as an attentive, relaxed, and alert presence, derived from human consciousness and experiences. Being aware means continually monitoring internal and external environments; it is possible to be aware of stimuli without making them the centre of attention. Whereas attention is a more focused, conscious awareness of self and ongoing experiences, thereby providing heightened sensitivity to experiences (Pike and Hald, 2011; Skjaerven, 2010). Consider the significance of mindfulness, discussed in Chapter 11.

Human bodily experience of our body and the sense of its parts belonging to us is called self-attribution or body ownership. Lopez et al. (2008) suggest bodily experiences could be a promising approach for the development of a comprehensive, neurobiological model of self-consciousness. Two important bodily experiences – namely embodiment and body ownership – associated in the processing of bodily information, seem to be key phenomenological aspects for bodily self-consciousness.

Altered internal body sensation has been linked to several clinical conditions, for example anxiety (Ainley et al., 2012). During mental illness, the patient's own body perception can change (anorexia nervosa, psychosis, dissociation, body dysmorphia, dementia). Altered perceptions can be perceived as an illusion which can be challenging for health care professionals to understand (Lopez et al., 2008). Recognising where in the body–mind this fits is even more challenging. It is helpful to take a step back and consider how neuroanatomical pathways can contribute to different bodily experiences of embodiment and body ownership and an ongoing feeling of being located inside the body. Consider how autoscopic phenomena (out-of-body experience and feeling-of-a-presence) have been demonstrated in neurological patients and in healthy subjects in whom integration of multisensory and vestibular bodily information is experimentally disturbed (Lopez et al., 2008).

The robust, well-designed study of Thakkar et al. (2011) compared outpatients with a diagnosis of schizophrenia to healthy controls, using a rubber hand illusion. From the findings, potential mechanisms are hypothesised in the contribution of psychotic symptoms: altered proprioception, multisensory integration of conflicting signals, weaker or more flexible internal model of their own body, impairment in a sense of personal initiation of one's own actions (agency) and disturbed body ownership. Healthy volunteers can also experience illusory 'out-of-body experiences' when the visual perspective is changed (Petkova and Ehrsson, 2008). This study informs us about the processes of the entirety of body ownership and ongoing feeling of being located inside the whole body (embodiment) by matching multisensory (visual, tactile, pressure, movement, proprioceptive) and motor signals from the first-person perspective.

Interoceptive sensitivity (internal body sensation) is an essential component of recent models of self, where the sense of bodily self results from the integration and interaction of both interoceptive and exteroceptive sensory imputs (Ainley et al., 2012). Mental representations of our physical appearance are modulated by integrating multisensory inputs which provides a plausible mechanism for constructing and updating our self-representation – the concept of 'I' (Tajadura-Jiménez et al., 2012) the other me. This discourse potentially supports the promotion of body–mind awareness within a therapeutic context.

## Embodiment in movement

Different theories of human movement traditions reflect diverse philosophical views and opinions about the importance of structural, neural, psychological, social, cultural and environmental aspects. The theoretical constructs of Scandinavian physiotherapists were strongly influenced by Jacque Dropsy, who interpreted a person's reduced awareness, contact and relationship as dysfunctional movements, which were lacking vitality, flow, rhythm and unity. Changing awareness changes movement which changes contact and relationship, evidenced by both studies and experience (Hedlund and Gyllensten, 2010; Kolnes, 2012; Skjaerven, 2010).

From the literature discussed, the commonalities emerging from therapeutic movement which impact on embodiment and body ownership are: subtle movement with a focused sensory awareness on the internal felt sense and external contact within the movement. The physical therapist's embodied presence and own movement awareness were preconditions for guiding patients and noticing subtle nuances of movement in self and others (Kolnes, 2012; Skjaerven, 2010).

- When listening to a person in great distress, does your stomach feel tight or fluttery?
- If a person displays anger, are your jaws clenched? Are your legs wanting to run?
- Consider your own embodied experience and how this might inform your clinical practice.
- How would clinical or peer supervision be important to monitor this?

Patients highlight the importance of being able to recognise how small changes in movement quality enable big changes. Overall, therapeutic movement develops a functional integration between awareness building, learning, reflecting, ownership, posture, breathing patterns, muscle tension, felt body sense and balance, connecting a person's life, history and feelings, the personal experience of embodiment, strengthening the patient's experience of mastery in everyday situations (Skjaerven, 2010). By bringing attention and awareness to the doing and being and experience of movement, the physical and mental aspects of self are developed. The focus is on the ease, stability and intention though simple, achievable movement (Gyllensten et al., 2009).

Extensive, robust qualitative and pragmatic methodology, together with externally evaluated outcome measures designed specifically to capture the quality and meaning of touch and movement awareness, has enabled a growing evidence base and consolidation of these theoretical principles (Meurle-Hallberg and Armelius 2006; Skjaerven, 2010).

## Embodiment in touch

The whole body is the organ of touch where tactility is a profound and primary whole person experience, central to the phenomenological viewpoint (Nathan, 2007). Specifically in mental health, Alexander Lowen highlights how the feeling of identity arises from a feeling of contact with the body, when there is no body contact a person feels *out of touch* with reality (cited in Montagu, 1986: 261), highlighted in psychosis, self-harm, trauma/dissociation.

From the nursing perspective, there has been a diversity of descriptions of touch in the literature, as either *doing for* the physical body or *being with* a recipient (Edvardsson, 2003) or *procedural* touch versus *expressive* touch (Nathan, 2007). The experience of using touch in dementia nursing practice has clinical implications for developing rapport, described by the nurses as 'in a bubble in a moment of equality', 'being centred in the moment', 'equal, … connected', 'an experience which transcends the moment of touch and influences one's way of caring', 'makes professionals feel valuable but also valuable as people' and 'concepts of body and self merge together' (Edvardsson, 2003). The interpretation of body–mind integration is expressed differently by health care professionals: *positive interchange of body and mind and empathic understanding*, compared to clients: *sharing spirituality and feeling of connection* (Chang, 2001). Staff also noted *touch influencing the stability of body–mind, as integrated interconnectivity*.

Healing by light touch is ubiquitous across cultures, whilst Kerr et al. (2007) suggest the general traits are administered in a behaviourally relevant context, in which the person anticipates the possibility of healing. Considering mental health services, Eiden (1998) explores the polarisation of the use of touch between the inherent use of touch in body psychotherapy (based on Reich) and with the no touch approach of general psychotherapy and many NHS mental health services (which can be reasoned from the perspective of risk assessment). The client can experience touch as an anchor, a sense of holding, container or boundary to facilitate the safe experience of emotion, conveying the message, 'I am present with you.' This prevents overwhelming and enables exploration of the perceptions to find personal meaning, facilitating an embodied body–mind integrative process (Eiden, 1998; Sumner and Haines, 2010). 'Touch is the authentic voice of feeling' (Montagu, 1986).

### Embodiment in trauma and dissociation

The James–Lange physiological theory of emotion and Antonio Damasio's sense of self, based on somatosensory awareness, have been much contested, especially in the light of cognitive theories. However, these physiological theories are re-emerging as clinicians and neurologists, such as Scaer (2001) and Levine (2010), clinically observe the direct and continuous interconnection between internal somatosensory awareness, perception, the dysfunctional autonomic nervous system, breathing and cardiovascular changes and body dissociation after trauma. Scaer (2001) challenges the psychologically constructed terms somatisation and conversion and argues towards inclusion of a biological-body context moving beyond the concept of mind–body medicine to a mind–brain–body continuum (see also Blechert et al., 2007). Clinical reasoning is supported towards working more directly and sensitively with the felt sense of the body in severe trauma (Björnsdotter et al., 2010; Craig, 2009; Sumner and Haines, 2010; Van der Kolk, 2006). If we consider that trauma mechanisms are a continuation of stress, this discourse becomes applicable to everyone (Levine, 2010).

Current advances in neuroanatomy support the clinical observations of autonomic dysregulation in severe trauma, post-traumatic stress disorder and somatic dissociation (polyvagal theory; Levine, 2010; Porges, 2007); the sensory-affective role of the C-tactile (CT) light touch system, associated with interoception (Björnsdotter et al., 2009; Craig, 2009); visceral neurotransmitters (Mailoo et al., 2011); high sympathetic activity coupled with low parasympathetic cardiac control, with respiratory abnormalities (Blechert et al., 2007); and cortical changes (Tajadura-Jiménez et al., 2012; Van der Kolk, 2006). This supports just one aspect of the many body–mind rationales.

# Theory applied to practice

Consider how the appropriateness of a physical intervention is determined by the individual need of the person at that time; need to be distracted or engaged, calmed or stirred, grounded or roused, increase cardiovascular output or mastery, self-activated at home or social engagement, structural framework or creativity.

A range of physical interventions are presented in Table 21.1. The brief notes are to demonstrate the diversity of interventions and the integration of physical, psychological and functional outcomes to broaden therapeutic parameters and to reflect on the effects of activities rather than attempt to fit diagnosis with a specific activity. The study methodologies have not been critiqued within the table and it is advised that individual papers are critically appraised to benefit from the depth of discussions within the studies.

**TABLE 21.1**  Interventions relating to the body, having holistic and diverse outcomes

| Intervention | Participants | Outcome | Comments | Reference |
|---|---|---|---|---|
| Individualised yoga programme + standard care (2x weekly) Control: standard care (MD and dietician every 2nd week) | Young people Eating disorders | Preoccupation with food decreased sig. Both groups reduced anxiety and depression | Yoga group maintained improvement at 1 month follow-up with no weight loss | Carei et al. (2010) |
| Feldenkrais movement awareness therapy group sessions | Non-specific neck and shoulder pain All female | Felt more present in their body Grounded Improved posture with ease Empowered Gentle with self | Lost their fear to feel and reflect on the body Helped in the process of change Connection between doing and feeling | Öhman et al. (2011) |
| Shiatsu longitudinal, 6/12 observational, pragmatic study Received advice, on exercise, diet, posture, points to work on at home or other ways of self-care | n = 633 Eclectic reasons for having shiatsu Over 18 yrs | Improved body awareness. More in touch with emotions. Body–mind connection Changes to lifestyle resulting from shiatsu – more rest and exercise | Awareness and expression of thoughts and feelings affecting body Incl. levels of confidence and resolve | Long (2009) |
| Dance | Service users in acute setting | Realistic sense of connection between body and mind + inner + outer experience | Led to social inclusion both inside and outside the hospital | Froggett and Little (2012) |

| Intervention | Participants | Outcome | Comments | Reference |
|---|---|---|---|---|
| Physical activity Compared level of physical activity, functional exercise capacity and body image and self-esteem | Schizophrenia Low (L) (high (H) Perceived sports competence and perceived physical fitness (PSCPF) | L-PSCPF: poorer participation Shorter distance walked (20.4%) Physical self-perception lower than H-PSCPF | | Vancamfort et al. (2011) |
| Physical therapy as a treatment review | Schizophrenia | Aerobic, strength exercise + yoga reduce anxiety, distress + psychological symptoms | Results limited re. heterogeneity of studies, but potential value | Vancamfort et al. (2012) |
| Yoga – 1 week, Detailed description | Tsunami survivors | Sig. decrease in related fear, sadness, anxiety, disturbed sleep, breath rate | Measures taken 1 month post yoga | Descilo et al. (2009) |
| Patanjali (hatha) yoga 1 hr daily Detailed description Control: waiting list 1 month after flood | Flood survivors PTSD | Yoga: sig. dif. in sadness reduction Control: increase in anxiety | Follow-on from above study More emphasis on breathing intervention | Telles (2010) |
| Movement, imagery, meditation, breathing exercises | PTSD Young people Kosovo | Reduced PTSD symptoms | | Gordon et al. (2008) |
| Body-orientated body psychotherapy activities 10 weeks Detailed manual Dance and sensory awareness | Chronic schizophrenia (specific inclusion criteria) Described perceptions of disembodiment and somatic disintegration, abnormal somatic sensations | Body perception became accurate Recognised and articulated unusual body perceptions Identified and expressed emotions Uncoordinated movements improved | Adherence better than control. Unusual perceptions triggered by simple stretch Difficulty engaging with weights No effect between body perception and negative symptoms | Rohright et al. (2008) |

*(Continued)*

**TABLE 21.1**   (Continued)

| Intervention | Participants | Outcome | Comments | Reference |
|---|---|---|---|---|
| Movement Body awareness | Anorexia In- and outpatients | Improved awareness and handling of body signals (greatest comments) | Inpatient; more problems with self-identity, wish for contact with their body and control of the body was more central | Kolnes (2012) |
| Basic body awareness therapy (BBAT) | Stress-related behaviour and somatoform disorders | Negative self-image, anxiety, depression, paranoid ideation *is linked to:* impaired body capacity measured<br><br>Inc. respiratory control Flexed postural pattern Decreased flexibility of neck and shoulders | Goals: stable, relaxed posture, grounded, coordinate movement with breathing, well-defined in movements and interpersonal relations, to be mentally present or mindful | Meurle-Hallberg and Armelius (2006) |
| Light, gentle touch, not affiliated to any specific therapy Four sessions | Combination of psychological distress and illness and physical symptoms | Significantly improved stress, anxiety, depression and ability to cope | Greatest benefits were seen with those with the severest symptoms | Weze et al. (2006) |
| Body awareness therapy for at least 1 year Normal support | Schizophrenia Living in community | Improved: affect regulation, body awareness, self-esteem, ability to think, social interaction | Felt more vitalised and feelings of interest In-depth qualitative responses | Hedlund and Gyllensten (2010) |
| Body awareness therapy (BBAT)+ treatment as usual (TAU)– Control –(TAU) long-term effects | Psychiatric outpatients *N* = 77 patients with mood, stress-related somatoform, behavioural or personality disorders | BBAT: sig. improved body awareness, attitude to body, fewer symptoms, improved self-efficacy, compared to control, from baseline to 6/12 | BBAT significantly less use of psychiatric treatment from health care professionals (not psychiatrist) sig. less use of social services | Gyllensten et al. (2009) |

| Intervention | Participants | Outcome | Comments | Reference |
|---|---|---|---|---|
| Simplified tai chi + qigong pre- and post-psychotherapy sessions 1 year duration Further studies now taking this forward | 4 refugee survivors of trauma with complex PTSD No adverse events to intervention | Facilitated psychotherapy sessions due to less hyper-vigilance and increased introspection Improved physical, mental, psychological and spiritual well-being | Good discussion of evidence and clinical reasoning Felt more attuned to bodies Cannot attribute improvement specifically to intervention, but participants found it therapeutically helpful | Grodin et al. (2008) |
| 6-month tai chi/qigong 3 x one-hour classes per week Intervention described in depth | Older adults chosen for ability to articulate their experiences N = 8 | 'Both an inner and outer experience' 6 reported a positive spiritual experience Improved mind–body connection Increase in general self-awareness | Motivated by a variety of positive multi-dimensional mind–body–spirit effects that are holistic and broad in scope | Yang et al. (2011) |
| Intervention in detail: 25 min. massage, inner awareness Mindful attention to body experience and articulation and education | Female with severe childhood sexual abuse history N = 10 Compared with wait list control | 1  Experience of 'a more secure sense of self' 2  Positive influence on psychotherapy progress 3  Profound personal insight 4  Sig. positive change in psychological and physical well-being compared to control | Therapist facilitated body–mind integration through touch and dialogue Findings suggested body-orientated therapy Reduced dissociation typically associated with PTSD, and increased emotional awareness and personal empowerment | Price (2006) |

*(Continued)*

**TABLE 21.1**   (Continued)

| Intervention | Participants | Outcome | Comments | Reference |
|---|---|---|---|---|
| Reflexology | Female mental health service users | Trousdell (1996) 'more valued, empowered and more able to stay in the moment, rather than worrying about the past or future … becoming more assertive'. | Mackereth (1999) New found interest in personal health Improved mood and energy levels Supportive, nurturing, sensing Grounding in relation to dissociation 'Safe touch' in relation to abuse | Trousdell (1996) Mackereth (1999) |
| Acupressure: manual pressure of forehead Acupuncture point called yintang; compared to a sham point | Healthy subjects experiencing pain from controlled needle insertion | Compared to controls: Sig. reduced pain Reduced low/ high frequency ratio of heart rate variability (HRV), implying a reduction in sympathetic activity | Several other studies demonstrate sedation and anxiety reduction by acupressure at this point | Aria et al. (2008) |

There is a substantial body of evidence linking physical health and mental illness, and physical activity is associated positively with mood, disease prevention and productivity (Biddle and Mutrie, 2008; Faulkner and Taylor, 2005). The therapeutic use of physical activity in mental health services has been comprehensively reviewed by Callaghan (2004) together with a pragmatic view of the nursing role. Building on the evidence of exercise as an effective treatment for mild to moderate depression (Daley, 2008), the *Moving on up* report (Mental Health Foundation, 2009) describes the factors identified in successful exercise referral schemes: careful planning and availability of individualised support, pacing of an exercise programme, a variety of exercise activities to cater for different interests and levels of fitness, closer working with health care staff to provide prompt, clear referrals and ability to judge the 'right time' in a person's recovery. A structured group physical activity programme is highlighted as a low intensity psychosocial intervention in the NICE CG90 (2009) depression guidelines.

There are considerable perceived barriers to many exercise activities, however it is a patient's *perception* of fitness which enhances self-concept (Knapen, 2005).

**Potential Psychological factors**
Self-image
Personal resources
Finances,
Motivation
Self-initiation/staff support
Concentration
Memory
Mood
Safety concerns

**Potential Physical factors**
Tiredness/fatigue
Weight management
Pain management
General fitness
Cardiovascular, respiratory,
Musculo-skeletal function
Medication side effects
Sleep patterns
Balance/co-ordination
Difficulty level of activity

**Potential Social factors**
Trust in staff
Social skills
Group inter-relationships
Fear of discrimination,
Relevance and enjoyment of activity
Past history & experience of exercise
Culture,
Lifestyle

**Potential Motivation for Activities**

| | |
|---|---|
| Functional: | gardening |
| Cardiovascular fitness: | jogging, walk |
| Sport: | table tennis |
| Social: | football |
| Hobby: | skate board |
| Creative: | dance |
| Grounded: | Qigong |
| Altruistic: | dog walking |
| Family: | decorating |
| Expression of emotions: | boxing, dance |
| Self-image: | pilates |
| Sense of self: | Feldenkrais, |
| Weight loss: | gym aerobic ex. |
| Strength gain: | weights |
| Mastery: | juggling, Tai chi |
| Awareness of body: | yoga, Feldenkrais |

**Body-mind Approach**
Breath awareness
Emphasis of movement:
   Slow, rhythm, flow
Mindful awareness of the
   feel and position of body,
Aware of being a whole…
   unity
Imagery
Self-reflection,
Non-critical, creative, fun

**Potential Outcome:**
More awareness of body-
   mind-emotion connection
Sense of self in relation
   to environment, self
   and others
Relaxation
Insightful thoughts
Potential Subjective
   evaluation

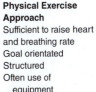

**Physical Exercise Approach**
Sufficient to raise heart
and breathing rate
Goal orientated
Structured
Often use of
   equipment
Measurable goals

**Potential Outcome:**
Physical fitness,
Improved mood,
Mastery, social inclusion
Thought distraction
Perceived control
Potential Objective
   evaluation

**Potential Healthcare Professionals:**
*(depending on skills & resources)*
Fitness/sports instructor
Physiotherapist
Occupational therapist
Mental health nurse
Body psychotherapist
Complementary therapist
Sensorimotor psychotherapist
Self

**FIGURE 21.2**   Considerations when promoting Physical Activity from a Mental Healthcare Perspective

McDevitt et al, (2006) Biddle and Mutrie (2008), Faulkner and Taylor (2005), Skjaerven et al (2010) and clinical experience

McDevitt et al. (2006) explores the fine balance between staff providing activities for service users with severe mental illness, against facilitating personal initiative. As motivation is key, it can be argued that the health care professional with the most understanding of the patient may be the key person to motivate, individualise and promote an achievable activity with personal meaning and relevance.

When targeting mental health outcomes, through physical activity, consideration of the different approaches discussed needs to be individualised and clinically reasoned. There are no definitive prescriptions. Evidence, skills and experience of clinicians serve as signposts (see Figure 21.2).

As in all our clinical practice, compassionate, person-centred care, guided by personal resources and meaning of the patient take centre stage, alongside biopsychosocial support. As health care professionals with an understanding of mental health, we can journey with the patient, perceiving and promoting therapeutic body–mind implications in all activities (Van der Kolk, 2006). Sometimes mental distress exacerbates the body-focus, increasing pain and tension, or cuts off the body-focus leading to a numbed dissociation. Illness transcends the mind–body dichotomy (Stam, 1998).

> When the body is well and healthy it becomes transparent – we are not specifically aware of our, head …. We are busy … reaching out. During illness our attention is directed inwards; we are more than aware of aching joints, pounding head and bloated abdomen, reducing outside worldly contact. This dysfunction gives the body a dys-appearance. (Leder, 2005: 111)

**CASE EXAMPLE**

When in overwhelm; it is easier to feel your way out than think your way out. (Sumner and Haines, 2010)

### Case Study

This brief overview describes the clinical reasoning underpinning several physiotherapy sessions with Linda, whilst she is staying on an acute mental health ward and post discharge.

Linda had a past history of physical and sexual child abuse, anxiety, depression with ongoing self-harm resulting in several hospital admissions.

On the ward Linda presented with episodes of panic, somatic dissociation and psychosis. Linda found conversation and social interactions challenging, leading to a preference of staying in bed and not engaging in ward activities. There was much distress over taking any medication.

Linda's physical presentation included: diverse muscle pains; shakey legs; neck ache and cold hands and feet; difficulty walking, with shortness of breath; fear of falling with a stooped, flexed posture; abdomen feels full and sick.

'I should be able to sort this out on my own ... I've always been able to stand up for myself, now I'm just a pushover to be controlled by others ... as soon as I stand I feel like my legs will give way and I disappear. I feel I need to walk ... it helped in the past.'

## Treatment and related clinical reasoning

**Deep Foot massage** addressed the immediate need of 'cold feet' to give instant comfort and feedback. Feet may be perceived as the least invasive part of the body to touch, whilst maintaining eye contact. The feet can easily be drawn away, promoting empowerment. Linda recognises this is similar to reflexology, which she accepts as safe and therapeutic. This begins the process of introducing a positive, safe, somatic sensation (Trousdell, 1998) which improves somatic awareness to the feet, facilitating balance. This is continued as self-management by rolling feet over tennis balls.

**Self Acupressure** was taught to the palm (solar plexus reflex connection to relax diaphragmatic area), wrist (PC6 acupuncture point to reduce nausea and reduce hyperventilation) and forehead Yintang acupuncture point (Aria et al., 2008) to reduce sympathetic nervous system arousal. Linda expressed interest in the concept of regulating her stress response by her own action finding it self-soothing and meaningful without it being harmful.

**Standing with spine against the wall, knees flexed** gains a positive experience of standing without fear of falling. By feeling the spine touching the wall, physical feedback, a safe support and body awareness are enhanced. The following promote a mindful approach:

- noticing how relaxation gives greater physical contact on the wall, which in turn lengthens the spine reducing pain.
- noticing, feeling and owning the tension (increasing strength) in the upper leg muscles (quadriceps) as part of her body, enabling 'standing up to life'.
- noticing pressure changes of the ribs on the wall, how, with lower abdominal breathing, the shoulders can drop and open, easing neck pain.
- flat palms on the moving abdomen, noticing breathing rhythm and how this affects feelings.

**Tai Chi and Yoga** were accepted as normal, healthy activities by Linda. Skills learnt at the wall were transferred to the open space of her ward room. Focus was on multisensory integration of slow, fluid arm movement, breath, posture and connection to the ground. Balance exercises instigated a sense of mastery, self-efficacy ... and often humour, whilst extra attention focused the mind in the body, as distraction from negative self-talk. This progressed to stepping forward and backwards, focusing on control and balance and how to move forward in life.

Alongside her walking and breathing rhythms, Linda worked at maintaining awareness of her feet on the ground and massaging her hands to maintain physical awareness, preventing further somatic dissociation and panic. Dog walking facilitated this process.

*(Continued)*

*(Continued)*

**Progress post discharge**

Walking has progressed to joining a walking group and leisure centre. Linda has developed confidence both in her body and social relationships, utilising exercise and reflexology to prevent self-harm. She has had no further admissions and is now feeling sufficiently resilient and resourced to address further psychological issues.

A further resource can be viewed at www.mind.org.uk/help/ecominds/mental_health_and_the_environment.

---

# Treatment during inpatient admission

The physiotherapist carried out a series of physical interventions with Linda.

## Deep foot massage: Reasoning

- Addressing immediate need of 'cold feet' to give instant comfort and feedback.
- Least invasive part of the body to touch, whilst maintaining eye contact.
- Non-verbal, safe – she can easily withdraw feet.
- Linda recognises this is similar to reflexology.
- Begins the process of introducing a positive, safe somatic sensation.
- Improves proprioception (body awareness) to feet to facilitate balance.
- Continue as self-management (rolling feet over tennis balls).

## Acupressure: Reasoning

Linda expressed interest in the concept of regulating energy flow by her own action and found finger acupressure of palm, and wrist and forehead self-soothing and meaningful without it being harmful. This includes an evidenced acupressure point for reducing sympathetic nervous system activity (Arai et al., 2008).

## Standing, spine against the wall, knees flexed: Reasoning

- Gain a positive experience of standing without fear of falling.
- Acknowledging the feeling of pressure as support, focusing on where the spine touches the wall for physical feedback.
- Noticing how relaxation promotes more physical contact, which in turn lengthens the spine, reducing pain.

- Noticing and feeling the tension (increasing strength) in the upper leg muscles (quadriceps) as part of her body, enabling 'standing up to life'.
- Noticing pressure changes of the ribs on the wall, how, with lower abdominal breathing, the shoulders can drop and open, easing neck pain.
- Flat palms on the moving abdomen. Noticing breathing rhythm, potential changes of sensations.

### Tai chi and yoga: Reasoning:

- Accepted as normal, healthy activity by Linda.
- Skills learnt at the wall, transferred to open space of bedroom. Focus on multi-sensory integration of slow arm movement, breath, posture and connection to the ground. Balance exercises instigated a sense of mastery, self-efficacy … and often humour.
- Extra attention focused the mind in the body, as distraction from negative self-talk.
- Introduce stepping forward and backwards, focusing on control and balance and how resilience to being pushed is empowering.
- Alongside walking and breathing rhythms, word rhythms were connected to integrate different body feelings; *I am safe, I will get through this.*
- All the above were developed as coping strategies helping to prevent somatic dissociation, anxiety and panic whilst 'outside'.

## Progress

Walking has progressed to joining a walking group and leisure centre. Linda has developed confidence both in her body and social relationships, not needing to self-harm. She has had no further admissions, and now is feeling sufficiently resilient and resourced to address further psychological issues.

## Summary

Rather than use the terms biopsychosocial, well-being, holistic or complementary therapy as an overarching cliché, consider how our body is reflecting our world, experience, meaning and interactions. Having some understanding of the body–mind, gives us a way of connecting, understanding and being with the person.

Each healthcare professional has a duty of care towards the *whole* body-mind person. Considering the previous evidence and discussions, an informed, caring,

*(Continued)*

*(Continued)*

appropriate use of touch, movement and perceived meaning in the lived experience of the person's body may be integral to therapeutic rapport building and indeed therapy and recovery (Skjaerven et al., 2003).

Consider, within the nursing role, how you acknowledge and bring to attention the inner physical sensations and movement of the person's body together with a mindful approach to the changes in your own body. Potentially, the most minimal and subtle changes in body awareness can bring about therapeutic strides, for example:

- a safe, reassuring touch on the upper arm may help the person to *feel* human contact and *feel* safe themselves.
- bringing attention to the physical contact of spine against the chair or feet on the floor facilitates grounding and being present.
- a slight change of posture, finger stretches or a few deeper slower breaths can positively change how the person feels inside.
- minimal activity such as walking to the local shop can be done mindfully by paying attention and reflecting on how the body may feel and change.
- when engaging with someone who is distressed, consider what areas of your body feel tense or just different and how this relates to both your thoughts and feelings of the other person.

# References

Ainley, V., Tajadura-Jiménez, A., Fotopoulou, A. and Tsakiris, M. (2012) 'Looking into myself: the effect of self-focused attention on interoceptive sensitivity', *Psychophysiology*. doi: 10.1111/j.1469-8986.2012.01468.x.

Aria, Y.C., Ushida, T., Osuga, T., Matsubara, T., Oshima, K. and Kawaguchi, K. (2008) *Anesthesia and Analgesia*, 107: 661–4.

Blechert, J., Michael, T., Grossman, P., Lajtman, M. and Wilhelm, F.H. (2007) 'Autonomic and respiratory characteristics of posttraumatic stress disorder and panic disorder', *Psychosomatic Medicine*, 69 (9): 935–43.

Biddle, S.J.H. and Mutrie, N. (2008) *Psychology of Physical Activity* (2nd edn). London: Routledge.

Björnsdotter, M., Morrison, I. and Olausson, H. (2010) 'Feeling good: on the role of C fiber mediated touch in interoception', *Experimental Brain Research*, 207 (3–4): 149–55.

Boadella, D. (1997) 'Awakening sensibility, recovering motility: psycho-physical synthesis at the foundations of body-psychotherapy: the 100-year legacy of Pierre Janet (1859–1947)', *International Journal of Psychotherapy*, 2: 45–56.

Bonfioli, E., Berti, L., Goss, C., Muraro, F. and Burti, L. (2012) 'Health promotion lifestyle intervention for weight management in psychosis: a systematic review and meta-analysis of RCT's', *BMC Psychiatry*, 12 (78): 1–12.

Borrell-Carrió, F., Suchman, A.L. and Epstein, R.M. (2004) 'The Biopsychosocial Model 25 years later: principles, practice and scientific inquiry', *Annals of Family Medicine*, 2 (6): 576–82.

Callaghan, P. (2004) 'Exercise: a neglected intervention in mental health care?', *Journal of Psychiatric and Mental Health Nursing*, 11 (4): 476–83.

Carei, T.R., Fyfe-Johnson, A.L., Breuner, C.C. and Brown, M.A. (2010) 'Randomized controlled clinical trial of yoga in the treatment of eating disorders', *Journal of Adolescent Health*, 46 (4): 346–51.

Cassidy, C. (2004) 'What does it mean to practice an energy medicine?', *Journal of Alternative and Complementary Therapies*, 10 (1): 79–81.

Chang, S.O. (2001) 'The conceptual structure of physical touch in caring', *Journal of Advanced Nursing*, 33 (6): 820–7.

Craig, A.D. (2009) 'How do you feel – now? The anterior insula and human awareness', *National Review of Neuroscience*, 10 (1): 59–70.

CSP (Chartered Society of Physiotherapy) (2008) *Recovering Mind and Body: A Framework for the Role of Physiotherapy in Mental Health and Wellbeing.* London: CSP.

Daley, A. (2008) 'Exercise and depression: a review of reviews', *Journal of Clinical Psychology in Medical Settings*, 15: 140–7.

Descilo, T., Vedamurtachar, A., Gerbarg, P.L., Nagaraja, D., Gangadhar, B.N., Damodaran, B., Adelson, B., Braslow, L.H., Marcus, S. and Brown, R.P. (2010) 'Effects of a yoga breath intervention alone and in combination with an exposure therapy for post-traumatic stress disorder and depression in survivors of the 2004 South-East Asia tsunami', *Acta Psychiatria Scandinavica*, 121 (4): 289–300.

Edvardsson, J.D., Sandman, P.O. and Rasmussen, B.H. (2003) 'Meanings of giving touch in the care of older patients: becoming a valuable person and professional', *Journal of Clinical Nursing*, 12: 601–9.

Eiden, B. (1998) 'The use of touch in psychotherapy', *Self and Society*, 26: 1–3.

Evans, H. (2007) 'Craniosacral touch and the perception of inherent health', *Journal of Holistic Healthcare*, 4 (4): 19–23.

Froggett, L. and Little, R. (2012) 'Dance as a complex intervention in an acute mental health setting: a place "in-between"', *British Journal of Occupational Therapy*, 75 (2): 93–9.

Garbacz, E. and Marshall, S. (2000) 'Classical Chinese medicine: the science of biological forces', *Medical Acupuncture*, 12 (2): 21–8.

Gilbert, P. (2002) 'Understanding the biopsychosocial approach: conceptualization', *Clinical Psychology*, 14: 13–17.

Gordon, J.S., Staples, J.K., Blyta, A., Bytyqi, M. and Wilson, A.T. (2008) 'Treatment of posttraumatic stress disorder in postwar Kosovar adolescents using mind-body skills groups: a randomized controlled trial', *Journal of Clinical Psychiatry*, 69: 1469–76.

Grodin, M.A., Piwowarczyk, L., Fulker, D., Bazazi, B.A. and Saper, R.B. (2008) 'Treating survivors of torture and refugee trauma: a preliminary case series using Qigong and T'ai Chi', *Journal of Alternative and Complementary Medicine*, 14 (7): 801–6.

Gyllensten, A.L., Ekdahl, C. and Hansson, L. (2009) 'Long-term effectiveness of basic body awareness therapy in psychiatric outpatient care: a randomized controlled study', *Advances in Physiotherapy*, 11 (1): 2–12.

Hedlund, L. and Gyllensten, A.L. (2010) 'The experiences of basic body awareness therapy in patients with schizophrenia', *Journal of Bodywork and Movement Therapies*, 14: 245–54.

Kerr, C.E., Wasserman, R.H. and Moore, C.I. (2007) 'Cortical dynamics as a therapeutic mechanism for touch healing', *Journal of Alternative and Complementary Medicine*, 13 (1): 59–66.

Knapen, J., Van de Vliet, P., Coppenolle, H.V., Peuskens, J., Pieters, G. and Knapan, K. (2005) 'Comparison of changes in physical self-concept global self-esteem', *Psychotherapy and Psychosomatics*, 74: 353–61.

Kolnes, L.J. (2012) 'Embodying the body in anorexia nervosa: a physiotherapeutic approach', *Journal of Bodywork and Movement Therapies*, 16: 281–288.

Laing, R.D. (1969) *The Divided Self.* London: Penguin.

Leder, D. (2005) 'Moving beyond "mind" and "body"', *Philosophy, Psychiatry, and Psychology*, 12 (2): 109–13.

Levine, P. (2010) *In an Unspoken Voice: How the Body Releases Trauma and Restores Goodness.* Berkeley, CA: North Atlantic Books.

Long, A. (2009) 'The potential of complementary and alternative medicine in promoting well-being and critical health literacy: a prospective, observational study of shiatsu', *BMC Complementary and Alternative Medicine*, 9 (19): 1–11.

Lopez, C., Halje, P. and Blanke, O. (2008) 'Body ownership and embodiment: vestibular and multisensory mechanisms', *Neurophysiologie Clinique/Clinical Neurophysiology*, 38: 149–61.

McDevitt, J., Snyder, M. and Miller, A. (2006) 'Perceptions of barriers and benefits to physical activity among outpatients in psychiatric rehabilitation', *Journal of Nursing Scholarship*, 38 (1): 50–5.

Mackereth, P.A. (1999) 'An introduction to catharsis and the healing crisis in reflexology', *Complementary Therapies in Nursing and Midwifery*, 5: 67–74.

Mailoo, V., Chow, G. and Kennish, S. (2011) 'Psychoneuroimmunology of infection: implications for occupational therapy', *International Journal of Therapy and Rehabilitation*, 18 (11): 643–50.

Mental Health Foundation (2009) *Moving on up*. London: Mental Health Foundation.

Meurle-Hallberg, K. and Armelius, K. (2006) 'Associations between physical and psychological problems in a group of patients with stress-related behaviour and somatoform disorders', *Physiotherapy Theory and Practice*, 22 (1): 17–31.

Meurle-Hallberg, K., Armelius, B.Å. and Von Koch, L. (2004) 'Body patterns in patients with psychosomatic, musculoskeletal and schizophrenic disorders: psychometric properties and clinical relevance of Resource Oriented Body Examination (ROBE-II)', *Advances in Physiotherapy*, 6: 130–42.

Montagu, A. (1986) *Touching, the Human Significance of the Skin* (3rd edn). New York: Harper and Row.

Nathan, B. (2007) 'The sense of touch – a philosophical surprise', *Journal of Holistic Healthcare*, 4 (4): 24–31.

Naylor, C., Parsonage, M., McDaid, D., Knapp, M., Fossey, M. and Galea, A. (2012) *Report on Long-term Conditions and Mental Health: The Cost of Co-morbidities: A Joint Publication by the King's Fund and Centre for Mental Health*. London: London School of Economics.

NHS (2009) *Transforming Services for Health, Wellbeing and Reducing Inequalities*. London: Department of Health.

NHS Confederation Briefing (2009) *Healthy Mind, Healthy Body: How Liaison Psychiatry Services Can Transform Quality and Productivity in Acute Settings*. No. 179, April. London: Department of Health.

Nicholls, D. and Gibson, B. (2010) 'The body and physiotherapy', *Physiotherapy Theory and Practice*, 26 (8): 497–509.

Northey, A. and Barnett, F. (2012) 'Physical health parameters: comparison of people with severe mental illness the general population', *British Journal of Occupational Therapy*, 75 (2): 100–5.

Öhman, A., Åström, L. and Malmgren-Olsson, E.B. (2011) 'Feldenkrais therapy as group treatment for chronic pain: a qualitative evaluation', *Journal of Bodywork and Movement Therapies*, 15 (2): 153–61.

Oschman, J.L. (2003) *Energy Medicine in Therapeutics and Human Performance.* Oxford: Butterworth Heinemann.

Oschman, J.L. (2006) 'Trauma energetics', *Journal of Bodywork and Movement Therapies*, 10: 21–34.

Petkova, V.I. and Ehrsson, H.H. (2008) 'If I were you: perceptual illusion of body swapping', *PLoS ONE*, 3 (12): 9.

Pike, C. and Hald, L. (2011) 'Neuropsychological effects of IRECA during recovery from acute stress: experimental investigation of an applied mindfulness technique'. Presentation at the Holistic Psychology Annual Conference.

Price, C. (2006) 'Body orientated therapy in sexual abuse recovery: a pilot-test comparison', *Journal of Bodywork and Movement Therapies*, 10: 58–64.

Porges, S.W. (2007) 'A phylogenetic journey through the vague and ambiguous Xth cranial nerve: a commentary on contemporary heart rate variability research', *Biological Psychology*, 74 (2): 301–7.

Röhricht, F., Papadopoulos, N., Holden, S., Clarke, T. and Priebe, S. (2008) 'Therapeutic processes and clinical outcomes of body psychotherapy in chronic schizophrenia – an open clinical trial', *The Arts in Psychotherapy*, 38: 196–203.

Russ, T., Stamatakis, E., Hamer, M., Starr, J.M., Kivimaki, M. and Batty, G.D. (2012) 'Association between psychological stress and mortality: individual participant pooled analysis of 10 prospective cohort studies', *British Medical Journal*, 345: e4933. doi: 10.1136/bmj.e4933.

Scaer, R.C. (2001) 'The neurophysiology of dissociation and chronic disease', *Applied Psychophysiology and Biofeedback*, 26 (1): 73–91. Available at: www.traumasoma.com/excerpt1.html) (accessed on: 20 August 2012).

Skjaerven, L.H., Gard, G. and Kristofferson, K. (2003) 'Basic elements and dimensions to the phenomenon of quality of movement – a case study', *Journal of Bodywork and Movement Therapies*, 7 (4): 251–60.

Skjaerven, L.H., Kristoffersen, K. and Gard, G. (2010) 'How can movement quality be promoted in clinical practice: a phenomenological study of physical therapy experts', *Physical Therapy*, 90 (10): 1479–92.

Stam, H.J. (1998) *The Body and Psychology.* London: Sage.

Sumner, G. and Haines, S. (2010) *Cranial Intelligence: A Practical Guide to Biodynamic Craniosacral Therapy.* London: Singing Dragon.

Tajadura-Jiménez, A., Grehl, S. and Tsakiris, M. (2012) 'The other in me: interpersonal multisensory stimulation changes the mental representation of the self', *PLoS ONE*. doi: 10.1371/journal.pone.0040682.

Telles, S., Singh, N., Joshi, M. and Balkrishna, A. (2010) 'Post traumatic stress symptoms and heart rate variability in Bihar flood survivors following yoga: a randomized controlled study', *BMC Psychiatry*, 10 (18): 1–10.

Thakkar, K.N., Nichols, H.S., McIntosh, L.G. and Park, S. (2011) 'Disturbances in body ownership in schizophrenia: evidence from the rubber hand illusion and case study of a spontaneous out-of-body experience', *PLoS ONE*, 6 (10): e27089.

Trousdell, P. (1996) 'Reflexology meets emotional needs', *International Journal of Alternative and Complementary Medicine*, November: 9–12.

Vancampfort, D., Hert, M.D., Maurissen, K., Sweers, K., Knapen, J., Raepsaet, J. and Probst, M. (2011) 'Physical activity participation, functional exercise capacity and self-esteem in patients with schizophrenia', *International Journal of Therapy and Rehabilitation*, 18 (4): 222–30.

Vancampfort, D., Probst, M., Skjaerven, L.H., Catalán-Matamoros, D., Lundvik-Gyllensten, A.L., Gómez-Conesa, A., Ijntema, R. and De Hert, M. (2012) 'Systematic review of the benefits of physical therapy within a multidisciplinary care approach for people with schizophrenia', *Physical Therapy*, 92: 11–23.

Van der Kolk, B.A. (2006) 'Clinical implications of neuroscience research in PTSD', *Annals of the New York Academy of Sciences*, 1071: 277–93.

Walach, H. (2007) 'Mind-body-spirituality', *Mind and Matter*, 5 (2): 215–40.

Weze, C., Leathhard, H.L., Grange, J., Tiplady, P. and Stevens, G. (2006) 'Healing by gentle touch ameliorates stress and other symptoms in people suffering with mental health disorders or psychological stress', *eCAM Advance Access*. doi: 10.1093/ecam/nel052.

Wilde, M. (1999) 'Embodiment now', *Advances in Nursing Science*, 22 (2): 25–38.

Yang, Y., DeCelle, S., Reed, M., Rosenburg, K., Schlagal, R. and Greene, J. (2011) 'Subjective experiences of older adults practicing taiji and qigong', *Journal of Aging Research*. doi: 10.4061/2011/650210.

Young, C. (2006) 'One hundred and fifty years on: the history, significance and scope of body psychotherapy today', *Body, Movement and Dance in Psychotherapy*, 1 (1): 17–28.

# Index